Evolution of the Nervous System

Evolution WITHDRAWN
of the Nervous System

HARVEY B. SARNAT, B.S., M.S., M.D.

Assistant Professor of Neurology
St. Louis University School of Medicine
St. Louis, Missouri

MARTIN G. NETSKY, A.B., M.S., M.D.

Professor of Neuropathology
University of Virginia School of Medicine
Charlottesville, Virginia

New York
OXFORD UNIVERSITY PRESS
London   Toronto   1974

To our wives

Preface

The structure of the human nervous system may be studied in at least three ways. The first is to study the spatial relations of fiber tracts and other structures in the mature human brain. This method is the only one to which most physicians, and indeed many neurologists and neurosurgeons, are usually exposed; it has the most immediate application to clinical diagnosis.

The second approach is to study embryonic development and cerebral maturation after birth. This analysis of ontogenesis is particularly important to the physician concerned with the clinical problems of anomalous development of the nervous system.

The third way of exploring neuroanatomy is through the dimension of time as revealed by analysis of evolution. The millions of years required for the evolution of species make direct experimental studies difficult. This method is thus the most abstract because the processes under study usually cannot be observed directly. In addition, much must be inferred from the comparative study of species evolving along lines different from man, arising from common ancestral forms now extinct. The study of comparative anatomy, however, provides a background for understanding how the nervous system of man came into being. The functional capabilities of phylogenetically older systems are demonstrated in lower vertebrates, as well as their inadequacies for increasing the range of functions needed by evolving species, including man. Numerous laboratory experiments have the goal of isolating functional systems for study by creating lesions in the brains of experimental animals. Nature, however, has isolated these systems in simple species lacking the later modifications.

Although we base our analyses on structure, the chapters are for the most part arranged by functional units. Considerations of structure based on electron microscopy are generally omitted. This technique has added enormously to our knowledge of the similarity of cells of various species, but has resulted in relatively little information on the diverse results of the process of evolution.

Monographs on comparative neuroanatomy are limited to the excellent books by Papez (1929) and by Kappers, Huber, and Crosby (1936). The former is a laboratory manual; the latter contains an enormous amount of detailed information, but is out of date. Interest in the subject has greatly increased in recent years. New journals have appeared, and the annual publication rate of the *Journal of Comparative Neurology* recently has been doubled. Data, moreover, are scattered throughout many other publications dealing with biology, evolution, clinical medicine, and the neurosciences.

In this book, we present a survey of the comparative anatomy and trends in evolution of the central nervous system of vertebrates as they relate to man and to the neurologic sciences. Invertebrates are cited only as they bear on our main theme; these species diverged from the lines of vertebrate evolution, hence they cast little light on the nervous system of man except at the synaptic, cellular, and subcellular levels. We stress concepts but also offer citations of papers where specific questions may be answered. Some generalizations, not allowing for exceptions in particular species, are made in the interest of brevity, clarity, and continuity of thought. It has also been necessary to speculate on various aspects of development, but such speculations are clearly indicated. Applications to human problems are made as often as possible in the hope that neuroscientists and clinicians may be better able to understand the problems of the brain and spinal cord. Our purpose has been to provide a means not otherwise readily available to achieve better understanding of the evolutionary aspect of the normal and abnormal nervous system of man.

January 1974   H.B.S.
                                                                      M.G.N.

Acknowledgment

The authors express their gratitude to Professor Alex Tumarkin, emeritus director of the Department of Otorhinolaryngology, The University, Liverpool, England, for many valuable suggestions resulting from his review of Chapter 5 on the evolution of hearing. We are also grateful to Dr. Paul A. Young, chairman of the Department of Anatomy, St. Louis University School of Medicine, St. Louis, Missouri, for his review of the manuscript.

Several individuals who assisted us technically deserve special mention for performing an exceptionally high quality of work: Ms. Gloria Clark, laboratory technician, Ms. Susan Sparrow, medical illustrator, and Ms. Anne Russell, medical photographer. We also appreciate the efforts of our editor, Mr. Jeffrey House, Ms. Vivian Marsalisi, assistant managing editor, and the staff of Oxford University Press in the realization of this publication.

We thank the following publishers and individuals for permission to use their illustrations:

The American Physiological Society, and Snider and Eldred. *Journal of Neurophysiology 15*: 27, 1952. Figure 1B.

The Cambridge University Press, Coghill. "Evolution and the Problem of Behavior," 1929.

The Ciba Foundation, and Tumarkin, chapter in "Hearing Mechanisms in Vertebrates," 1968, Figures 5 and 8.

S. Karger; and Ebbesson, Jane, and Schroeder. *Brain, Behavior and Evolution 6*: 92, 1972, Figures 5, 13, 15, 20, 25, 28.

Macmillan Publishing Company and Crosby, Humphrey and Lauer, "Correlative Anatomy of the Nervous System," 1962, Figure 161.

E. C. Crosby; Kappers, Huber and Crosby: "The Comparative Anatomy of the Nervous System of Vertebrates Including Man," 1936, Figure 50.

New York Academy of Science and Lende, Figure 10; Karten, Figure 5; Stringelin and Senn, Figure 1, all from Annals of the New York Academy of Sciences, volume on "Comparative Evolution of the Vertebrate Nervous System," 1969.

Pergamon Press and Hebb and Ratkovic, chapter in "Comparative Neurochemistry," 1964, Figure 1.

The University of Chicago Press, Herrick. "The Brain of the Tiger Salamander," 1965, Figure 50.

W. B. Saunders Company and Romer. "The Vertebrate Body," 1970, Figures 120, 357, 374, 380, 383, 403, Table I.

Wistar Institute Press and the following authors and journals: Abbie *Journal of Comparative Neurology* 70: 9, 1939, Figures 8-14; Bone, *ibid.* 115; 27, 1960, Figures 1, 2, 7B; Larsell, *ibid. 86;* 395, 1947, Figure 1; Winkler and Seidenstein, *ibid. 111:* 469, 1959, Figure 9; Woodard, *ibid. 115:* 65, 1960, Figure 2.

This work was supported, in part, by NIH training grant in neuropathology #NS 05383 to Dr. Martin G. Netsky; NIH training grant #NS 05120 to the Department of Neurology, University of Virginia School of Medicine; and by USPHS-NINDS Special Research Fellowship Award in Pediatric Neurology #1F 11 NS 02535 to Dr. Harvey B. Sarnat.

Finally, I (H.B.S.) wish also to mention my personal gratitude to two teachers and investigators who first inspired my interest in comparative zoology and neuroanatomy, respectively. They are Dr. Lyell J. Thomas, Professor Emeritus of Zoology at the University of Illinois in Urbana, and Dr. Luis M. H. Larramendi, presently Professor of Anatomy at the Pritzker School of Medicine of the University of Chicago.

Contents

Illustrations

Tables

Evolution of the Nervous System

1
Evolution, neurology, and the phylogenetic series

Meaning of evolution

Evolution signifies constant change in all forms of life. Mutations in cultures of bacteria, and in colonies of some insects, evolve within days and offer some insight into the dynamic process requiring millions of years for the development of vertebrate species. The principle of evolution is that *presently living species have each evolved from earlier, but not from contemporary species.* The unavailability of extinct ancestors for direct examination makes the evolution of all vertebrates, including man, largely speculative. Nevertheless, study of the comparative anatomy of the nervous systems of contemporary species reveals relatively constant patterns of structure with seemingly infinite variations. In this book, then, an attempt is made to identify those features common to the nervous system of all vertebrates and thus to reconstruct the probable sequence of evolutionary change leading to the development of the human brain. In many ways, the brain of man is more similar to than different from the brain of "lower" animals.

It is frequently suggested that high intelligence, from the evolutionary standpoint, may be equated with superiority. In his essay "The evolutionary advantages of being stupid," Robin (1973) shows that in some circumstances a small cerebral mass may be more advantageous than a large one. For example, the freshwater turtle survives prolonged underwater dives of more than a week. The small brain requires relatively little energy and is capable of functioning normally with zero oxygen tensions in the blood. It is capable of meeting the energy requirements

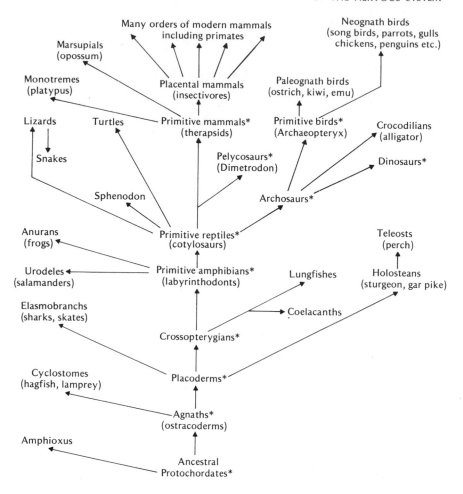

*Extinct

Figure 1-1   Simplified scheme of vertebrate evolution. Modified from Romer (1970).

entirely from anerobic glycolysis. Other diving animals with progressively larger brains tolerate lack of oxygen for shorter periods. The bottle-nosed porpoise, a highly intelligent mammal, has a maximal diving time of only five minutes. The turtle has survived, largely unchanged as a stupid animal, for more than 200,000,000 years; it can hardly be regarded as an unsuccessful animal. If oxygen supply in the ambient environment should ever become limited, the turtle, with its small, slowly functioning brain, would inherit the Earth, while man became extinct. This example emphasizes that the line of evolution leading to man is not necessarily the best for all animals and that each path of specialization offers both advantages and liabilities.

Phylogeny refers to the relation of individual species of vertebrates to all other species, living or extinct, with respect to their place in evolution. These relations are schematically illustrated in Figure 1-1. It is technically inaccurate to speak of "lower" and "higher" vertebrates, because all contemporary species have evolved, each along a different path of specialization or generalization. The arbitrary place that each class of vertebrates and each species occupies on the phylogenetic scale is based on many anatomic features of body and brain. Some vertebrates lower in this scale have particular structures better developed than do other animals considered higher, including man. Many examples are offered in this text. The terms lower and higher vertebrates remain convenient designations for grouping and comparing species, and are thus used in this book. It is hoped that the terms will be understood in the sense that the authors intend, in accordance with the scheme in Figure 1. Unless otherwise stated, reptiles, birds, and mammals are considered the higher vertebrates.

"Primitive" is another troublesome word because it denotes the yet undifferentiated condition of a structure in the embryo; it is sometimes used by comparative anatomists to designate a lesser degree of differentiation of a structure in one species, relative to the corresponding structure in another. Primitive structures are thus presumed to have evolved slowly from their ancestral counterparts. We do not regard the human brain as primitive, yet many regions are more highly differentiated in other vertebrates than in man. For example, fishes have large and well-developed gustatory centers in the medulla (Chapter 4); those of man could be called primitive by comparison. The zona incerta (Chapter 12) is a poorly differentiated area in man, but it is even less well organized or absent in other species. Is the zona incerta primitive in man? The answer to this question is not yet available. A primitive animal thus is one with predominantly generalized or poorly differentiated structures, although some features may be highly specialized.

Organ systems may regress during evolution, particularly in species whose specialization requires no further development of a given organ. It is often difficult to distinguish primitive from degenerative features. Among cyclostomes, for example, myxinoids have a less well differentiated brain, but a more advanced spinal cord, than petromyzonts. Similarly, salamanders have extremely generalized and poorly developed cerebral structures, comparable in many respects to those of cyclostomes. Are these features of salamanders the result of regression from the condition occurring earlier in a more highly developed ancestor, or are salamanders simply laggards who have changed little from their primitive ancestor?

Homology is defined as the study of comparable anatomic structures in different species; these structures can be traced in evolution to a similar structure in common ancestors. The frequent adaptation of homologous structures to new functions in later species *limits the definition of homology to one of structure and excludes function*. Organs of similar function but different anatomic derivation are termed analogous. Criteria for establishing homology differ with various organ systems. Homology of skeletal muscles, for example, is based upon origin, insertion, and innervation.

Homologies in the central nervous system are less easily defined (Campbell and Hodes, 1970). The anatomic position of a mass of gray matter within the neuraxis depends on the relative development of surrounding structures. The hippocampus, for example, is dorsally situated in the forebrain of most animals but becomes displaced ventrally in primates by the development of the neocortex. Other factors influencing anatomic position include cellular migration (i.e., the facial nucleus may lie in the roof or in the floor of the medulla in different species) and specialization (i.e., the descending trigeminal tract extends caudally to the lumbar region of the spinal cord in the frog).

In view of these variations, homology in structures of the central nervous system is based on fiber connections and relations to surrounding or distant structures. It therefore can be best appreciated by considering the brain and spinal cord as a whole and by studying comparative embryonic development.

When neurons performing a common function move closer together, as the phylogenetic scale is ascended, synaptic relations among the cells within these nuclei become increasingly complex. The general trend of evolution toward greater differentiation and complexity increases the capacity for interpretation of sensory data and for translation into behavioral responses. In another sense, there is an evolutionary trend toward simplicity in developing faster and more direct neural pathways to decrease conductive and synaptic delays. Examples include the development of the corticospinal tract and of a direct reticulospinal tract to supplement the polysynaptic pathway.

Repeated observations linking the sequence of embryonic development to evolution have interested biologists for decades. "Ontogeny recapitulates phylogeny" has become an almost universally accepted principle. Actually, embryos of higher species pass through stages in which they resemble the embryos rather than the adult forms of lower species. Embryology has contributed much to the verification of theories of evolution, but will illuminate the problem even more with the further study of embryonic development, particularly in lower species. Mammalian embryos "recapitulate" early stages of phylogenesis so quickly and transiently that only later stages can be easily understood. The earliest evolution of cerebral centers associated with special sensory organs is thus more likely to be revealed by study of the larval lamprey than by the study of the embryo of the pig.

Perspective of evolution in clinical neurology

Inspired by the evolutionary philosophy of Herbert Spencer, John Hughlings Jackson (1884) developed a theory that "dissolution" (degeneration) follows a course inverse to that of evolution. According to this theory, the entire nervous system in disease is exposed to a noxious influence, but the highest centers, being phylogenetically newest, are the least resistant. Jackson also hypothesized that after destruction of a cerebral center some symptoms resulted from the overaction of other structures released from the influence of the destroyed center. He came close to predicting the later physiologic demonstration of inhibitory synapses.

Many metabolic and degenerative diseases of the human nervous system may be viewed through the perspective of evolution. Olivo-pontocerebellar degeneration often spares the phylogenetically oldest portions of the cerebellar vermis while selectively involving the neocerebellum and related structures, such as the chief inferior olivary nucleus, and the pontine and arcuate nuclei. Developmental hypoplasias of the neo-cerebellar hemispheres may be associated with systemic degeneration of other phylogenetically new structures in postnatal life (Norman and Urich, 1958). Friedreich's ataxia is a disease involving mainly the dorsal spinocerebellar tracts, dorsal columns, corticospinal tracts, and neocere-bellum. These structures are almost exclusively elements of the nervous system of mammals and are either absent or rudimentary in lower vertebrates.

Subacute combined degeneration of the spinal cord involves tracts of phylogenetically recent origin. In Pick's disease, a form of "presenile" dementia, the atrophic regions of cerebral cortex generally are phyloge-netically more recent acquisitions, but the older primary sensory and motor cortices are relatively spared (Malamud, 1957). The globoid cell leukodystrophy of Krabbe is a metabolic disease associated with deficien-cies of specific enzymatic activity and has a characteristic morphologic pattern. The subcortical white matter is severely affected, but many phylogenetically older tracts of the forebrain are spared, including olfac-tory tracts, fornix, mammillothalamic fasciculus, and stria medullaris, as well as such older tracts of the brainstem as the medial longitudinal fas-ciculus (Norman et al., 1961).

These examples suggest that *both morphologic differentiation and changes in metabolism occurred with the evolution of species.*

One problem of homology is exemplified by the optic nerve. This structure, found throughout the phylogenetic series of vertebrates, is not actually a peripheral nerve. In most vertebrates, the fibers synapse mainly in the optic tectum of the midbrain, the homolog of the human superior colliculus. In mammals, however, relatively few fibers project to the su-perior colliculus; most of the optic nerve fibers in mammals synapse in the thalamus. Are the optic nerves of mammals and those of fish homolo-gous structures? Does hereditary optic atrophy of Leber represent an-other example of human disease selectively involving phylogenetically new structures? These questions will be considered in Chapter 8.

In contrast to the inverse evolutionary pattern of some heredodegen-erative diseases, anomalies of nervous system development often selec-tively affect the phylogenetically oldest structures and spare the recent acquisitions. There are several reasons for this phenomenon. Structures differentiating early in evolution tend to lie in the midline or paramedian regions of advanced vertebrates; the later developed structures lie more laterally, particularly in the forebrain and cerebellum. Many developmental anomalies are associated with absence, failure of fusion, and other defects of midline structures, such as occur in the Dandy-Walker malformation (Brodal and Hauglie-Hannsen, 1959; Hart et al., 1972), or with failure of forebrain cleavage in the midline in cases of holoprosencephaly or arrhinencephaly (Yakovlev, 1959).

Toxic or teratogenic factors affecting the fetus in early stages of development may selectively involve those structures developing earliest, both embryologically and phylogenetically. Among anomalies resulting from failure of normal migration of neuroblasts, involvement of recent structures greatly exceeds that of older ones. This situation may be related, in part, to the greater distance of migration of laterally lying neurons from the periventricular regions. The longer period available for exposure to noxious agents, at a time when cells are particularly vulnerable, is also a factor.

In addition to these theoretic considerations, comparative anatomy has practical applications to research in which experimental animals are used. The value of extrapolating observations made in other species to man, or from one animal species to another, is limited, however. Comparative studies are justified by considering critically whether generalizations can be achieved. The versatility of the nervous system in adapting to new needs by altering the function of old systems and by developing new ones is well illustrated in evolution. This versatility has important implications in understanding injury to the immature nervous system of the human fetus and infant, and the regenerative and compensatory mechanisms that minimize such injuries.

Terminology

Certain terms of reference are widely used in comparative anatomy. In some cases, we have chosen neuroanatomic terms that enhance understanding of structure or function rather than use the more familiar but less precise clinical word. The foremost example is the term "cranial nerves." This phrase refers to a group of heterogenous fibers, not all of which are cranial and not all of which are nerves. The arbitrary grouping of these neural elements is clinically useful because most emerge from the brainstem. The cranial nerves may be reclassified, for our purposes, into groups having common phylogenetic origin and understandable relations to one another.

Confusion has arisen from the lack of consistent terms in the literature of comparative neuroanatomy, in part because of disagreement among authors with regard to homology and in part because neologisms coined by different authors may refer to the same structure in the same species. Synonymous terms are then used interchangeably in the literature. Preferred terms also change with time; comparison of older with more recent writings may be confusing. The posterior quadrigeminal body, for example, is now more commonly known in man as the "inferior colliculus"; the homologous structure in fishes and amphibians is called the "torus semicircularis," as well as the area posticum and area tegmentalis profundus. Terms, such as "torus semicircularis," may be descriptive only of the species to which they are applied and therefore are not suitable for all classes of vertebrates, even if agreement in homology is achieved. In this book, the most widely accepted current nomenclature has been used, and we have attempted to be consistent in applying the same names to homologous structures in different species. Generally accepted terms in human neuroanatomy are given wherever applicable. English is used in preference to the more cumbersome and less familiar Latin names.

The importance of precision in defining words in common usage is recognized, but this consideration may restrict the meaning of some words in clinical medicine. In a few cases, words of restricted definition, when applied to man alone, have been broadened in meaning in this text. Our purpose is to emphasize the similarities rather than the differences between man and other vertebrates. Broadened definitions differing from conventional use are so indicated in the text.

Theory of neurobiotaxis

The factors influencing the organization of the nervous system have been of great interest, both to research workers in basic neuroscience and to clinicians. The migration of neurons within the central nervous system was observed by Cajal (1900) in his studies of fetal brain. He explained this movement as follows: "If, during embryonic development, new axons pass to some region of the central nervous system, ganglion cells may approach these axons in two different ways, either by sending forth dendrites, or by a migration of the cell body itself." As an example, he used the migration of the external granular layer of the cerebellar cortex into the deeper part of the folia during postnatal maturation. Kappers (1908, 1916, 1919) compared the brains of various vertebrates, and independently arrived at the same conclusion as Cajal, but with regard to phylogeny rather than ontogeny. He termed the phenomenon "neurobiotaxis," and formulated the hypothesis that if several centers of stimulation of neurons are present, the outgrowth of the chief dendrites and eventually the shifting of the cells takes place in the direction of greatest stimulation. The axon thus is usually lengthened. The cell body moves away from the centers which it is stimulating in turn.

The theory of neurobiotaxis invokes the idea of function and bioelectric fields influencing the orientation and migration of neurons. Kappers, Huber, and Crosby (1936) offered a detailed discussion of the earlier concepts contributing to the development of the theory. Burr (1932) was influenced by the ideas of Coghill (1929) and stated that "areas of high rates of cell division direct growing nerve fibers." The proponents of this concept thought that neurobiotaxis complemented their theory in explaining the organization of the central nervous system.

The accessory abducens nucleus of birds provides innervation of the nictitating membrane or "third eyelid." Terni (1921, 1922) suggested that this nucleus migrates laterally, away from the paramedian position of the main abducens nucleus, in accord with the theory of neurobiotaxis. This location provides for faster closure of the lid after noxious stimulation of the cornea, by establishing proximity of the accessory abducens nucleus to the descending trigeminal nucleus. Levi-Montalcini (1964) tested this theory by extirpating the rostral part of the medulla of two-day-old chick embryos. The descending trigeminal nucleus did not form, but the accessory abducens nucleus migrated normally, suggesting that the migration was not dependent upon a direct influence of the descending trigeminal nucleus. She regarded this finding as evidence against the validity of the theory of neurobiotaxis, but conceded that her observations were in agreement with those of Kappers, Huber, and Crosby (1936) that in the central nervous system, neurons "migrate always in a direction opposite to the axonal outgrowth." Harkmark (1954) has also discussed the difficulties in experimentally proving the theory of neurobiotaxis with regard to development of the rhombic lip in embryos.

Whether the forces that cause neuronal migration in phylogeny are the same as those acting in embryology is still an unsettled question. It will probably remain so until more is known about the ontogenesis of the nervous system. Neurobiotaxis remains an attractive but unproved theory. If indeed it is valid, it is almost certainly only one of several factors influencing neuronal migration, including mechanical, bioelectric, and chemical or humoral forces.

Table 1-1. Geologic periods after the time when fossils first became abundant (Romer, 1970).

Era (and duration)	Period	Estimated time since beginning of each period (in millions of years)	Epoch	Life
Cenozoic (age of mammals; about 65 million years)	Quaternary	2+	Holocene (Recent)	Modern species and subspecies: dominance of man.
			Pleistocene	Modern species of mammals or their forerunners; decimation of large mammals; widespread glaciation.
	Tertiary	65	Pliocene	Appearance of many modern genera of mammals.
			Miocene	Rise of modern subfamilies of mammals; spread of grassy plains; evolution of grazing mammals.
			Oligocene	Rise of modern families of mammals.
			Eocene	Rise of modern orders and suborders of mammals.
			Paleocene	Dominance of archaic mammals.
Mesozoic (age of reptiles; lasted about 165 million years)	Cretaceous	130		Dominance of angiosperm plants commences; extinction of larger reptiles and ammonites by end of period.
	Jurassic	180		Reptiles dominant on land, sea, and in air; first birds; archaic mammals.
	Triassic	230		First dinosaurs, turtles, ichthyosaurs, plesiosaurs; cycads and conifers dominant.
Paleozoic (lasted about 340 million years)	Permian	280		Radiation of reptiles, which displace amphibians as dominant group: widespread glaciation.
	Carboniferous	350		Fern and seed fern coal forests; sharks and crinoids abundant; radiation of amphibians; first reptiles.
	Devonian	400		Age of fishes (mostly fresh water); first trees, forests and amphibians.
	Silurian	450		Invasion of the land by plants and arthropods; archaic fishes.
	Ordovician	500		Appearance of vertebrates (ostracoderms); brachiopods and cephalopods dominant.
	Cambrian	570		Appearance of all major invertebrate phyla and many classes; dominance of trilobites and brachiopods; diversified algae.

Introduction to the phylogenetic series

A brief description of the classes of vertebrates is offered as a background for later discussion of the evolution of specific structures in the central nervous system. Table 1-1 summarizes the geologic periods in the evolution of life on Earth.

Protochordates (tunicates, acorn-worms, amphioxus). These small, marine animals are jawless and feed by filtering. Amphioxus particularly has general features of body scheme resembling the early embryonic stages of vertebrates, including a dorsal notochord which does not develop into a vertebral column. Dorsal to the notochord is a hollow neural tube resembling the vertebrate spinal cord. The rostral end of the neural tube is differentiated into a rudimentary brain in amphioxus. The central nervous system of this creature is considered in detail in Chapters 2 and 3 because it has the fundamental structures from which evolved the nervous systems of all vertebrates. Protochordates are probably similar to the ancestors of the earliest true vertebrates. They are instructive to study because they demonstrate the limited extent to which the brain develops without stimuli from organs of special sense.

Cyclostomes (class Agnatha) are an ancient class of primitive, jawless fish which included the filter-feeding, bony, armor-plated ostracoderms of the Ordovician, Silurian, and early Devonian periods of more than 425 million years ago (Table 1-1).

Surviving members of the class Agnatha include the myxinoids (slime hag, hagfish) and petromyzonts (lamprey), all of which are jawless parasitic fishes who prey on teleosts or are scavengers of dead fish. In the larval stages, however, they are non-parasitic filter-feeders. Cyclostomes have primitive, cartilaginous skeletons, lack appendages and scales, and have a few specialized structures, such as the tongue-like rasping structure in the round adhesive mouth of petromyzonts. As with most other features of their bodies, the central nervous system and special sense organs are unique, suggesting a combination of primitiveness and retrogression.

In spite of the simplicity of their nervous system relative to those of more advanced vertebrates, cyclostomes are advanced significantly over amphioxus because they have organs of special sense. Hypothetic transitional forms between amphioxus and cyclostomes almost certainly existed, but they are extinct.

Placoderms were fish of the Devonian period and had bony plates of armor. They probably evolved from ostracoderms, and advanced greatly by developing a simple jaw. Living representatives of this class have not survived. We can only speculate on the organization of their central nervous system.

Elasmobranchs (plagiostomes). Fossil records indicate that these fishes with entirely cartilaginous skeletons, represented today by sharks, skates, and rays, evolved from placoderms. They have a simple jaw and a chondrocranium. The central nervous system is more complex than that of cyclostomes and is in many ways closer to that of amphibians than to teleostean fishes.

A related group of cartilaginous fish, the class Holocephali, evolved separately from placoderms and are represented today by the chimaeras.

Teleosts and other bony fish. The most diverse, most advanced, and most prolific order of bony fishes, including many thousands of species, are the teleosts. The common perch is a representative species. Teleosts evolved in the Jurassic period from another group of more primitive bony fish known as the holosteans, represented today by the sturgeon, gar pike, and bowfin. The earliest pre-teleostean bony fishes (actinopterygians) arose in the Silurian period.

Ancestral Devonian fishes probably swallowed air at the surface of the water. This air either passed through the intestinal tract or was regurgitated. A blind pouch evolved on the ventral surface of the esophagus. This pouch became the swim bladder in most teleosts. A trapped bubble of swallowed air was used in hydrostatic depth control and secondarily as a resonating membrane in the auditory system (Chapter 5). Another group of Devonian fishes, the crossopterygians, used the evolving esophageal pouch as an organ of respiration to enable the animals to survive out of water. The lung thus evolved, and the crossopterygians are the ancestors of all living terrestrial vertebrates.

Teleosts achieved the highest level of adaptation to an aquatic environment and have evolved countless variations of body form for highly specialized ways of life. This diversity is reflected in variations of the central nervous system, but a general plan of organization of the teleostean nervous system is common to all.

Amphibians. In the Devonian period, the most common bony fishes were the crossopterygians, a predatory group. They became extinct in the

Carboniferous period, but before disappearing, a new group developed, the coelacanths. These creatures were fishes with stub-noses, feeble jaws and teeth, and fleshy lobed fins. They were considered extinct since the days of dinosaurs, but in 1939 a strange fish caught off the coast of Madagascar proved to be a coelacanth! Many more have subsequently been studied. Coelacanths remain the closest living relatives of the crossopterygians who first successfully left the water or survived the drying of ponds and lakes. Modern lungfishes (Dipnoi) also evolved from crossopterygians. Before becoming extinct, the crossopterygians gave rise to another form that became the first true amphibian, the labyrinthodont.

Modern amphibians are of three orders. Urodeles, represented by newts and salamanders, probably most closely resemble the stem amphibian labyrinthodonts. They have undergone modifications in a direction opposite to that of the most other modern animals. Rather than elaborately developing certain body structures for specialization, urodeles dedifferentiated or regressed to a more generalized body. Their skeleton degenerated by losing bones from the skull and by retaining embryonic cartilages. Regression is evident, too, in the central nervous system, where nuclei of the brainstem are poorly differentiated, and the embryonic condition of neurons crowded into the subependymal zone is retained in the adult. The usual migration to the periphery does not occur. A few species, such as *Necturus,* even retain embryonic gills, and achieve sexual maturity without metamorphosing into true adults. Another interpretation is that urodeles are simply laggards who failed to evolve from their ancestral form.

Apoda, a second order of amphibians with complete loss of limbs, lives as a small, blind, worm-like burrower and is probably an aberrant line of retrogressive evolution.

The third order of modern amphibians, anurans, are the tailless forms, such as the frog or toad. In the larval stages (tadpole), anurans have tails and resemble urodeles in cerebral structure. Anurans first appeared in the Jurassic period. These amphibians have some regressive features, particularly in the skeleton, but in general they have undergone great specialization by shortening of the trunk, loss of the tail, and enlargement of the hindlimbs for jumping. The brain of the frog is not the simple, generalized, embryonic type, as in the salamander.

The transformation of the nuclei of the lateral line nerves of fishes into the cochlear nuclei of terrestrial vertebrates in the development of the auditory system is an example of phylogenetic adaptation of an old structure to new function (Chapter 5). This evolutionary process is repeated ontogenetically in the metamorphosis of frogs. Anurans thus offer an opportunity to study this process, and they illustrate the repetition of phylogeny in ontogeny.

Reptiles. A major feature distinguishing reptiles from amphibians is the amniotic egg. It can be laid on land and therefore the animals are freed from dependence on proximity to water. Other differences are in the skeleton and skin, which afford the animal better protection and makes it unnecessary for it to be always in or near water. The primitive stem reptiles (cotylosaurs) evolved from early amphibians in the Carboniferous period. They gave rise to many lines of descent, including several orders of dinosaurs, turtles, lizards, and some early mammal-like reptiles. Crocodiles and alligators are the closest living relatives of dinosaurs, both groups having descended from archosaur reptiles (thecodonts) of the Triassic period. The concept of common origin of alligators and dinosaurs is supported by the similarity of skeletal structure. The rear legs of alligators are longer than the forelegs; the tail is long and thick. These features suggest that the ancestors of crocodilians once walked upright and balanced with their heavy tail, as did the "terrible lizards," flesh-eating bipedal dinosaurs.

Dinosaurs are often regarded as an unsuccessful experiment by Nature because they became extinct. These creatures, however, dominated the Earth for more than 165 million years, in contrast to the 65 million years that mammals have lived, and the less than 2 million years that man has existed. In some ways, dinosaurs were more advanced than modern reptiles and the earliest mammals—they had an air-conducting ear, for example (Chapter 5). Dinosaurs probably became extinct because of the onset of an ice age that few modern mammals could survive. Reptiles were especially susceptible to extinction in freezing climates because of the vulnerability of eggs laid on land. In addition, evidence is accumulating that dinosaurs were warm-blooded and that this "advanced" physiologic feature was detrimental to such large creatures in the ice age (Chapter 9).

Snakes are derived from lizards; the limbs are lost and the vertebral column lengthens. Comparison of reptiles within the same class reveals extreme contrasts in development of axial and appendicular musculature. These differences are reflected in the structures of the central nervous system related to motor function. Turtles have well-developed muscles in the extremities, but the axial muscles are atrophic or almost absent because the immobile spine is fixed to the external shell; snakes have large powerful muscles of the trunk associated with an extremely mobile spine but lack extremities altogether. Alligators are slow and clumsy on land; lizards are quick and agile runners.

Birds. Birds descended from the archosaur reptiles of the Jurassic period, as did dinosaurs and crocodilians. Birds are still closely related to reptiles, except for homeostasis of temperature and the presence of feathers. *Archaeopteryx,* an ancestral species of bird of the late Jurassic period, had reptilian teeth, clawed fingers on the wings, and a long reptilian tail. Fossils indicate that it bridged the gap between dinosaur-type archosaurs and modern birds.

Paleognaths and neognaths are two major groups of modern birds. The paleognaths represent the early stages of avian evolution, and include the kiwi, ostrich, emu, and cassowary. All other birds are neognaths; the many orders have various specializations. The avian central nervous system has unique, specialized features. In some ways, the brain of birds is as complex as that of mammals, although the forebrain is differently organized. Birds are not extensively discussed in this book because they are not in the line of evolution leading to man.

Mammals. Mammals are descended from reptiles, but the reptilian line leading to them evolved early from stem reptiles. Their relation to living reptiles is remote. A group of reptiles with cranial structure suggestive of primitive mammals, known as the pelycosaurs (a representative species in *Dimetrodon*), flourished in the early Permian period. Succeeding them in late Permian and early Triassic periods were the therapsids, the most common animals of their day. The therapsids were carnivorous runners with four legs who, as in their mammalian descendants, had elbows and knees under, rather than away from the body, for better support and greater speed. The largest of several species of therapsids were as long as ten feet. By the late Triassic period, many features of the therapsid skull, jaw, dentition, and limbs closely approached the pattern of modern mammals. In spite of their advanced structure, the therapsids did not successfully compete with the dinosaurs, and became extinct. There survived, however, small mouse-size therapsids from which evolved the oldest true mammals in the Cretaceous and early Tertiary periods.

There are three subclasses of presently living mammals. Monotremes are represented by the Australian platypus and spiny anteater. They are primitive mammals who still lay eggs in reptilian fashion. They are specialized in so many ways that they cannot themselves be regarded as ancestors of placental mammals. Marsupials include the kangaroo, opossum, koala bear, and Tasmanian wolf. They bear their young alive, but lack a placenta. The young therefore are born immature and are kept in a pouch on the abdomen of the mother until they can survive in the external environment. Placental mammals, of which man is a member, are the most numerous and advanced group. As a result of the nutritive placenta, the embryo of these mammals is more mature before birth than that of marsupials.

A diversity of specialized orders of placental mammals flourish today. The ancestors from which these various orders were derived are the insectivores. Insectivores still survive today, not much changed from the ancestral forms. They include shrews, moles, and hedgehogs.

Primates. The presently living tree shrews of Malaya link the insectivores with the primitive primates. The lowest true primates may be the lemurs of Madagascar. A succession of primate types through tarsiers, monkeys, baboons, and apes represent various stages in the development of those features of anatomy characterizing primates.

Man may represent the highest stage of primate development on this planet. Although suggestions have been made at various times in recent human history that man is regressing intellectually, morphologic evidence does not corroborate cerebral degeneracy of the species.

2
Plan of vertebrate nervous system

Patterns of organization in vertebrate nervous systems

The central nervous systems of all vertebrates have a common structural organization. The basic plan is best seen in the embryonic stages of advanced vertebrates and in the adult forms of some primitive species. The nervous system of adult vertebrates, however, has more variations among species than are found in any other organ of the body.

The salamander brain is a useful model for all vertebrate brains. The nervous system of urodelan amphibians is dedifferentiated or retrogressive to the extent of having lost highly specialized features and having reverted to a simple, embryonic organization without major migrations of neurons. These animals, however, retain rudimentary forebrain structures intricately developed in higher terrestrial vertebrates. It was for these reasons that Herrick (1948) exhaustively studied the brain of the salamander as representative of the generalized brain of the vertebrates.

The separation of neurons into categories of somatic and visceral, as well as sensory and motor, is morphologically most distinct in the spinal cord. These types of functional neurons with distinguishing histologic characteristics are segregated into specific regions of the cord. The somatic sensory neurons are dorsal, the somatic motor are ventral, and the visceral columns lie in between (Chapter 3). This arrangement persists in the medulla oblongata, a rostral extension of the spinal cord, but is distorted by expansion of the fourth ventricle. The relations of sensory and motor nuclei in the medulla are changed in many vertebrates by a secondary migration during embryogenesis. The original pattern persists in the salamander.

The primitive arrangement of a ventricular system surrounded by gray matter and with white matter lying outside the gray matter is retained in the spinal cord of all vertebrates and in the medulla of the salamander. Elsewhere, in most adult vertebrates, secondary migration of neurons reverses the relations of gray and white matter.

The pons, an arbitrary subdivision of the medulla, is distinguished only in mammals by the presence of pontine nuclei and fibers of the cortico-ponto-cerebellar and corticospinal tracts. These structures form the basis pontis and the branchium pontis (middle cerebellar peduncle). The tegmental portion of the pons is continuous with the medulla. Nuclei of cranial nerves such as the abducens and facial may lie either in the pons or the medulla, depending on the species.

The midbrain is a transitional area from the functionally reflexive spinal cord and medulla to the correlative and associative diencephalon and forebrain. It resembles the medulla in that it has primary sensory nuclei (part of the trigeminal complex) and somatic motor nuclei (oculomotor and trochlear). It also has a correlative region, the optic tectum, which integrates vestibular, tactile, and visual information. The tectum may, however, be of diencephalic origin (Chapter 8). In lower vertebrates, a specialized caudal part of the tegmentum of the midbrain is known as the isthmus. It contains several functionally important nuclei of the suprasegmental motor system, the reticular formation, and the ascending gustatory system. It is a distinct sector of the developing human brain in the stage of the neural tube, but in the mature brain of man, nuclei of the isthmus are dispersed among other structures of more recent phylogenetic origin.

Throughout phylogeny, neurons of similar form and function are arranged into compact aggregates termed "nuclei." Superficial sheets of laminated structure are designated "cortex." The cerebral cortex is sometimes called the "pallium," but this latter term is more appropriate for the entire wall of the hemisphere, including ependyma and pia mater. The nuclei, or functional centers, may be morphologically well demarcated from surrounding structures by interposed fiber tracts, by the numerical density of the cellular population, or by distinctive cellular appearance. Alternatively, they may have poorly defined borders and blend imperceptibly with surrounding nuclei. Nuclei are often poorly differentiated in lower species and have greater organization and distinction in further evolved species. The trend in evolution is toward differentiation and specialization, hence to more complex organization of structures. Dedifferentiation also may occur in evolution, either generalized as exemplified by the salamander brain, or when individual structures are no longer important to the animal. An example of the latter is the evolution of the olfactory system in birds, aquatic mammals, and man; in these animals, the system is less prominent and is dedifferentiated when compared with some lower species relying more upon olfaction.

Anatomic differentiation into nuclei, however, is not the only means of specialization in the central nervous system. The reticular formation exemplifies a group of neurons, highly developed and specialized physiologically, but with little morphologic distinction (Chapter 11). Physiologic data suggest that the organization of much of the limbic system is similar to that of the reticular formation.

The vertebrate body is bilaterally symmetric. The brain is also a paired organ with few exceptions such as the pineal body, the habenulae (Chapter 9), and the functional asymmetry of portions of the human cerebral cortex (Chapter 12). Few midline structures are unpaired; most structures that seem to be in the midline, such as the cerebellar vermis, contain neurons belonging to the right or left sides of the brain with respect to position within the nucleus and to fiber connections.

Centers in the central nervous system usually subserve function of the opposite side of the body. The suggested reason for this phenomenon is explained in Chapter 3. The anatomic basis is the decussation of fibers before reaching their destination, particularly those of long descending and ascending tracts. The crossing of fibers occurs along the course of the axon, near its origin, in its center, or, as it approaches its termination; the site of decussation usually is constant in a given tract.

Commissural fibers interconnect corresponding areas of the two sides of the brain.

Systemic neural pathways are series of neurons, synapsing in sequence, for relay of impulses (either information or instructions) from one part of the nervous system to another. The impulse transmitted by each neuron in the series is related to previous ones received by that neuron, often from several sources. The neural pathway is not limited to one neuron acting at a time; many neurons transmit in parallel along the same tract. Collateral fibers to adjacent neurons serve a synchronizing function. The reflex arc is a simple neural circuit involving a sensory neuron synapsing with a motor neuron, or with an intermediate neuron interposed between the two. Most neural pathways are more complex, involving multiple synapses and the correlation of sensory information from several sources before synthesizing the motor response. In contrast to the simple reflex arcs characteristic of all vertebrates and found even in amphioxus, many invertebrates, such as the sea anemone, respond to stimuli by a prolonged change in the pattern of spontaneous activity. This type of organization is not necessarily primitive, however; the cerebral cortex of man reacts similarly at times (Pantin, 1952).

Nuclei with intermediate synapses in a neural pathway are often spoken of as "way-stations." This term implies that the intermediate neuron or center (nucleus) does nothing more than relay the unchanged impulse to the next neuron in the series. If this concept were correct, the neural pathway would be inefficient because of the imposition of synaptic delays. It would be better served by a long, direct axon from the primary neuron. Intermediate neurons, however, alter or correlate an impulse, before transmitting a new and different impulse to the next center in the series. Many diencephalic centers in the human brain are commonly thought of as way-stations to the cerebral cortex. If the brains of lower vertebrates are examined, however, these same diencephalic centers are seen to be among the highest correlative centers, where sensory information is compiled and motor responses are initiated. That ability is not relinquished by the development of still "higher" centers; the diencephalon in man is capable of associative function (Chapter 9), but the expression may be inhibited by centers such as the cerebral cortex. An example might be the interpretation of a material as edible food, and a sensation of hunger arising in the diencephalon. The hypothalamus and epithalamus initiate digestive activity, but are inhibited by the cerebral cortex because social or other factors make eating inappropriate at that time.

Figures 2-1 and 2-2 are diagrams of suprasegmental control of somatic motor function in a lower vertebrate and in a higher mammal, respectively. The basic motor system of lower vertebrates is not replaced but becomes supplemented by the development of new structures. The relative importance of mesencephalic and diencephalic centers diminishes as the corpus striatum and cerebral cortex evolve, but the phylogenetically old motor system remains intact and is little changed.

The development of limbs in terrestrial vertebrates was the most important factor in the evolution of new centers of motor control and coordination in the telencephalon and the cerebellar hemispheres. The phylogenetically old motor centers were adequate for mass movements of axial muscles but could not achieve the precision required by animals

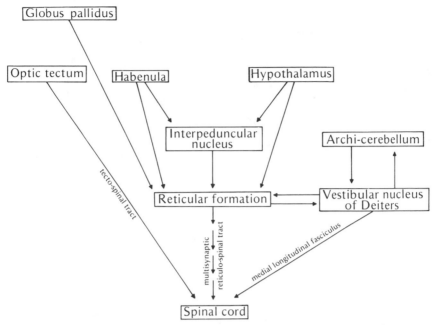

Figure 2-1   Diagram of the suprasegmental motor system of a lower vertebrate.

with extremities. The fins of fish are mainly rudders; propulsion through water is by movement of the trunk and tail.

Somatotopic organization is the arrangement of neurons within a nucleus or cortex, or the arrangement of axons within a tract, for sequential function. For example, the primary sensory and motor gyri of the human cerebral cortex contain adjacent groups of neurons arranged in sequence, corresponding to the disposition of the parts of the body. Those neurons serving the proximal portions of the upper extremity lie dorsal to those dealing with successively distal parts of the arm. Somatotopic organization has been demonstrated also in the cerebellar cortex and nuclei, in the cochlear nuclei with respect to a progressive sequence of tones, in the visual cortex with regard to projection of the retinal fields, and in the ventral horns of the spinal cord for sequential arrangement of motor neurons innervating successive groups of muscles. The dorsal spinal columns in man exemplify somatotopic organization of fiber tracts. Although somatotopic organization has not been investigated in all parts of the central nervous system, it is probably present throughout.

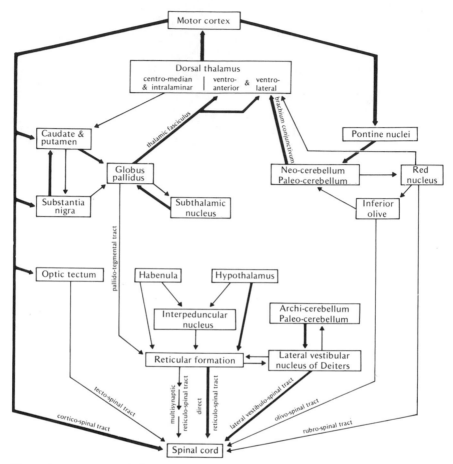

Figure 2-2   Diagram of the suprasegmental motor system of a mammal. The basic system of the lower vertebrates has been retained and supplemented, not replaced. The most important pathways are indicated by heavy lines.

It serves to maintain an orderly relation of neurons and fibers to other neurons in near and distant centers. Somatotopic organization is present in lower vertebrates as well, and is a basic feature of the organization of the vertebrate nervous system.

Somatotopic organization is often called "representation." The dorsal part of the postcentral gyrus in man is a motor area subserving the opposite leg by initiating and controlling movement of that leg. The cerebral cortex does not, however, "represent" (i.e., symbolize or replace) the leg any more than do the sciatic nerve or femoral artery (Gooddy, 1956).

Lamination is an arrangement of alternating layers of neurons, and of processes and synapses. It is another pattern of organization and is found throughout phylogeny. It arranges synaptic pathways in the most efficient manner for convergence and for correlative function. Lamination is characteristic of some but not all nuclear groups. It is found in the most primitive vertebrates, within parts of the hypothalamus and the olfactory bulbs. Lamination is a constant feature in the visual system and in the cerebellar cortex.

In the cerebral cortex, layers of neurons differ in various areas and form the basis of the study of cytoarchitectonics. Early investigators attempted to correlate function with neuronal types and morphologic pattern, and thus create a functional map of the cerebral cortex. While structure and function are somewhat correlated, functions are not as anatomically limited as they were once thought to be.

Gyri and sulci in the cerebral cortex of many mammals increase the surface area without augmenting the total volume and hence the total size of the brain. The development of this pattern of infolding can be studied in late fetal and early postnatal stages. The same principle applies to the creation of the folia of the cerebellar cortex in reptiles, birds, and mammals. Generally, the larger the brain, the greater the number of gyri.

In some areas of the nervous system, "glomeruli" are found, consisting of glial-enclosed nests of terminal axons and dendrites with synapses. These synaptic centers are associated with unique, specialized types of neurons, such as the granular cells of the cerebellum, cells of the olfactory bulb, some neurons of the hypothalamus, and those of the interpeduncular nucleus. Processes of ependymal and glial cells sometimes participate in the formation of glomeruli. The term "glomerulus" was originally applied by early histologists to the olfactory glomeruli as "circumscribed islands of gray matter" (Cajal, 1909-1911).

The importance of the synapse in neural pathways has been recognized increasingly since the discovery that synapses may be either excitatory or inhibitory, and that chemical substances serve as synaptic transmitters. The distribution in the brain of chemical substances active in synaptic transmission is similar in most vertebrates but also proportionate to the extent of development of each cerebral structure. Neurons

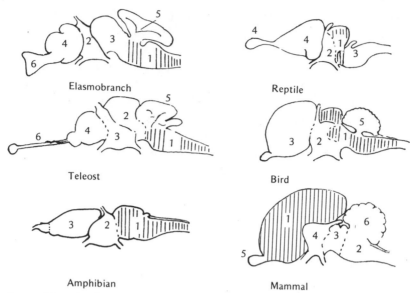

Figure 2-3 Distribution of choline acetylase, the enzyme catalyzing the formation of acetylcholine, in the brains of different vertebrates. Numbers indicate gradient of concentration; shaded areas and low numbers have the largest amounts of enzyme (Hebb and Ratković, 1964).

containing acetylcholine are present in the shark and in lower mammals, as well as in man (Hebb and Ratkovic, 1964; Krnjevic and Silver, 1965). The presence of this substance in the medulla of these animals and also in the cerebral cortex of man indicates that this transmitter is fundamental throughout phylogeny, but is also used in synaptic transmission in phylogenetically young structures (Fig. 2-3). Catecholamines are widely distributed in the brains of fishes and of terrestrial vertebrates of all classes (Brodie et al., 1964). Amphibians differ from other vertebrates by having mainly epinephrine rather than norepinephrine in the central nervous system (Brodie et al., 1964). Serotonin (5-hydroxytryptamine) is also found in most parts of the brain of submammalian species (Welsh, 1964) and of mammals (Amin et al., 1954); the ratio of serotonin to catecholamines is much higher in some lower vertebrates than in mammals (Brodie et al., 1964).

Electrotonic synaptic transmission without the use of chemical substances may occur in the thalamus of fishes (Bennett, 1966). A similar mechanism is found in the ciliary ganglion of birds (Martin and Pilar,

1963). The membranes of the two cells forming the synapse are locally thickened and in close apposition.

Brain of amphioxus

The central nervous system of amphioxus consists almost entirely of a spinal cord (Fig. 2-4). The organization is primitive, partly regressive, but surprisingly specialized in other ways (Bone, 1960). General somatic sensory nerves are distributed to epidermis and muscle, and somatic motor nerves innervate the myotomes (Chapter 3). A small, poorly differentiated brain lies at the rostral end of the spinal cord (Franz, 1923; Kappers et al., 1936). Special sense organs have not evolved in amphioxus; receptors for smell and taste, lateral line organs (Chapter 5), labyrinth, and eyes are absent. Amphioxus is a living example of a chordate nervous system lacking the specialized centers to process special sensory

Figure 2-4   Rostral end of amphioxus. The notochord is ventral to the spinal cord and extends farther rostrally than does the brain. Clusters of pigmented cells occur within both the spinal cord and the diminutive brain at fairly regular intervals. Ventral structures are the buccal cavity with surrounding cirri and branchial or gill arches. Whole mount. Acetocarmine, X 62.

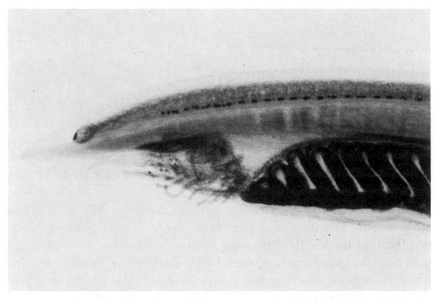

information that comprise large portions of the brains of true vertebrates.

The central nervous system of amphioxus arises, as in vertebrate embryogenesis, as an ectodermal medullary fold which closes in a progressively rostral direction, but the closure is incomplete. The neural tube retains communication with the surrounding sea water through an anterior cleft or neuropore. Early observers thought this cleft was an "olfactory groove." Pigmented cells in the neural tube were also first believed to be light receptors.

Paired nerves arise from the ventral surface of the cephalic end of the brain, homologous with the vertebrate terminalis nerve, the first in the series of branchial nerves (Chapter 4). A groove lined with a specialized, ciliated epithelium lies in the ventral wall of the brain just behind the entrance of the terminalis nerves. It is similar to the sensory epithelium of the infundibular region, the saccus vasculosus (Chapter 9) of fishes (Boeke, 1908). This groove, probably homologous with the infundibulum of vertebrates, may be regarded as a landmark to demarcate the diencephalon. Olfactory nerves and centers, and habenulae are absent. The thalamus and hypothalamus are undifferentiated. They consist of a few neurons around the third ventricle; the neurons are sparse and do not form a layer.

It is difficult to ascertain the limits of the midbrain in amphioxus, or even if a midbrain exists. The usual landmarks of the midbrain of vertebrates are absent. The lack of eyes is associated with the absence of optic, oculomotor, and trochlear nerves, and the optic tectum. The tegmental nuclei of the mesencephalon are also totally undifferentiated.

The cerebellum is lacking. Paired nerves, frequently with two rootlets and dorsal rami, arise dorsally behind the infundibulum and just rostral to the first myotome. They are sensory in character and are probably homologous with the dorsal part of the ophthalmic division of the trigeminal nerve. The five paired nerves lying caudally are primitive branchial nerves, both sensory and motor in function, and probably are the forerunners of branches of the trigeminal nerve. Vestibular nuclei do not exist.

The boundary between medulla and spinal cord is difficult to determine because primitive branchial arches occur along the entire rostral two-thirds of the length of the animal. The segmental nerves associated with them might all be considered branchial nerves of the medulla, which in higher vertebrates merge into the facial, glossopharyngeal, vagal, and accessory nerves. Another interpretation is that the more caudal nerves of the branchial arches are spinal nerves associated with arches that disappear with evolution.

It is instructive to observe in amphioxus how little the organization of the brain differentiates from that of the spinal cord because special sensory organs do not develop.

Brain of a hypothetic ancestral vertebrate

At least two features absent in amphioxus created conditions favorable to further cerebral evolution in an early ancestral vertebrate. One development in the latter was the labyrinth, an organ for orientation in space, discussed in Chapter 5. The other important development was that of sensory organs for distant information.

Eyes and olfactory receptors developed early in the evolution of vertebrates. These structures are already differentiated in the most primitive of living vertebrates, the cyclostomes. Tactile perception and taste give information about the immediate environment, but sight and olfaction also inform about the distant or remote environment. The importance of distant information is evidenced by the evolution of the phylogenetic series of vertebrates, contrasted with the failure of creatures lacking distance receptors to evolve further, exemplified by amphioxus.

The anatomic organization of the nervous system established in the hypothetic ancestral vertebrate was repeated and expanded by all subsequent vertebrates. That basic pattern involved specialization of the hindbrain for receiving information about the immediate environment, and of the midbrain and forebrain for receiving information about the distant environment. Sensory impulses related to touch, temperature, taste, and balance thus entered the medulla for quick reflexive responses by motor nuclei. Information from distance receptors, however, entered the midbrain from the eyes, or the forebrain from the olfactory epithelium. Because the distance from the object perceived by sight or smell was greater, more time was available before motor responses were required, so that a longer delay in conducting impulses to medullary motor centers was not a disadvantage. Remote information also required more interpretation before responses were made, and the forebrain therefore became associative while the medulla remained reflexive. With the further evolution of the forebrain, all sensory information eventually was relayed rostrally for interpretation and correlation, but the primitive medullary reflexes persisted, even in man.

Hearing is another special sense in part related to distance. It can inform about the remote environment. In contrast to the organization just outlined, its primary centers are in the medulla (the pons of mammals). Hearing, however, is a secondary adaptation of the lateral line and vestibular systems that were not originally intended to perceive sound (Chapter 5). Hearing, except perhaps the detection of low frequency vibrations, is absent in the lowest vertebrates, as it almost certainly was in the ancestral vertebrate. In accordance with the basic organization of the nervous system, auditory impulses entering the medulla are transmitted rostrally to the midbrain, both for interpretation and for reflexive responses. The separation of distant information from that relating to the immediate environment was thus preserved.

Although the transitional animal between creatures resembling amphioxus and the most primitive living vertebrates has been long extinct, it produced important advances which made possible the evolution of vertebrates: the development of a labyrinth and of distance-receptors. The details of the early evolution of eyes and olfactory apparatus and their central connections can be only suspected from the study of ontogenesis of living vertebrates. The factors inducing the original development remain obscure.

The spinal cord of the larval lamprey *Ammocoetes* probably resembles the hypothetic transitional vertebrate closer than any other living animal. The first detailed description of the nervous system of this creature was made by Tretjakoff (1909a, b), and the brains of adult cyclostomes were described by Johnston (1902) and Jansen (1930). The application of newer techniques to the study of metamorphosis of larval cyclostomes may reveal stages in the development of cerebral sensory systems not apparent from the study of ontogenesis in higher vertebrates.

Evolution of meninges

The meninges of lower vertebrates differ considerably from those of man and other mammals (Sterzi, 1901, 1902; Geldern, 1923; Kappers et al., 1936). Early ancestral vertebrates probably had a layer of undifferentiated mesenchyme between the neural tube and the epidermis, similar to that of amphioxus or early embryonic stages of modern vertebrates. From this mesenchyme, a cartilage-forming perichondrium or a bone-forming periosteum developed and gave origin to the skeletal elements of skull and spine. The primitive meninx of cyclostomes (Fig. 2-5) is a

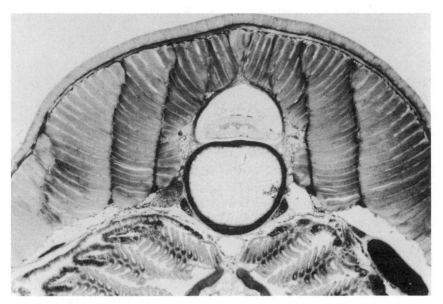

Figure 2-5 Coronal section of midbody of *Ammocoetes* (larval lamprey) to show relations of notochord, myotomes, spinal cord, primitive meninx, and perimeningeal fat and loose connective tissue. Luxol fast blue and cresyl violet, X 62.

layer of loose mesenchyme with a high glycogen content; it contains blood vessels and melanocytes. This matrix surrounds the brain and spinal cord. It has been studied electron microscopically and histochemically (Rovainen et al., 1971). An absence of septa penetrating the cord is associated with lack of vascular supply to the interior of the cord. In elasmobranchs, meningeal septa of connective tissue and accompanying vessels grow into the cord from the primitive meninx, but remain separated from the nervous elements by glia. This arrangement persists throughout phylogeny.

Cyclostomes and elasmobranchs have a protective layer of fatty and mucoid perimeningeal tissue, and a fibrous perichondrium attached to the loose primitive meninx by collagenous lateral ligaments. Smaller dorsal and ventral ligaments are also present in elasmobranchs. Perimeningeal adipose tissue of man lies in the space between the dura and the periosteum of the vertebral column. It may be a phylogenetic remnant of this perimeningeal buffer tissue.

In some teleostean fishes, the outer layer of the primitive meninx becomes condensed into a fibrous layer that comprises the dura mater in higher vertebrates. The arachnoid and pial membranes are still undifferentiated in fishes, and arachnoidal cavities or a subarachnoid space do not exist. The cerebrospinal fluid is therefore limited to the ventricular cavities and central canal. The choroid plexus in cyclostomes and some other lower vertebrates forms an evaginated sac protruding from the roof of the third and fourth ventricles, and mesencephalon. These sacs contain much cerebrospinal fluid. A subarachnoid space develops in higher vertebrates. It contains cerebrospinal fluid, and the choroid plexuses are infolded within the ventricles.

The primitive meninx of amphibians and reptiles has two layers of condensation. The outer layer is the dura or pachymeninx; the inner layer is the leptomeninx. Large lateral ligaments and smaller dorsal and ventral ligaments are attached to the dura. In reptiles, a wide peridural space contains perimeningeal tissue and veins.

In birds, the dura is further differentiated and a subdural space is more evident. The perimeningeal space is not as large as in reptiles. The leptomeninx is incompletely differentiated into arachnoid and pial membranes, and a small amount of cerebrospinal fluid is present in arachnoidal spaces around the medulla and cervical and thoracic regions of the spinal cord (Hansen-Pruss, 1923).

The arachnoid and pia mater are fully developed in marsupial and placental mammals. The pia becomes a thin membrane adherent to brain, particularly where blood vessels penetrate, and forms the external wall of the potential perivascular space of Virchow-Robin. The subarachnoid space contains a large volume of cerebrospinal fluid. The dura mater has two layers, but the outer layer is really periosteum and not of true meningeal origin.

Globus (1937) proposed that human meningiomas arise from undifferentiated cell rests of primitive meninx, which occur in ontogenesis as well as in phylogenesis. The variety of tissues derived from primitive meninx accounts for the differences in cellular elements and their products in various meningiomas. Some of these tumors even have a core of undifferentiated mesenchyme (Fig. 2-6). Embryonal remnants resembling arachnoid are frequently seen in human meninges surrounding both normal and malformed brains. Psammoma bodies are structures associated with meningeal neoplasms; they may accompany these embryonal remnants (Globus, 1937).

Lipomas are tumors of fatty tissue. They may occur in man anywhere

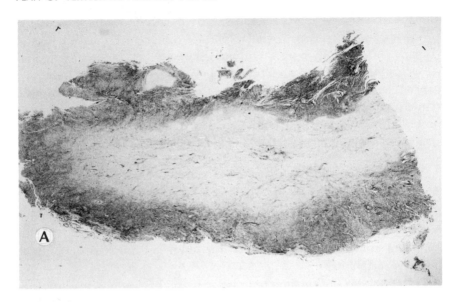

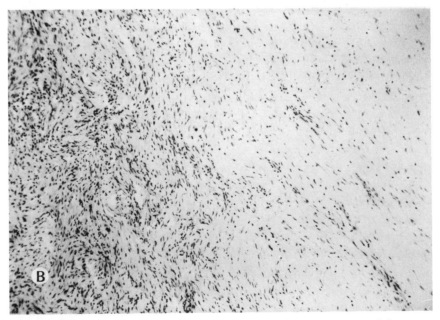

Figure 2-6 Unusual meningioma from a 57-year-old woman. Portions of the tumor resemble primitive meninx. (A) A central zone of poorly differentiated loose mesenchyme is bordered on both sides by condensed, moderately cellular connective tissue. (B) The loose and dense components blend microscopically. Hematoxylin and eosin, (A) X 9; (B) X 120.

along the neuraxis, but are found most frequently in the regions of the corpus callosum, tectum of the midbrain, tuber cinereum, and cauda equina. They may arise from the leptomeninges or from multipotential mesenchymal cells of the embryonic primitive meninx. An alternative explanation is that lipomas in these locations are of perimeningeal origin, reminiscent of lower vertebrates in whom the central nervous system is protected by a layer of fat and mucoid tissue around the meninges instead of by the fluid-filled subarachnoid space of mammals.

Phylogeny of ventricular system

The central nervous system of all vertebrates is a hollow, fluid-filled tubular structure which undergoes many modifications (Fig. 2-7). This tubular feature distinguishes it from the solid-core nervous systems of higher invertebrates.

The reason for this configuration is found in observations on ontogenesis. The neural tube develops embryologically as an infolding of surface ectoderm. The dorsal lips of the tube meet, then fuse in a caudorostral direction until the entire structure is closed. The ventricles of the brain and the central canal of the spinal cord are the result of formation of a neural tube and usually remain in continuity, even in adults.

Amphioxus, as already mentioned, still retains an anterior neuropore permitting free communication between the ventricle and the surrounding water. The single large ventricle expands posterior to the infundibulum and then narrows again further caudally to form a fissure-like lumen in the spinal cord. The rostral end of the single ventricle probably corresponds to the third ventricle of vertebrates. The posterior enlargement is associated with thinning of the roof of the brain in that region and probably corresponds to the fourth ventricle of vertebrates. The absence of a telencephalon explains the absence of lateral ventricles in this animal. The primordial pattern of the ventricular system of vertebrates is thus established even in protochordates. The cerebral aqueduct (iter, aqueduct of Sylvius) first develops in amphibians.

The spinal cord of all vertebrates has a central canal. The canal may be flattened or modified by the shape of the cord itself, and disappears at the caudal end of the cord. The central canal is relatively large in lower vertebrates and in young animals. In man, the central canal is large and patent in infants and children, but in adults often is obliterated by the proliferation of ependymal cells. Whether this is an aging process,

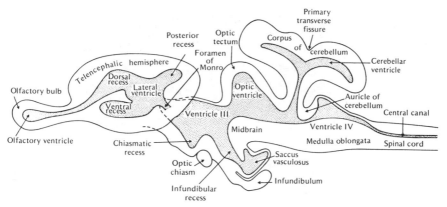

Figure 2-7   Diagram of ventricular system (stippled) of a shark. Midsagittal section of brainstem and parasagittal section through left cerebral hemisphere are depicted. Extensions of ventricular system into cerebellum and optic tectum are present only in lower vertebrates. The olfactory ventricle is obliterated in adult man.

the result of minor trauma, the clinically unexpressed presence of viruses in the cerebrospinal fluid, or other pathologic factors is not certain.

The shape of the fourth ventricle is related to the development of the cerebellum and medulla. In lower vertebrates such as elasmobranchs, the fourth ventricle extends dorsally within the center of the body of the cerebellum (Fig. 2-7). In petromyzonts, the roof of the fourth ventricle is formed by an expanded sac-like choroid plexus.

The third ventricle is present throughout phylogeny, with several extensions, such as the pineal, chiasmatic, and infundibular recesses. The infundibular recess in fishes is elaborated into paired narrow extensions into the inferior lobes of the hypothalamus, and into the saccus vasculosus (Chapter 9).

The third ventricle is continuous with a mesencephalic ventricle in most vertebrates. Dorsal extensions of the mesencephalic ventricle separate the optic tectum from the tegmentum of the midbrain. These extensions, the optic ventricles, are absent in mammals and in some reptiles and birds, but prominent in most other animals. Their disappearance in mammals accompanies the definitive formation of the cerebral aqueduct.

The cerebral aqueduct is lacking in fishes. In anuran amphibians, it is partially formed in the posterior part of the midbrain by the fusion of the torus semicircularis of the two sides. It communicates anteriorly with a mesencephalic ventricle and is continuous with the third ventricle. A

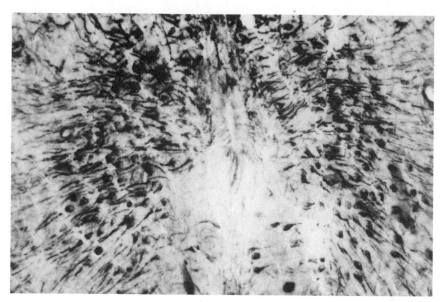

Figure 2-8   Central canal of spinal cord of adult bullfrog showing concentric layers of ependyma and subependyma. Each cell has a process radiating into parenchyma of cord. Frozen section. Esterase stain, X 25 (Sarnat et al., 1974).

definitive cerebral aqueduct traverses the midbrain between the third and fourth ventricles in some reptiles and birds and in all mammals.

The development of the lateral ventricles is dependent upon the differentiation of telencephalic structures, particularly the cerebral cortex. They are, therefore, best developed in higher mammals, particularly primates. Fishes have an "everted" telencephalon (Chapter 12) in which the lateral ventricles lie on the surface of the brain rather than within it. The occipital horn of the mammalian lateral ventricle is the phylogenetically newest development. It is barely present in most primates except man in whom it is the most variable portion of the ventricles.

The olfactory ventricles are small cavities within the olfactory bulbs. They extend back through the olfactory tracts into the lateral ventricles. In man, the olfactory ventricles and their caudal extension are usually obliterated, although patent in the fetus.

The circulation of cerebrospinal fluid in submammalian vertebrates is poorly understood. When Evans blue dye in albumen is injected into the lateral ventricle of the forebrain in sharks, the dye fills the entire ventricular system, including the extensions into the olfactory bulbs and the cerebellar ventricle, but does not spread along the external surface of the brain (Klatzo and Steinwall, 1967). This observation is consistent with the absence of a communicating subarachnoid space in lower vertebrates.

Ependyma and its derivatives

A ciliated neuroepithelial lining of the ventricles of the brain and central canal of the spinal cord is a constant feature throughout vertebrate phy-

Figure 2-9 Hemisection of spinal cord of oppossum. Many glial cell bodies are in the white matter and have processes radiating both toward the gray matter and also peripherally. Frozen section. Esterase stain, X 20 (Sarnat et al., 1974).

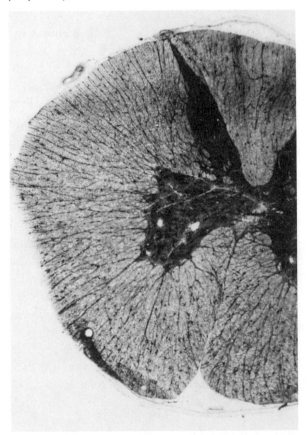

logeny. Cilia are lacking only in small, specialized regions of ependyma, such as the vascular organ of the lamina terminalis, subfornical and subcommissural organs, hypophyseal median eminence and area postrema at the transition of fourth ventricle into spinal canal, as demonstrated by the scanning electron microscope (Weindl and Joynt, 1972). In amphioxus, the ependymal cells serve as the principle glial component of the central nervous system (Bone, 1960). Ependymal cells are probably derived from the same cells of ectodermal origin which differentiate into neurons and neuroglia.

Processes extend into the cerebral parenchyma from the bases of ependymal cells and may be multiple and highly branched (ependymal astrocytes) or single, long, and unbranched (tanycytes) (Horstmann, 1954). In submammalian vertebrates, ependymal basal processes are generally present throughout the ventricular system, as demonstrated in the frog (Oksche, 1958; Paul, 1967) and turtle (Fleischhauer, 1957). The spinal ependyma and subependyma of lower vertebrates surround the central canal in concentric layers. Each cell has a radiating process (Figs. 2-8 and 2-9). Some processes reach the surface of the cord; others terminate in the gray matter, probably in relation to neurons (Sarnat et al., 1973).

Among placental mammals, the ependyma differs regionally, particularly in the third ventricle and its various recesses, in the rat (Colmant, 1967) and cat (Fleischhauer, 1961). Nearly all ependymal cells in the hypothalamic region of the adult mouse, rat, rabbit, and cat have basal processes differing considerably in length, caliber, spinous structures, and patterns of branching, as demonstrated by impregnation techniques (Bleier, 1971). Tanycytes of this region have been studied in the adult rat by electron microscopy (Brawer, 1972). Ependymal processes are not found in the thalamic portion of the third ventricle, but in neonatal and young animals, these processes are numerous in the rostral and ventral portions of the walls of the lateral ventricles, extending into the septum and caudate nucleus. These are rarely seen in adult animals (Bleier, 1971). Electron microscopy of the cerebral aqueduct reveals both branched and unbranched basal processes of the ependyma in newborn and one-week-old rabbits, but not in adult animals (Tennyson and Pappas, 1962). In the salamander, processes of ependymal cells in the midbrain participate with neuronal processes in the formation of glomeruli in the interpeduncular nucleus (Herrick, 1948; Chapter 9).

The termination of processes of ependymal cells in mammals is largely upon neurons and capillaries and within tangles of glial cell processes (Bleier, 1971). In amphioxus, bundles of ependymal cell processes terminate in end-feet upon the outer surface of the spinal cord (Fig. 2-10; Bone, 1960). Blood vessels do not penetrate the spinal cord. The failure of spinal neurons to migrate from a location near the ependyma in amphioxus (Fig. 2-10) may be related to a nutritive function of the ependyma. The presence of glycogen in spinal ependymal cells and their processes throughout phylogeny (Fig. 2-11) further suggests that these cells may provide a supplemental energy reserve for spinal neurons, particularly in lower vertebrates lacking a dense vascular network in the central nervous system (Sarnat et al., 1973, 1974; see Evolution of Sources of Nutritive Supply, page 51).

The importance of the spinal ependyma in the regeneration of the spinal cord after amputation of the tail of the salamander was demonstrated by Egar and Singer (1972). The caudal end of the regenerating cord is a simple ependymal tube. More rostrally, ependymal cells of the

Figure 2-10 Section of spinal cord of Amphioxus to show processes of ependymal cells extending to surface of cord. Neurons are near ependyma and do not migrate. Large cells with melanin in cytoplasm are near ventral part of central canal that extends to dorsal surface. White structures in parenchyma of cord are large ascending and descending fibers. Luxol fast blue and cresyl violet, X 125.

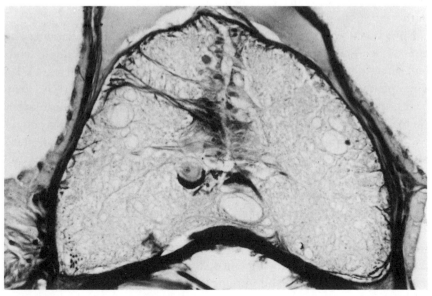

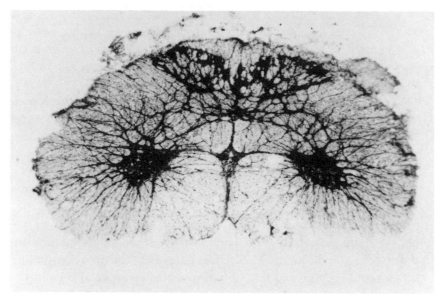

Figure 2-11   Distribution of glycogen in ependymal and glial cells in spinal cord of shark. Many radiating processes extend to and from the periphery of the cord. Frozen section. Phosphorylase stain, X 20 (Sarnat et al., 1974).

enlarged central canal have many basal processes that enclose tunnel-like pathways guiding regenerating axons caudally.

Ependymal cell processes of the infundibulum have a characteristic appearance and pattern of branching in mammals, terminating as end-feet directly upon the walls of hypophyseal portal vessels (Bleier, 1971). The ependymal cells and their processes in the infundibular recess may transport substances between the cerebrospinal fluid of the third ventricle to the nerves and capillaries of the hypothalamus and adenohypophysis (anterior pituitary), possibly functioning as part of the pituitary regulatory system or a short feedback loop to the neurons of the hypothalamus (Lofgren, 1959; Bleier, 1971).

Subependymomas of adult man are tumors arising from the ventricular wall, the septum pellucidum, or central canal of the spinal cord. These masses are composed of a mixture of ependymal cells and subependymal astrocytes. The cells are not anaplastic, and the tumor is thought to be either a benign neoplasm (Boykin et al., 1954) or a hamartoma (Russell and Rubinstein, 1971). The tumors are occasionally multiple, particularly in the fourth ventricle and may be an incidental finding at necropsy. It is conceivable that the astrocytes of this growth may actually be ependymal cells retaining branched basal processes, in locations normal for lower vertebrates and human fetuses, but not for adult man.

The choroid plexus is formed by the intraventricular proliferation of ependymal cells during embryonic development, resulting in numerous neuroepithelial infoldings and tubules projecting into the ventricles (Fig. 2-12; Shuangshoti and Netsky, 1966a). It includes some connective tissue and a rich vascular network, both derived from the overlying meninges during early ontogenesis. In all vertebrates, choroid plexus secretes and resorbs cerebrospinal fluid, but this function may be quantitatively more significant in lower vertebrates and in human embryos. The choroid plexus of lampreys contains 60 per cent of the total cerebral blood volume, in contrast to only 4 per cent in the rat (Heisey, 1968). Histochemical differences between developing and mature choroid plex-

Figure 2-12   Diagram of choroid plexus and paraphysis in a lower vertebrate such as lamprey (Netsky and Shuangshoti, 1970).

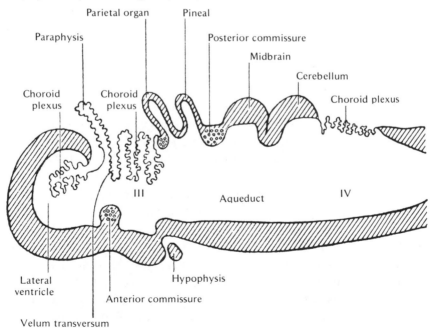

uses in man also have been reported. Glycogen is particularly prominent in the telencephalic choroid plexus of fetuses and disappears after birth. This change suggests differences in function of the choroid plexus at different stages of maturity. The loss of glycogen may be related to the change from anaerobic to aerobic metabolism associated with breathing at the time of birth (Shuangshoti and Netsky, 1966a).

The paraphysis is an extraventricular choroid plexus, containing similar neuroepithelial-lined villi (Kappers, 1955; Shuangshoti and Netsky, 1966a, b). It arises from the diencephalic roof in the area of the velum transversum. The paraphysis is best developed in lower vertebrates. It is variably present in the human fetus, but not as the complex tubular formations present in urodelan amphibians and other lower vertebrates (Shuangshoti and Netsky, 1966a, b). The vascular plexus of the paraphysis differs from that of the choroid plexus in being composed entirely of venous sinusoids in the salamander (Herrick, 1948). Differences in secretory activity between the paraphysis and intraventricular choroid plexus have been demonstrated (Kappers, 1950).

The velum transversum is also a modified choroid plexus which, together with the lamina terminalis, forms an arbitrary border between diencephalon and telencephalon. The velum transversum is distinct in lower vertebrates; in some urodelan amphibians it serves as the choroid plexus of the third ventricle. The exact distribution of choroid plexus within the ventricles differs among vertebrates, but is probably not significant for the evolution of the human brain.

The subcommissural organ (of Dendy) is a site of focally thickened ependyma, beneath the posterior commissure. The cells are tall, ciliated, and columnar. The organ is present in all vertebrates. A long, non-neural fiber of Reissner, formed by a fusion of processes from many ependymal cells of the subcommissural organ, extends through the cerebral aqueduct, fourth ventricle, and spinal canal to the caudal end of the spinal cord. In man, the fiber of Reissner disappears after infancy.

Nerve fibers connecting the pineal body and subcommissural organ have been described (Kappers, 1965; Mollgaard and Moller, 1973). Oksche (1962) postulated that the photosensory frontal organ (parietal eye) of frogs affected the pineal body to regulate a secretory function of the subcommissural organ. It had been proposed for many years that the subcommissural organ secreted a substance into the cerebrospinal fluid. Palkovits (1965) reported that a watery extract of the subcommissural organ of rats had an antidiuretic effect and influenced the absorption of sodium, potassium, and water from the small intestine by acting indirectly on the adrenals.

Comparative histology of neuroglia

The main component of the neuroglia of amphioxus is ependyma (Schneider, 1879; Mueller, 1900; Achucarro, 1918; Bone, 1960). The ependymal cells lining the central canal have long processes extending to the surface of the spinal cord and terminate as end-feet upon the limiting membrane of the cord (Figs. 2-10 and 2-13). Other cells extend as chains near the dorsal roots within the cord and also peripherally along the dorsal roots. These cells were interpreted by Bone (1960) as primitive cells of Schwann. The presence of Schwannian cells within the central nervous system is not a unique feature in amphioxus. In man, intramedullary

Figure 2-13   Diagram of ependymal, glial, and notochordal cells in the spinal cord of Amphioxus (1) ependymal cells; (2) glial cells; (3) primitive cells of Schwann. See text for details. (Bone, 1960).

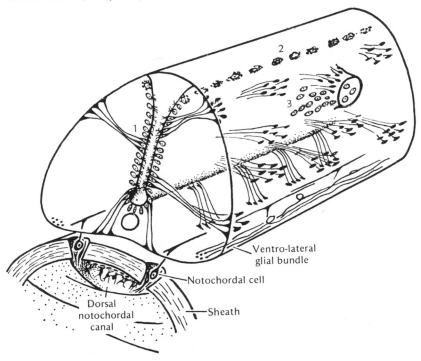

Ventro-lateral glial bundle

Notochordal cell

Dorsal notochordal canal

Sheath

proliferation of cells of Schwann in the spinal cord occurs in normal patients as microscopic nodules, probably as a response to physical or metabolic injury (Adelman and Aronson, 1972). A third type of non-neural cell in the roof of the spinal cord (Fig. 2-13) may be the only true glial cell in amphioxus (Schneider, 1879; Bone, 1960).

A progressive differentiation of neuroglia from neuroepithelium occurs in cyclostomes, elasmobranchs, and teleosts, as demonstrated by impregnation techniques (Mueller, 1900). Some sharks have numerous ependymal cells, with long processes having large end-feet in contact with small blood vessels. These cells may be intermediate in the evolution of the astrocyte (Horstmann, 1954). Tanycytes also occur in the hypothalamic region of mammals, and are discussed in the section on ependyma in this chapter. Other elasmobranchs and teleostean fishes (Acucharro, 1918), however, have more characteristic astrocytes (Horstmann, 1954). The astrocytes and oligodendroglia typical of mammals (Glees, 1955) are also present in amphibians and in birds (Bairati and Maccagnani, 1950).

A unique type of astrocyte is found in the optic tectum of birds (Bairati and Maccagnani, 1950). The cerebellar cortex, another laminated structure, also has a specialized type of astrocyte in the layer of cells of Purkinje, in all vertebrates with well organized cerebellar folia. This cell of Bergmann has a long, straight process reaching the pia to form marginal end-feet on the superficial limiting membrane (Glees, 1955). The process of the cell of Bergmann serves as support for the dendrites of the cell of Purkinje.

Phylogenetic changes in vascular system

Amphioxus lacks vessels in the central nervous system. Arteries do not penetrate the spinal cord of the lamprey, although a few small vessels enter the brain. Simple capillary loops supply the spinal cord of myxinoids.

Arterial blood reaches the head of fishes through a pair of arteries arising from the anterior end of the dorsal aorta. These vessels extend forward along both sides of the head and are primordial carotid arteries. They enter the skull near the pituitary gland and give origin to the ophthalmic artery to supply the retina on each side, similar to the condition in higher vertebrates.

The orbital artery is a major branch of the carotid artery of fishes; it arises outside the skull and supplies much of the face and jaws. This vessel persists in most terrestrial vertebrates as the homologous stapedial artery, so named because it arises near the stapes. The lingual artery is another branch of the carotid artery in amphibians and reptiles, and it is homologous with the external carotid artery of mammals. It is a small artery that supplies blood to the tongue and throat in reptiles, and in lower mammals its distribution includes the lower jaw, and, in some species, also the maxilla. In higher mammals, the external carotid artery is larger and incorporates branches of the stapedial artery; the latter vessel is correspondingly smaller or is completely lost in some species, including man. (In man it is present in the embryo, however.) A new and shorter route thus develops for supplying blood to the jaws and face of higher mammals (Romer, 1970).

In some mammals, such as the dog, arterial anastomoses are large and numerous between branches of the external carotid artery and those of the internal carotid (de la Torre et al., 1959). This feature protects the animal from cerebral infarction after occlusion of the internal carotid artery. In man, this collateral circulation is usually vestigial and inadequate for significant shunting of blood.

The intracranial circulation of representative species of each class of vertebrates has been described by Gillilan (1967, 1972). The brains of most submammalian vertebrates are supplied exclusively by a pair of internal carotid arteries. Within the skull, each internal carotid divides into a caudal and rostral division. In fishes, the caudal branch is the larger and supplies the medulla, cerebellum, and optic tectum. Amphibians, reptiles, and birds have progressive enlargement of the rostral branch to nourish the expanded forebrain; most of the blood thus flows rostrally in the advanced species. Cerebral branches of the internal carotid artery are homologous with similar branches in mammals; they include anterior, middle, and posterior cerebral arteries and the anterior choroidals. The primordia of these vessels are already differentiated in some amphibians. Many snakes have an aberrant condition in which one carotid artery supplies both sides of the brain.

The basilar artery is formed by the union of the caudal rami of the internal carotid arteries of the two sides. In most birds, either the basilar artery arises from only one carotid artery or the bilateral carotid contributions are unequal in size (Pearson, 1972). The basilar artery extends along the ventral surface of the brainstem, giving origin to segmental branches that supply the medulla. The diameter of the basilar artery decreases as it extends caudally. In most reptiles and birds, it does not end blindly, but is continuous with the ventral spinal artery. Only snakes have an additional source of blood to the caudal end of the basilar artery through the artery of the first cervical nerve, a vessel not homologous with the vertebral artery of mammals.

In the 5-week (9 mm) human embryo, the internal carotid artery divides into two terminal branches: a small anterior and a large posterior trunk that continues into the basilar artery (Earle et al., 1953). This condition is reminiscent of that in adult fishes. The trigeminal artery is the communication between the internal carotid and basilar arteries in somewhat older human embryos. It is considerably proximal to the posterior communicating artery, and atrophies in later fetal life; in a few normal individuals, the trigeminal artery persists as the major source of blood to the posterior cerebral circulation in adult life (Fig. 2-14). It is also found in some infants with holoprosencephalic brains (Zingesser et al., 1966). This vessel in man is thus a phylogenetic carry-over of the usual condition in submammalian vertebrates. The otic and hypoglossal arteries are additional fetal shunts between the carotid and basilar arteries in man.

A major advance in the cerebral circulation of lower mammals is the development of paired vertebral arteries. These vessels terminate in the caudal end of the single basilar artery and the direction of blood flow in the basilar artery is thus reversed. The major blood supply to the posterior cerebral arteries differs among species, coming from the basilar, the internal carotid, or from both arteries. The arterial circle of Willis at the base of the brain is lacking in many lower mammals because the anterior communicating and posterior communicating arteries are absent. Collateral circulation between the internal carotid and vertebrobasilar systems, and between the carotids of the two sides is therefore lacking in those animals. This feature of the intracranial circulation has been used in the experimental study of cerebral infarction in the gerbil (Levine and Sohn, 1969; Kahn, 1972). Most birds, in contrast, have an anastomosis between the two internal carotid arteries (Pearson, 1972).

The superior cerebellar arteries are paired vessels arising at the rostral end of the basilar artery in most vertebrates. They are the principal source of blood to the cerebellum of reptiles, but birds and mammals also have a pair of inferior cerebellar arteries arising from the basilar artery to augment the blood supply to the enlarged cerebellum. In some advanced mammals including man, the inferior cerebellar artery is re-

placed by two vessels, the posterior inferior cerebellar and anterior cerebellar arteries. These two vessels in man are reciprocal in size and vary
among individuals.

The arterial distribution to most parts of the brain is relatively constant in reptiles, birds, and mammals. For example, the optic tectum in
most vertebrates is supplied by branches of the basilar, posterior cerebral arteries, and superior cerebellar arteries, as it is in man. Lenticulo-
striate arteries supply the corpus striatum; the unique portions of that
structure in birds also receive arterial blood from branches of the middle

Figure 2-14   Right carotid arteriogram of a patient with persistent embryonic trigeminal artery. This large communication shunts blood from the internal carotid artery
to the basilar and hence posterior cerebral arteries; the place of origin of the trigeminal artery from the internal carotid is considerably proximal to that of the posterior
communicating artery. The left vertebral artery in this case was small and almost vestigial; the right vertebral artery was not injected. This anomaly in man is reminiscent
of the usual condition in submammalian vertebrates, in which vertebral arteries do
not develop, and the basilar artery receives blood from the internal carotid vessels.

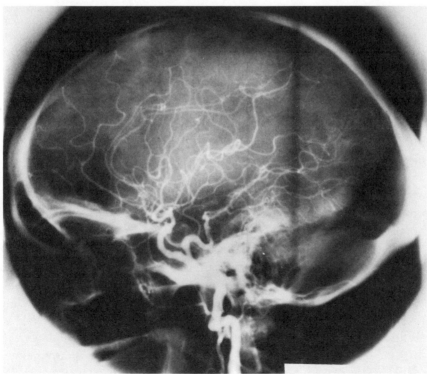

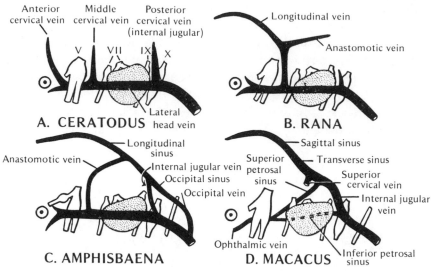

Figure 2-15 Phylogenetic development of intracranial venous drainage. Roots of some cranial nerves are indicated by Roman numerals; the position of the eye is shown by a circle with central dot; the stippled structure is the otic capsule. The lateral head vein disappears in mammals, and all blood is drained from the brain by the paired internal jugular veins. (A) *Ceratodus*, lungfish; (B) *Rana*, frog; (C) *Amphisbaena*, lizard; (D) *Macacus*, monkey. (Romer, 1970).

cerebral arteries (Pearson, 1972). The highly developed avian structures, the hyperstriatum and ectostriatum, are thought to incorporate the primordial neocortex of reptiles (Chapter 12).

Vertebrates have two intrinsic patterns of small intracerebral vessels (Gillilan, 1967, 1972). In most species, arterioles terminate in a continuous capillary plexus that is densest in nuclear regions. Cyclostomes, lungfishes, some amphibians, many lizards, and marsupial mammals differ from other vertebrates in that arterioles end in capillary loops rather than in plexuses. Each penetrating arteriole of the loop is accompanied by a venule; each pair of vessels constitutes an end-system. Marsupials also have a few capillary plexuses in some regions of the brain, including the infundibular stalk, choroid plexuses, and area postrema. The first evidence of specialization in the vascular arrangement in phylogeny is the formation of a perineuronal plexus in the optic tectum of amphibians (Gillilan, 1967).

In all classes of vertebrates except mammals, a pair of lateral head veins arise from an expanded venous sinus within the orbit. These lateral head veins course posteriorly outside the skull and receive tributaries from the brain. They eventually return blood to the heart by entering the common cardinal veins in fishes, or the superior vena cava in lung-fishes and terrestrial vertebrates. A series of venous sinuses progressively develop within the skull (Romer, 1970; Fig. 2-15).

An important advance occurs in the intracranial venous circulation in mammals. The lateral head veins disappear and the major intracranial veins become enclosed by the dural membranes to form intercommunicating venous sinuses. Venous blood from the orbit and face enters the intracranial sinuses to mix with venous blood from the brain and leave the head through a pair of large internal jugular veins. This feature of the mammalian venous circulation is responsible for the occasional extension to the brain of superficial infections of the face, and may result in infectious thrombosis of the cavernous sinus in man. A pair of external jugular veins also drains blood from superficial parts of the head and joins the internal jugular to form the common jugular vein. This latter pair of vessels returns blood to the heart through the subclavian vein and superior vena cava.

Blood-brain barrier

In mammals, tight junctions between adjacent endothelial cells of cerebral blood vessels prevent circulating proteins from leaving the lumen of the vessel. These tight endothelial junctions comprise a part of the anatomic substrate of the "blood-brain barrier." They have been demonstrated electron microscopically in the mouse (Reese and Karnovsky, 1967), in the urodelan amphibian *Necturus* (Bodenheimer and Brightman, 1968), and in the goldfish (Brightman et al., 1971). Experimentally, this barrier prevents intravenously injected dyes that form complexes with serum proteins from diffusing into the parenchyma of the brain, although they do penetrate the choroid plexus and also may enter injured cerebral tissue.

Preliminary evidence thus suggests that a blood-brain barrier is present in all vertebrates. Sharks differ from most other vertebrates in having predominantly open gaps between endothelial cells in the brain, and relatively few tight junctions. The site of the barrier in sharks is the cell layer external to the capillary endothelium. The perivascular glial sheath in these animals is composed mainly of astrocytic cell bodies, rather than end-feet, as in most vertebrates (Klatzo and Steinwall, 1965). Both gap junctions and tight junctions are related to adjacent astrocytes, forming a circumferential barrier that prevents substances of high molecular weight from leaving the capillary (Brightman and Reese, 1969).

The open endothelial junctions in the brain of the shark are similar to the open junctions in the capillaries of mammalian skeletal and cardiac muscle (Karnovsky, 1967). The wide separations of 500 to 1000 Å between endothelial cells in human gliomas are much larger than the endothelial gap junctions of 40 Å in the normal shark brain (Brightman et al., 1971). In the shark, protein-dye complexes are prevented from diffusing into cerebral tissue, even after extensive thermal or chemical injury (Brightman et al., 1971). The numerous astrocytic processes in the neuropil are probably united by gap junctions rather than continuous tight junctions, however, because peroxidase injected into the cerebral ventricles is not prevented from passing through the extracellular space of the neuropil (Brightman et al., 1971). The preservation of the blood-brain barrier in the injured shark brain may be the result of astrocytic response to injury by forming belts of tight junctions that contain proteins within the injured region (Brightman et al., 1971); proliferation of glia around injured areas in shark brain is minimal or does not occur (Klatzo and Steinwall, 1965).

The choroid plexus of the shark resembles that of other vertebrates in having a fenestrated endothelium permeable to proteins and also an epithelium that prevents such substances from entering the cerebrospinal fluid. In other vertebrates, the transfer of protein also is blocked by tight junctions between epithelial cells of the choroid plexus (Brightman and Reese, 1969) and by lack of active transport of such products in pinocytotic vesicles (Brightman, 1967).

The area postrema is a structure in the caudal angle of the fourth ventricle (obex) and is composed of neurons and glial cells, in addition to an ependymal surface and numerous blood vessels continuous with those of the choroid plexus. The structure is present in elasmobranchs as well as in mammals, and probably occurs in all vertebrates. The area postrema is unusually permeable to substances injected either intracisternally or intravascularly. The early uptake of a macromolecular marker such as peroxidase, as well as a micromolecular marker such as sodium, suggests a specialized function of the unique glial cells in sampling extracellular fluid; the area postrema then controls the choroid plexus by regulating blood flow through the release of catecholamines. This hypothesis of an osmoreceptive function of the area postrema for the feedback control of the choroid plexus was proposed by Torack (1973). The subfornical or subcommissural organ may be a similar osmoreceptor, related to the choroid plexus of the third ventricle.

Evolution of sources of nutritive supply

The nutrition of the spinal cord involves three stages of evolution (Sarnat et al., 1973, 1974). The lowest species, including amphioxus and cyclostomes, lack intramedullary blood vessels and have prominent ependymal processes extending to the surface of the spinal cord (Fig. 2-10). Fishes, amphibians and reptiles have relatively sparse capillary networks in the spinal cord and retain prominent ependymal processes that extend into the gray matter of the cord (Fig. 2-8). The ependymal cell bodies and processes are rich in glycogen, and the ependyma may transport nutrients from the cerebrospinal fluid of the large central canal of the spinal cord and from the vascular, glycogen-rich meningeal tissue. The ependyma of adult placental mammals, in contrast, is atrophic, lacks processes, and has sparse glycogen; the capillary network is extensive, however, and glucose and other nutrients are derived from this vascular source. An intermediate condition is found in the opossum. This animal has neither ependymal processes nor a dense capillary network, but has developed an extensive system of glial processes extending to and from the periphery of the spinal cord (Fig. 2-9). These cells may derive nutrients from the cerebrospinal fluid of the spinal subarachnoid space, a compartment not developed in lower vertebrates.

The spinal central canal is large and patent in human fetuses. Basal ependymal processes and glial processes extend to the surface of the spinal cord (von Lenhossék, 1891; Cajal, 1909-1911). The elaborate development of the spinal ependyma in the human fetus and its atrophic condition in adult life are also likely related to the reciprocal increase in vascularity of the spinal cord that occurs with maturation. The relationship suggests that the spinal ependyma is an important source of energy reserve in both the human embryo and in lower vertebrates. An additional interpretation is that both lower vertebrates and human fetuses are more dependent upon anaerobic glycolysis for energy than are adult placental mammals, who use the more efficient metabolic pathway of oxidative phosphorylation of glucose.

The nutritive function of the ependyma is still an unproved hypothesis, however. Despite the phylogenetic differences in the morphology and glycogen content of ependymal cells, the mechanisms regulating the concentration of glucose in ventricular fluid relative to that in blood may be similar in sharks and in mammals (Oppelt et al., 1963).

3
Spinal cord and motor unit

Comparative gross structure of spinal cord

The dorsal position and cylindrical structure of the spinal cord of amphioxus are fundamentally similar to the position and structure in vertebrates. Advanced invertebrates such as arthropods, in contrast, have paired neural cords on the ventral side of the body. These cords are chains of segmental ganglia joined by longitudinal fibers.

Although amphioxus has a more primitive nervous system than any living vertebrate, homologous structures are recognized in the cord. The dorsal and ventral roots of this animal emerge alternately from the spinal cord. They do not join as they do in higher vertebrates, but remain separate peripherally. Dorsal roots emerge between successive myotomes, ventral roots in the middle of the myotomes. The roots then enter the segmental muscles (Fig. 3-1). A unique feature in amphioxus is a shift forward of one side of the body with respect to the other, so that corresponding nerve roots and myotomes of the two sides also alternate.

The segmental organization of the spinal cord is a secondary feature imposed by the arrangement of the body in segments. Axons of motor neurons are grouped into ventral roots in amphioxus because the myotomes they innervate are segmental. Sensory fibers are combined as dorsal roots because they pass from the skin to the spinal cord between successive myotomes. Segmentation is an efficient arrangement for sequential contraction of myotomes; it is useful for defensive reflexes and is essential for propulsion in water or on land.

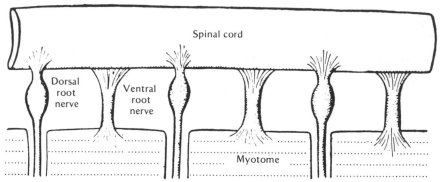

Figure 3-1 Relation of spinal roots and myotomes on one side of spinal cord of amphioxus and cyclostomes. Alternating arrangement of separate dorsal and ventral roots is related to sensory fibers passing between myotomes, and motor fibers entering centers of myotomes (Romer, 1970).

Sensory innervation of the skin is also segmental in all vertebrates. Overlap between adjacent segments is constant in phylogeny. It occurs in the shark (van Rijnberk, 1916) as well as in man, so that loss of one dorsal root does not result in a band of cutaneous anesthesia (Fig. 3-2). Such redundancy is found in many parts of the nervous system. The chance of survival is greater than when the disabling effect of focal injury is minimized.

Dorsal and ventral roots alternate in petromyzonts, as well as in amphioxus. The roots remain separate in petromyzonts, but unite into a common trunk in myxinoids, a feature characteristic of the spinal roots of all higher vertebrates. In myxinoids, elasmobranchs, and teleosts, the dorsal and ventral roots still emerge at levels slightly different from each other, but terrestrial vertebrates have dorsal and ventral roots emerging at the same level in each segment. In elasmobranchs, a small visceral efferent branch separates from the junction of dorsal and ventral roots, but white and gray communicating rami occur only in teleosts and terrestrial vertebrates to contribute to the ganglionated sympathetic chains (Chapter 10).

The number of paired spinal roots differs widely in phylogeny and is greatly altered by somatic specialization. Sharks have a hundred or more pairs of spinal roots; most frogs have only ten or eleven pairs. Caudal roots are absent in animals without tails, including man, but may be numerous and large in animals with prominent tails. The number of caudal segments is greatest in reptiles, in whom the tail is a continuation of the segmental somites, but posterior sacral and caudal spinal segments are also well developed in cats and in arboreal monkeys with prehensile tails.

The extinct ostracoderms had a spinal cord extending to the tip of the tail. In anuran amphibians, the larval tail is resorbed during metamorphosis. The caudal segments of the spinal cord undergo atrophy and become the ependymal and gliotic remnant called the filum terminale. Many fishes and mammals also have a filum terminale. The reptilian and avian spinal cord, however, extends the entire length of the spinal canal; a filum terminale is absent. The unequal length of the spinal cord and canal in mammals is related not only to atrophy or hypoplasia of caudal segments during embryogenesis but also to continued growth of the vertebral column after the spinal cord has attained its greatest length.

The most caudal region of the spinal cord in amphioxus is devoid of neurons and is composed entirely of ependyma. The central canal of this region is expanded, in contrast to the small or obliterated central canal in the filum terminale of vertebrates. The regenerating spinal cord after amputation of the tail of the salamander is reminiscent of the condition in amphioxus. An expansion of the central canal and a caudal growth of ependyma precede the regeneration of neural structures (Egar and Singer, 1972; Chapter 2).

The caudal end of the spinal cord of many fishes contains large glandular epithelial cells. The ventral part of the spinal cord is often enlarged at the most caudal segment. Associated with these glandular cells are vascular septa of connective tissue of meningeal origin. The entire struc-

Figure 3-2 Segmental innervation of the skin of a shark. The white area between the two stippled zones indicates an isolated analgesic segment produced by the cutting of three successive dorsal spinal roots (van Rijnberk, 1916).

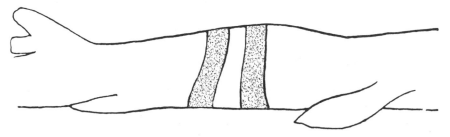

ture is called the hypophysis caudalis (Favaro, 1926). Its function is neurosecretory, similar to that of the preoptic area (Chapter 9).

The most rostral spinal roots are the spino-occipital nerves. The occipital nerves are outside the primitive skull of cyclostomes, but are included within the neocranium of elasmobranchs and higher vertebrates. Most of the ventral roots of spino-occipital nerves are secondarily lost in teleosts and some amphibians. In most terrestrial species, they coalesce to form the hypoglossal nerve (Chapter 7).

Cervical and lumbar enlargements of the spinal cord correspond to the development of extremities. These enlargements are lacking in fishes; the muscles associated with fins are used for stability rather than for propulsion through water. The lumbar enlargement predominates in frogs because of the powerful hind legs. In the ostrich, the lumbar region is larger than the cervical, but in birds that are strong fliers, the cervical region is the larger. Animals with extremities becoming secondarily atrophic or absent, such as snakes and whales, have small or absent cervical and lumbar enlargements. Turtles lack thoracic muscles. The corresponding part of the spinal cord is extremely thin.

Curtis and Helmholz (1911) found a decreased number of motor neurons in the ventral horns of the cervical region of the spinal cord in a newborn infant with congenital absence of upper extremities. In contrast to congenital absence of limbs, Taft (1920) reported a normal complement of ventral horn cells in appropriate segments of spinal cord of patients with limbs amputated many years previously.

The use of extremities for walking limits the efficient length of the animal, but the loss of extremities allows the body to lengthen, as exemplified by snakes. This elongation is accompanied by a greatly increased number of spinal segments associated both with muscles of the trunk and cutaneous dermatomes in most snakes. Many cervical segments occur in long-necked birds. An alternative arrangement is found in mammals with long necks. In the giraffe and horse the cervical vertebrae and associated segments of spinal cord are long but are not increased in number. A similar condition is found in the thoracic region of mammals with elongated bodies, such as the weasel and otter.

The cross-section of the spinal cord is round in most vertebrates. In amphioxus, it is triangular with a dorsal apex; the ventral surface is concave and conforms to the contour of the underlying notochord. This shape is similar to that of the embryonic spinal cord of many higher vertebrates. In cyclostomes, the spinal cord is flattened dorsoventrally.

Evolution of organization in spinal cord

Neurons are closely grouped around the central canal in the spinal cord of amphioxus and do not migrate. In the flattened spinal cord of cyclostomes, the neurons move laterally away from the primitive position of the neuroepithelium. Sensory and motor neurons, however, do not yet form dorsal and ventral horns of gray matter. These structures are first found in elasmobranchs and characterize the spinal cord of all higher vertebrates. The basic arrangement is a central canal formed by ependyma, surrounded by gray matter, and externally by tracts of ascending and descending fibers. This plan is established even in amphioxus and in cyclostomes, and it is maintained in the spinal cord throughout phylogeny.

The embryonic neural tube of vertebrates is divided on each side by a limiting sulcus extending longitudinally and separating the dorsal sensory region from the ventral motor region, except in cyclostomes. Functional columns are thus established. The dorsal and ventral zones each further subdivide into somatic and visceral columns (Fig. 3-3). Additional grouping of functionally similar neurons in the horns of the spinal cord occur in the cat (Rexed, 1952, 1954, 1965) and in the pigeon (van den Akker, 1970). The columns extend into the medulla, although the relations are altered by the expansion of the medullary roof of the fourth ventricle. The continuity of these functional columns is not dis-

Figure 3-3   Distribution of sensory and motor columns in (A) the spinal cord of the adult in most lower vertebrates, and (B) the medulla oblongata of the human embryo. The embryonic human spinal cord has a similar arrangement of columns as in the medulla. Motor centers arise in the basal plate, and sensory centers in the alar plate (Romer, 1970).

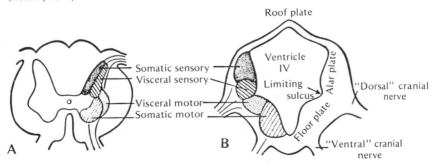

rupted in the spinal cord by secondary migration of neurons. Nuclei of the medulla migrate extensively, however (Chapter 7), and in most higher vertebrates the functional columns of the medulla are anatomically continuous only in the embryo.

Failure of neurons to migrate from the region of the central canal in amphioxus is probably related to nutritive factors rather than to a primitive state. Although horns of gray matter do not form in amphioxus, primary sensory neurons are dorsal in the spinal cord, motor neurons lie ventrally, and interneurons are intermediate in position. The fibers have already separated into dorsal and ventral roots. Dorsal roots contain somatic afferent fibers related to touch and proprioception, as well as visceral afferent fibers having terminations in mucous membranes and visceral efferent fibers to smooth muscle. The latter autonomic fibers are rearranged to emerge from the ventral roots in elasmobranchs and higher species (Chapter 10). Somatic efferent fibers compose the ventral roots in amphioxus, as they do in vertebrates.

Neurons giving origin to the dorsal root fibers lie within the spinal cord in amphioxus and do not yet aggregate in the dorsal roots to form ganglia. Intramedullary neurons giving rise to some or all fibers of the dorsal roots are also found in cyclostomes and teleosts and in immature forms of elasmobranchs, amphibians, and reptiles. In all other vertebrates including embryonic mammals, these neurons are insulated in ganglia among the fibers of the dorsal roots and lie outside the spinal cord. Primary sensory neurons are still intramedullary in the mesencephalic nucleus of the trigeminal nerve, however, even in man. In lower vertebrates, most primary sensory neurons of the spinal cord are bipolar, but some unipolar neurons occur in amphioxus and are the only type in advanced vertebrates.

The relation between the spinal cord and underlying notochord of amphioxus is extraordinary (Bone, 1960). The connective tissue sheath of the notochord is pierced at regular intervals by pairs of round cells with processes that enter the ventral surface of the spinal cord and branch into ascending and descending longitudinal fibers (Fig. 2-13). These cells have the staining qualities of neurons. They are surrounded by smaller cells with processes that enter the edges of a canal extending along the dorsal part of the notochord. Bone (1960) reluctantly concluded that the large unipolar notochordal cell with a bifurcating spinal process was a neuron, possibly relaying proprioceptive information from the bending movements of the notochord for the regulation of swimming movements. The need for such an arrangement is difficult to understand, because proprioceptive fibers from myotomes are present in amphioxus, similar to the condition in vertebrates. The larval lamprey, *Ammocoetes*, lacks such a connection between the notochord and spinal cord.

The intrinsic organization of the spinal cord was elucidated by study of developing larval amphibians (Coghill, 1913, 1914, 1929; Herrick and Coghill, 1915). The arrangement of neurons and pathways in these animals is fundamental in the evolution of the spinal cord and of the brain as well. The primary sensory neuron is the cell of Rohon and Beard (Fig. 3-4). It lies within the dorsal part of the spinal cord instead of in the dorsal root ganglion. Each segmental cell of Rohon and Beard has a large peripheral dendrite that bifurcates to supply the skin and also to enter the myotome. The axons ascend ipsilaterally to the medulla. They form a primitive pathway similar to the dorsal columns of mammals. The nonspecific sensory cells of Rohon and Beard occur in immature forms of lower vertebrates, but are supplemented or replaced in adult vertebrates by similar neurons specializing in either cutaneous sensation or proprioception. Similar primary sensory neurons form a sequential ascending pathway. The rostrally directed axon synapses with a dendritic branch of the next cell (Fig. 3-4) to propagate a sensory impulse from the body to the brain. This multisynaptic ascending pathway is also confined to the same side of the spinal cord as the primary sensory neurons that synapse with it.

A motor column in the ventral part of the spinal cord of *Amblystoma* (the urodelan amphibian studied by Coghill) is composed of stellate neurons with bifurcating axons. One branch passes into the ventral root to innervate the myotome of the same level; the other branch synapses with the next caudal motor neuron to propagate sequential contraction of muscle segments (Fig. 3-4).

The primary sensory and motor neurons are adequate for primitive reflexes of the spinal cord. Evidence for this fact is found in the monosynaptic tendon reflexes of man which participate in the control of muscle length and tone. The axon of the sensory neuron does not decussate. One other neuron is needed, however, for the developmnt of correlative centers, and hence for the evolution of the brain. This cell is an interneuron between primary sensory and motor neurons and lacks peripheral processes that pass outside the central nervous system. Such interneurons occur only in the rostral regions of the neural tube of developing larvae of *Amblystoma*. They connect the ascending sensory

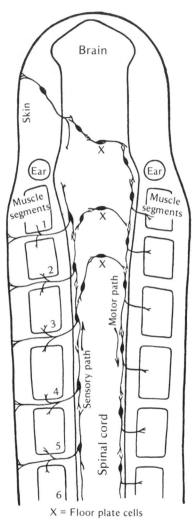

X = Floor plate cells

Figure 3-4   Components of the simple coiling reflex in the primitive spinal cord of a larval amphibian. The unspecialized primary sensory neuron, or cell of Rohon and Beard, has a dendrite with branches both to muscle and to skin. The axon ascends ipsilaterally in the spinal cord to synapse with decussating interneurons (floor plate cells) that relay the impulses to motor neurons on the opposite side of the spinal cord. Motor neurons not only innervate myotomes through axons that form the ventral spinal roots, but collateral fibers of these axons synapse with the next motor neuron to propagate an impulse caudally and cause sequential contraction of segmental myotomes (Coghill, 1929).

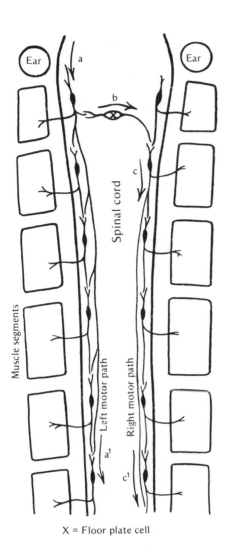

X = Floor plate cell

Figure 3-5   Diagram of the neural mechanism of cephalocaudal progression of movement away from the side of stimulus in *Amblystoma,* a larval amphibian. This organization is a slightly more complex derivative of the coiling reflex. Floor plate cells are decussating interneurons (Coghill, 1929).

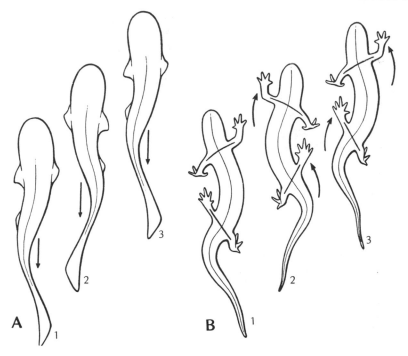

Figure 3-6 Illustration of the swimming movements of a (A) fish using the neural mechanism described by Coghill. Lower terrestrial vertebrates such as the (B) salamander utilize the same basic mechanism; the limbs are simple extensions of the axial muscles. Movements are in sequence with the muscles of the trunk (Romer, 1970).

and the contralateral descending motor chain of neurons. These decussating interneurons, the "floor plate cells" of Coghill, mediate a response to a stimulus anywhere on the side of the body or head by causing a sequential rostrocaudal contraction of myotomes on the opposite side (Coghill, 1929). The animal thus moves away from the side of stimulation (Fig. 3-5). The undulating movements of lower tetrapods is similar to the basic swimming movements of fishes (Fig. 3-6).

The spinal cord of amphioxus has several unique and specialized features extensively described by Bone (1960) who confirmed and expanded the earlier observations of Rohde (1888a, b) and Retzius (1891). Only those neurons and fibers relevant to the evolution of man will be discussed. Sensory neurons similar to the cells of Rohon and Beard are present, and motor neurons innervate the myotomes of amphioxus, as in

Amblystoma. In this primitive creature, however, the neurons most significant to evolution are the collosal cells of Rohde. These cells are large interneurons in the rostral and caudal segments of the spinal cord but are lacking in middle segments. Dendrites synapse with primary sensory neurons of both sides. The thick axons of the cells of Rohde decussate ventral to the central canal. Axons from caudal segments then ascend, and those from rostral segments descend, to synapse with motor neurons on the opposite side at levels other than the segments of origin (Fig. 3-7). This arrangement results in a coiling reflex to nonspecific cutaneous stimulation. Coiling of the entire body to any stimulus is the only response in amphioxus; local reflexes are totally lacking (Ten Cate, 1938). The same coiling response is also the first reflex to develop in larvae of *Amblystoma* and precedes the development of sequential movements away from stimuli (Coghill, 1929).

Crossed and uncrossed intersegmental fibers of the spinal cord are intrinsic spinal connections in all vertebrates. The number of fibers that ascend and descend increases greatly in phylogeny. The decussating interneuron is the basis of the primitive stepping and walking reflexes mediated entirely within the spinal cord. It coordinates movement of the trunk, tail, and extremities, and was demonstrated to be the mech-

Figure 3-7 Diagrammatic section of spinal cord of Amphioxus, showing cells of Rohde or decussating interneuron essential in the coiling reflex (Bone, 1960). This type of neuron is the forerunner of the crossed long pathways of the central nervous system of vertebrates.

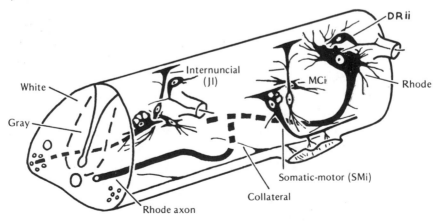

anism of swimming in *Amblystoma* (Coghill, 1929). The running of the decapitated chicken is well known; demonstrations of cats walking after transection of the upper cervical part of the spinal cord are also familiar. In man, the neonatal stepping reflex is mediated by an intrinsic system of the spinal cord, similar to that found in *Amblystoma*. The coordinated swing of the arms by adult man in walking is another phylogenetic carry-over of primitive reflexes of the spinal cord. The propriospinal pathways in mammals were described by Szentágothai (1964a).

The most rostral cell of Rohde is also similar to the giant cells of Mueller and Mauthner, in cyclostomes and teleosts, respectively (Chapter 7). The cells of Mueller and of Mauthner are neurons of the brain stem that have dendritic synapses with neurons of the vestibular and various sensory systems. They project thick axons directly to the caudal segments of the spinal cord for rapid reflexive movements of the tail. The most rostral cell of Rohde in amphioxus has an extremely large axon that descends to the caudal region ventrally in the midline of the spinal cord.

In higher vertebrates, most entering fibers of the dorsal roots continue to ascend or descend near the dorsal horn before terminating at other segmental levels. These fibers are largely confined to a bundle just lateral to the dorsal horn, the zone of Lissauer (dorsolateral tract).

Secondary sensory neurons of the spinal cord probably do not project to the primordial brain of amphioxus, except perhaps from the most rostral segments. The cells of Rohde, however, establish a pattern not only for propriospinal reflexive pathways, but also for the important secondary ascending sensory systems of the spinal cord in all vertebrates. In man, the primitive decussating interneurons with ascending axons have evolved to become such tracts as the spinothalamic and ventral spinocerebellar. In all vertebrates, the fibers composing these ascending tracts in the spinal cord decussate in a commissure ventral to the central canal, as they do in amphioxus. In evolution, amphioxus or a similar ancestor of man had the first decussation in the central nervous system.

Most fibers of the ascending sensory tract of cyclostomes still terminate within the spinal cord, but a few fibers ascend to the medulla. Spinobulbar fibers are numerous in elasmobranchs, and some spinomesencephalic fibers also occur. These ascending fibers arise from neurons in the opposite dorsal horn, particularly from the cervical region. The ascending sensory tract of lower vertebrates lies mainly in the lateral funiculus of the spinal cord. Pathways are less well demarcated as specific tracts than in higher species, however, and ascending fibers mix with descending fascicles from the medulla. Some ascending fibers also travel in the dorsal or ventral funiculi of the spinal cord in elasmobranchs and other lower vertebrates.

Spinobulbar and spinomesencephalic tracts are progressively larger in amphibians, reptiles, and birds. The correlative centers of the brainstem in which these tracts terminate are not completely known, but include the reticular nuclei and optic tectum. In mammals alone, ascending spinal tracts continue rostrally, to terminate in the thalamus (Chapter 8).

The crossed spinocerebellar tract is larger in teleosts than in elasmobranchs or amphibians, a finding consistent with the development of the cerebellum. The dorsal nucleus or column of Clarke gives rise to the uncrossed dorsal spinocerebellar tract in reptiles, birds, and mammals, but is not found in lower species (Chapter 6).

The substantia gelatinosa (of Rolando) is an aggregate of small neurons, unmyelinated fibers and glia. It caps the dorsal horns of the spinal cord in all terrestrial vertebrates, and is best developed in mammals. In spite of proximity to entering fibers of the dorsal root, only a few of these fibers terminate in the substantia gelatinosa; afferent impulses are received from interneurons in deeper parts of the dorsal horn (Truex and Carpenter, 1970). Much of the dorsal horn of teleosts has the consistency and appearance of the substantia gelatinosa, although it is homologous with more than just this structure of mammals.

The dorsal horns of gray matter of the spinal cord in fishes lie close to the midline. The two sides are continuous in some places. Near the central canal, a dorsal zone of proliferating subependymal glial cells separates the dorsal horns of the two sides. Dorsal columns of longitudinal fibers in fishes consist only of a few secondary sensory fibers that ascend dorsally near the midline.

Dorsal columns in anuran amphibians contain primary sensory fibers that ascend ipsilaterally, and terminate in the cerebellum (Joseph and Whitlock, 1968a; Lasek et al., 1968), although similar afferent cerebellar fibers arising in the dorsal root ganglia have not been found in other classes of vertebrates.

A system of fibers in the dorsal columns homologous with that of mammals is first found in reptiles. The fibers arise in the dorsal root ganglia and terminate in primordial gracile and cuneate nuclei in the lower medulla (Kappers et al., 1936; Joseph and Whitlock, 1968b). The dorsal columns are least well developed in reptiles lacking legs. In birds (van den Akker, 1970) and in mammals, the fibers are arranged somatotopically, those from caudal levels lying medial to those from progressively more rostral levels. In the upper thoracic and cervical regions, a thin septum divides the medial fibers (gracile fasciculus, column of Goll) from the lateral fibers (cuneate fasciculus, column of Burdach) in mammals.

The evolution and functional significance of the dorsal column and the medial lemniscus to which it ultimately gives rise are discussed in Chapter 8.

In all vertebrates, the somatic motor neurons lie on the same side of the spinal cord as the ventral roots to which they contribute fibers. A somatotopic arrangement of these cells is established. The motor neurons innervating flexor muscles lie dorsal to those subserving extensors, and neurons of distal muscles lie lateral to those of proximal muscles in mammals.

Large mammals tend to have larger motor neurons in the ventral horns than do smaller species because the length of the axon is greater in large animals, but the absolute size of these neurons is not proportionate to the size of the body. Physical and chemical factors may establish an upper limit to the size of motor neurons (Thompson, 1959).

The presence or absence of glycogen in the cytoplasm of motor neurons in various vertebrates does not follow a phylogenetic pattern. Its presence in the shark, lizard, pigeon, opossum, cat, and monkey suggests that the capability of motor neurons to synthesize and store glycogen is fundamental in evolution and that other factors determine whether glycogen is required for metabolism in these cells. The presence of glycogen in motor neurons of the tadpole, but not in those of the adult frog, indicates that even within a single species, different stages of maturation or environmental conditions may govern glycogenesis. Influencing factors may be the density of the surrounding capillary network and rate of vascular perfusion, the arrangement of ependymal processes transporting nutrients from the cerebrospinal fluid, and the relation of astrocytes to vessels and to neurons. Unlikely factors in neuronal glycogenesis are size of the animal, absolute size of motor neurons, physical activity and metabolic rate of the animal, and state of nutrition (Campa et al., 1973).

In some teleosts, muscles may specialize as electric organs. If these muscles are derived from somites, as in *Mormyrus*, the innervation continues to be from somatic motor neurons of the ventral horn. In fishes such as *Malopterurus,* the electric organ is derived from smooth muscle of the skin, and visceral efferent innervation is retained (Kappers et al., 1936).

The spinal cord of cyclostomes as with that of amphioxus is almost exclusively an autonomous structure. Rare fibers of the cells of Mueller, a few other fibers from the primordial vestibular nucleus of Deiters, and the reticular motor nuclei are the only pathways in cyclostomes for control of the spinal cord by the brain, but even these are lacking in amphioxus. The fibers of Mueller terminate upon motor neurons controlling the tail, but other motor cells along the entire course of the fibers of Mueller have dendritic arborizations in intimate relation with these large descending axons. A similar relation to the large descending fibers of the cells of Mauthner occurs in teleosts.

Long ascending and descending tracts are less compact bundles in lower vertebrates. Old tracts are more sharply demarcated than new tracts in advanced species. The corticospinal tract, being phylogenetically the most recent, is the most variable in man. It descends mainly in the lateral funiculus of the side of the spinal cord opposite the origin of the fibers, but is less compact a bundle in that location than is usually depicted in textbooks of neuroanatomy. The fibers often are diffusely scattered and mixed with those of other tracts. Some fibers of each corticospinal tract also descend in both ventral funiculi, and a few in the lateral funiculus on the same side of origin (Nyberg-Hansen and Brodal, 1963). The spinothalamic tracts are similarly scattered in the lateral and ventral funiculi of man, although confined to a smaller region.

The long descending tracts of man and other vertebrates were reviewed by Nathan and Smith (1955), Kuypers (1964), and Schoen (1964). The phylogeny of the dorsal columns was discussed by Norton (1969-1971). Specific tracts are further considered in other chapters of this book, in relation to the functional systems to which they belong. The comparative anatomy of the spinal cord was reviewed by Nieuwenhuys (1964).

A phylogenetic theory to explain cerebral centers
subserving the opposite side of the body

The coiling reflex in response to nonspecific cutaneous stimulation is the most primitive spinal reflex. It is the first reflex to appear in developing embryos of *Amblystoma,* and is present in amphioxus.

In the coiling reflex, impulses from the sensory neuron are conducted to motor neurons on the opposite side of the spinal cord, by an interneuron with a decussating axon. The decussation allows the animal to coil away from a noxious stimulus instead of around it. It thus differs from the truncal incurvation reflex of Galant in the newborn human infant. The decussating interneuron in the medulla initiates this series of muscular contractions on the opposite side of the body. It is the first cerebral "center" with a crossed efferent pathway, and is a primitive upper motor neuron.

The alternating contraction of myotomes on the two sides of the body, required for swimming and for ambulation in simple tetrapods also was necessarily mediated by decussating interneurons. Impetus was thus provided for preservation of the crossed arrangement.

Axons of the cells of Rohde in amphioxus either ascend or descend after decussation. In primitive vertebrates, some ascending fibers of similar decussating interneurons extend rostrally as the spinobulbar tract. Crude sensory information from each side of the body is thereby relayed to the medulla on the opposite side. Further rostral extension of axons of decussating interneurons during the phylogenetic process of cephalization (Chapter 12) forms the spinomesencephalic tract and finally the spinothalamic tracts (Fig. 3-8).

The crossed ascending sensory fibers no longer innervate lower motor neurons in the brainstem, but instead synapse with other similar interneurons that integrate sensory information from several sources before effecting an axonal discharge. These secondary cells are upper motor neurons, similar to the cells that mediate movement away from the stimulated side of the head in *Amblystoma*. The cell of Rohde in amphioxus or a similar decussating interneuron is therefore the ancestor of both ascending sensory and descending motor pathways of the central nervous system. In vertebrates, however, the decussating interneurons synapse with primary sensory neurons of only one side of the spinal cord or brain, unlike the cells of Rohde in amphioxus, that gather sensory information from both sides. The decussation of both afferent and efferent limbs of interneurons in the reflex arc is the basis for both sensory and motor centers of the brain subserving the opposite side of the body.

As the nervous system evolved, primary sensory neurons became specialized in conveying either muscle proprioception or cutaneous sensation. Some motor neurons remained unchanged. Others lost the collateral axon to other motor neurons or lost the peripheral axonal branch to

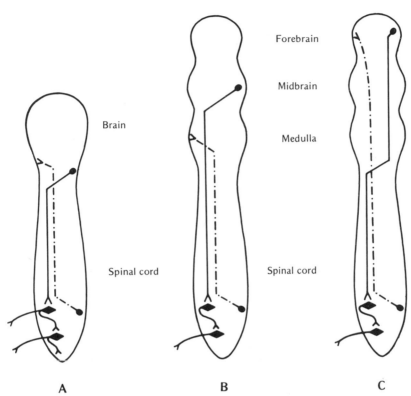

Brain

Forebrain

Midbrain

Medulla

Spinal cord

Spinal cord

A   B   C

Figure 3-8 Hypothetic evolution of decussated long tracts of the central nervous system. (A) Primitive condition, similar to that in Amphioxus; axons of interneurons in rostral part of spinal cord decussate and descend; those of caudal interneurons decussate and ascend to innervate primitive segmental motor neurons. Only caudal motor neurons are illustrated. This arrangement provides a mechanism for the defensive coiling reflex. (B) Condition in lower vertebrates: ascending axons cross and extend into medulla; other fibers arise in the brainstem and descend to the opposite side of the spinal cord. Examples are the spinovestibular and tectospinal tracts. (C) Condition in advanced vertebrates: further cephalization of crossed long pathways. Examples are the spinothalamic and corticospinal tracts. The various long tracts are not homologous, but have a similar origin from the primitive decussating interneuron. Primitive motor neurons (lower part of A) have branched axons innervating both muscle and adjacent spinal motor neurons. As these cells differentiate in evolution, loss of the axonal branch to other neurons results in pure motor neurons; other cells lose the peripheral axonal branch to give origin to local interneurons that do not have crossing fibers (lower part of B and C). These latter cells proliferate to form spinal interneurons and sensory nuclei in the brain.

muscle. These latter cells retained the central axonal branch to an adjacent neuron, becoming the associative interneuron with processes confined within nuclei of the brain. A few long ipsilateral pathways, such as the medial vestibulospinal tract of mammals, may originate from this type of neuron.

As cephalization progresses in phylogeny, more neurons and synapses are interposed between the primary afferent and efferent interneurons. Somatotopically organized nuclei develop as specialized function evolves. The basic pattern initiated by the evolution of the coiling reflex, however, remains unaltered. As motor activity is controlled by successively more complex correlative centers, the primitive coiling reflex is no longer the best or most appropriate response to stimuli. In animals possessing limbs with flexor and extensor muscles, it is particularly advantageous for the primary motor responses to be on the same side of the body that is stimulated, as in flexor withdrawal. The loss of the coiling reflex because of the double decussation in the more complicated reflex arc was therefore an advance in evolution.

The telencephalon has evolved as apparent paired evaginations of the diencephalon (Chapter 12). Afferent connections of the forebrain are from the diencephalon of the same side in most vertebrates, but they are crossed in the shark (Ebbesson and Schroeder, 1971). The basal ganglia and cerebral cortex therefore maintain a similar contralateral relation to the body in most vertebrates.

The axons of cells of Rohde in amphioxus and the similar decussating interneurons of *Amblystoma* cross ventral to the central canal. Even in man, the decussating interneurons of the spinothalamic tracts still decussate ventral to the central canal, and the decussations of the brain cross ventral to the ventricular system. Commissures relating corresponding areas of almost every part of the brain are a secondary development to integrate the cerebral control of the two sides of the body. Commissures thus differ from decussations of long tracts, and often do cross dorsal to the ventricles.

In the cerebellar system, the inferior olivary nuclei and deep cerebellar nuclei may also be regarded as decussating interneurons. Autoradiographic studies indicate that the olivary nuclei in the embryonic rat migrate ventrally from the rhombic lip but do not migrate across the midline (Ellenberger et al., 1969). In the adult, efferent fibers of these nuclei decussate and ascend to the cerebellar cortex of the contralateral side. Axons of the dentate nucleus similarly cross as they ascend. Pyramidal motor cells of the neocortex give rise to the corticospinal tract and are also reminiscent of the decussating interneuron.

The decussation of the optic nerves in the earliest vertebrates served the same function as the decussating interneuron of the tactile system; it provided a pathway for the defensive coiling reflex away from the visually stimulated (threatened) side. Just as the tactile coiling reflex was replaced later in evolution by local withdrawal reflexes, the development of the optic tectum and crossed tectospinal tract interposed a second decussation in the reflexive pathway to allow local ipsilateral defenses, such as closing of the eyelids or covering of the threatened eye with the foreleg. The optic chiasm probably developed before the evolution of the chambered eye or the perception of actual images (Chapter 8).

The dorsal columns (gracile and cuneate fasciculi) of advanced animals are fundamentally similar to the cells of Rohon and Beard in primitive species and are central extensions of peripheral nerves. The decussating interneurons in this ascending tactile and proprioceptive pathway are the cells of the gracile and cuneate nuclei that give origin to the medial lemniscus. A fundamental phylogenetic pattern is thus preserved even in the late evolution of more recent pathways.

Motor unit

The motor unit is defined as the combination of a single motor neuron in the spinal cord or brain stem, its axon extending into the ventral root and peripheral nerve, the neuromuscular junction, and all skeletal muscle fibers innervated by that motor neuron (Engel, 1967).

Fibers of skeletal muscle may be classified in two major categories by morphologic and histochemical characteristics. Type I or red fibers are more vascular and have numerous mitochondria; they contain high concentrations of oxidative enzymes and little phosphorylase or glycogen. Type II or white fibers are less vascular and have fewer mitochondria; they have low concentrations of oxidative enzymes and large amounts of phosphorylase (Campa and Engel, 1971). Intermediate subtypes of muscle fibers also are described.

Skeletal muscle in man contains a mixture of types. Even extraocular muscles are composed of at least two types of fibers (Peachey, 1971). All muscle fibers of a single motor unit are of the same type. In the fetus, muscle fibers do not differentiate into types until innervation is established. Several diseases of man selectively involve one type of muscle fiber, or motor neurons innervating one type (Engel, 1965; Fenischel and Engel, 1963).

The physiologic differences between the two types of muscle fibers are the twitch time (the time required for maximal contraction from a resting state), and properties of endurance and fatigue. Type I fibers have a slower twitch time than those of Type II, and they fatigue more slowly. The ability of a stork to stand on one leg for hours, an opossum to hang by the tail for long periods, the bat to grasp an object and remain inverted all day, and migrating birds to fly hundreds of miles without stopping is served by a predominance of Type I fibers.

The need for muscles with different qualities arose early in phylogenetic development. The characteristics of muscle fibers are similar in mammals and in birds (Dubowitz, 1969; Ogata and Mori, 1964).

Differences are found, however, in comparing muscle fibers of amphibians with those of mammals. In the toad, large white and small red fibers occur in the sartorius, gastrocnemius, and rectus abdominis muscles. The red fibers of small diameter have many mitochondria, and high concentrations of oxidative enzymes, but they are also rich in phosphorylase. The large white fibers have few mitochondria and are deficient in both kinds of enzymes (Dubowitz, 1969).

Teleosts have lateral red muscles and dorsal and ventral white muscles, but mixtures of fibers are found only in the intermediate zones. The mitochondria and enzymes occur almost exclusively in the red fibers, similar to the condition in the toad (Dubowitz, 1969). One fish, the tuna, has been found to use red muscle for routine swimming, and white muscle as a reserve of power for short bursts of intense activity, as in feeding or escape (Rayner and Keenan, 1967).

Dubowitz (1969) postulated that the reciprocal relation of the enzymatic content of Type I and Type II fibers in birds and mammals reflected a difference in metabolism of the two types of fibers. Type I, rich in mitochondrial oxidative enzymes, used the aerobic Krebs cycle for energy; Type II, rich in phosphorylase, depended upon the anaerobic Embden-Meyerhof pathways. This hypothesis is difficult to apply to the condition in lower vertebrates, particularly with regard to the metabolism of white muscle fibers, almost totally lacking in either type of enzyme.

In addition to the types of muscle fibers capable of twitch responses to stimulation, an extremely slow muscle fiber with a tonic type of contraction has been found in vertebrates of all classes except mammals (Peachey, 1961); intrafusal muscle fibers in mammals, however, may be of this variety (Boyd, 1961). Even myxinoids possess both slow (tonic) and fast (twitch) muscle fibers (Andersen et al., 1963).

The ultrastructure of the neuromuscular junction is similar in amphibians (Reger, 1958; Birks et al., 1960), reptiles (Robertson, 1956; Hess, 1965), birds (Hirano, 1967), and mammals (Reger, 1958; Teravainen, 1968). In the developing chick (Hirano, 1967) and rat (Teravainen, 1968), the junction forms between multinucleated muscle cells and multiple axons. Synaptic clefts isolating individual axonal terminations are secondarily formed by the infolding of sarcoplasm and teloglial sheath cells. Electron microscopic examination of the neuromuscular synapse in a primitive vertebrate such as the lamprey might reveal a morphologic pattern more similar to the embryonic than to the mature stage of terrestrial animals. In reptiles such as snakes, the extremely slow, tonic muscle fibers have several delicate, filamentous axons terminating on a single muscle fiber; the fast muscle fibers of snakes correspond to mammalian muscle; each receives one robust nerve ending (Hess, 1965).

An automatic mechanism to regulate muscle tone or degree of contraction in resting states, as well as during contraction, is probably needed by all vertebrates. Afferent fibers conveying proprioception from muscles are found even in amphioxus. In mammals, this mechanism involves stretch receptors (muscle spindles) within the muscle, and afferent neurons in the dorsal root ganglia that relay impulses from the stretch receptors to the spinal cord. Intrafusal muscle fibers are attached to each end of a stretch receptor and are innervated by small gamma motor neurons. The main contractile muscle fibers, both Type I and Type II, are the extrafusal muscle fibers, innervated by large alpha motor neurons of the motor unit. The arrangement in marsupials is similar to that in placental mammals (Jones, 1966). The physiology of this system in mammals was reviewed by Close (1972).

Anuran amphibians have a less complex system for control of muscle length. Each intrafusal muscle fiber in the frog extends the entire length of the muscle from tendon to tendon, in contrast to man, in whom at least one end is usually attached to the perimysium of an extrafusal fiber away from the tendon (Gray, 1957). Each intrafusal muscle fiber of the frog is innervated by branches of an axon that also innervates extrafusal muscle fibers. Gamma motor neurons are absent. The branched axons may be large or small and have either of two characteristic but different types of endings, corresponding to those of slow tonic or twitch extrafusal fibers. Both intrafusal and extrafusal muscle fibers thus may be slow tonic fibers or rapid twitch fibers, in contrast to mammals, in whom extrafusal muscle fibers are exclusively of the rapid twitch variety. In amphibians, therefore, instead of independent control of intrafusal and extrafusal fibers by separate motor neurons, the muscle spindles are automatically activated during all contractions (Gray, 1957; Eyzaguirre, 1957).

Descending fibers of the medial longitudinal fasciculus and of the lateral vestibulospinal tract terminate on both alpha and gamma motor neurons in mammals (Granit, 1970; Grillner et al., 1971). The presence of small and large neurons in the nucleus of Deiters in lower vertebrates as well as in mammals may be related to respective innervation of primitive gamma and alpha motor neurons (Pompeiano and Brodal, 1957a).

The corticospinal tract contains fibers belonging to both alpha and gamma systems (Kato et al., 1964; Granit, 1970). These fibers do not terminate directly on motor neurons of the ventral horns, but on intermediate neurons in the spinal cord (Nyberg-Hansen and Brodal, 1963). This anatomic observation has been corroborated by physiologic studies (Lundberg and Voorhoeve, 1961). The corticospinal tract has both facilitatory and inhibitory influences (Preston and Whitlock, 1960; Hern et al., 1962). The reticulospinal pathways also influence both alpha and gamma motor neurons (Granit, 1970). The convergence of direct and multisynaptic descending pathways upon both alpha and gamma neurons in mammals serves to combine general activation with a means of selective control not found in lower vertebrates (Granit, 1970).

4
Branchial nerves

Origin of branchial nerves

Branchial clefts are bilateral outpouchings of the pharynx in aquatic lower vertebrates. Water enters the mouth and is pumped out through the branchial clefts or gills. In amphioxus, the clefts filter particles of food, but they serve as gas exchangers between the body and the surrounding water in fishes and aquatic amphibians. The skeleton forms arches between successive branchial clefts. Each branchial arch contains striated pharyngeal muscle and a rich vascular supply. The sequence of dorsal nerve roots of the spinal cord continues rostrally; the branchial nerves are the dorsal roots of the medulla associated with the branchial arches (Fig. 4-1).

Amphioxus has more branchial clefts than do the cyclostomes. Teleostean fishes have the fewest gills on each side. The skeletal supporting structure of the first two branchial arches was altered early in phylogeny to form the maxilla and mandible. The third branchial cleft became smaller and is the spiracle of fishes; part of the skeleton of the third cleft became the hyoid bone, a supporting structure of the jaw. Gills disappear in terrestrial vertebrates, though evidence of their phylogenetic history is found in embryonic stages, even in man.

The branchial nerves are retained by advanced vertebrates in spite of the loss of gills. Specialization of these nerves began in the lowest vertebrates; as a result, they developed into the trigeminal, facial, glossopharyngeal, vagal, and accessory nerves. The acoustic nerve is derived from portions of the facial, glossopharyngeal, and vagal nerves. Although

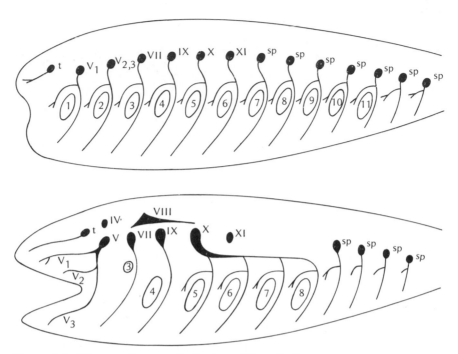

Figure 4-1 Diagram showing distribution of branchial nerves in a hypothetic ancestral vertebrate (top), similar to the arrangement in the embryos of living lower
vertebrates, and in modern jaw-bearing fishes (bottom). The changes include the
loss of the first two branchial clefts, reduction of the third branchial cleft to become
the spiracle, reduction in the total number of branchial clefts, fusion of the ophthalmic and maxillomandibular nerves (V) to form the trigeminal nerve, probable formation of the trochlear nerve (IV) from some visceral efferent fibers of the ophthalmic
nerve, formation of the acoustic nerve (VIII) from parts of the facial (VII), glossopharyngeal (IX) and vagal (X) nerves, increased distribution of the vagal nerve, and
loss of sensory function of the accessory nerve (XI). The most rostral branchial nerve
persists as the terminalis (t). Dorsal spinal nerves (sp) are no longer associated with
branchial clefts. Modified from Romer (1970).

predominantly special visceral sensory in function, the acoustic nerve
also has a general visceral efferent component (Rasmussen and Gacek,
1958; Ross, 1969), similar to other branchial nerves. The association of
goiter and congenital deafness, transmitted by an autosomal recessive
gene in man (Pendred's syndrome), may be related to the embryologic
origin of the thyroid from a branchial pouch, and of the acoustic nerve

from branchial nerves at the same level. The goiter probably results from deficient incorporation of iodine into organic molecules (Fraser, 1965).

Functional organization in medulla

The branchial nerves contain the same functional components as the dorsal spinal nerves. Primary sensory neurons lie within cranial ganglia on each branchial nerve, homologous with sensory ganglia of the dorsal roots. During evolution, each branchial nerve became specialized in the development of one or more of its components, while the other components atrophied or even disappeared. Each branchial nerve thus became unique, unlike the dorsal spinal nerves.

Medullary centers associated with the branchial nerves are organized by separation of functional components. Entering fibers regroup in accordance with their function rather than with the peripheral nerve carrying the fibers. The long rostrocaudal extent of most nuclei of the medulla facilitates the gathering of similar fibers of several branchial nerves.

Cutaneous (general somatic) sensibility

The trigeminal nerve became specialized early in phylogeny as the principal cutaneous sensory nerve of the face and head. It resulted from a fusion of two branchial nerves, corresponding to the ophthalmic and maxillo-mandibular branches. The separate origin of these branches can be recognized in amphioxus and in the embryos of some lower vertebrates. The trigeminus is a large nerve, even in the lowest presently living vertebrates (Fig. 4-2).

As the phylogenetic scale is ascended, the distribution of the trigeminal nerve progressively increases while the cutaneous sensory distribution of the facial, glossopharyngeal, and vagal nerves diminishes.

Fibers from the two major branches of the trigeminal nerve descend as separate bundles within the medulla of fishes. The ophthalmic branch is joined by cutaneous sensory fibers of the facial, glossopharyngeal and vagal nerves, and course caudally to the cervical region of the spinal cord. Fibers of the maxillo-mandibular branch lie dorsal to those of the ophthalmic branch and do not descend as far. The descending trigeminal tracts of the two branches become progressively less well demarcated

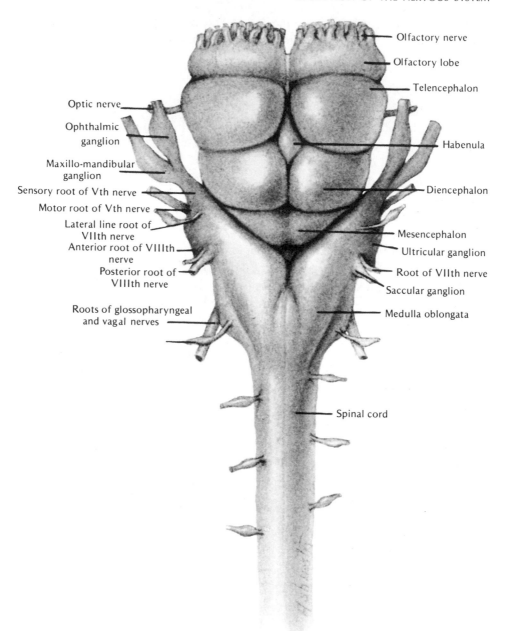

Figure 4-2   Drawing of dorsal surface of the brain of *Bdellostoma,* a myxinoid, to demonstrate the relative size of parts of the brain, and the great development of the trigeminal nerve even in this primitive species (Larsell, 1947).

from each other in higher vertebrates, although the somatotopic arrangement of fibers remains. The ophthalmic fibers establish continuity between the termination of trigeminal sensory fibers from the forehead and scalp and those of dorsal cervical roots from the back of the head. They also provide short reflexive pathways to cervical motor centers for retraction of the head in response to cutaneous stimulation of the forehead. Reflexive responses to maxillo-mandibular stimulation involve motor centers of the medulla for movement of the jaw and facial muscles.

Anuran amphibians have undergone extreme specialization. Their descending trigeminal tract extends as far as the lumbar region of the spinal cord. Because of the large surface area of the head of frogs and the great development of the hind legs for jumping, this arrangement provides for quick responses to cutaneous stimulation of the head.

Neurons similar to those of the dorsal horns of the spinal cord accompany the descending trigeminal tract. The neurons are few and are scattered in this region in lower vertebrates. They become more numerous in higher vertebrates and constitute a column of cells known as the descending trigeminal nucleus. The prominence of this nucleus in reptiles, birds, and mammals is associated with the development of Pacinian corpuscles and other cutaneous receptors. The descending trigeminal nucleus is continuous with the homologous substantia gelatinosa at the medullospinal junction in higher vertebrates.

The mesencephalic nucleus of the trigeminal nerve is associated with proprioceptive fibers from the muscles of mastication. It is absent in cyclostomes, but well developed in all vertebrates with jaws.

The chief sensory nucleus of the trigeminus is lacking in aquatic lower vertebrates, although an enlargement of the rostral end of the descending nucleus in teleosts may be a primordial chief sensory nucleus. In higher vertebrates, this part of the trigeminal nucleus differs functionally from the descending portion. It is associated with the more precise cutaneous sensations, such as two-point discrimination. The chief sensory and mesencephalic nuclei are probably homologous with the gracile and cuneate nuclei which receive dorsal root fibers from the spinal cord, also without intermediate synapse.

Highly differentiated sensory terminations occur in the beak and tongue of birds; the size of the trigeminal nerve is proportionate to the size of the beak. The chief sensory nucleus is well developed in birds, but the descending part is small.

The size of the sensory trigeminal nerve in mammals correlates not

only with the area of distribution, but also with the density of terminations within particular parts of the total area. The trigeminal nerve is
thus large in monotremes because it innervates a wide area, and is massive also in rodents because of a dense concentration of fibers in the
nose. The importance of the snout as an organ of exploration in many
mammals is associated with specialized structure of the snout in pigs
and moles, as well as with the development of sensitive whiskers in rodents and cats. Many mammals and even human infants use the mouth
as a primary organ of exploration, employing both tactile sensibility and
taste.

Direct connections of primary sensory fibers to motor centers become
less numerous as the phylogenetic series is ascended. Secondary fibers
from neurons of the descending trigeminal nucleus decussate and then
terminate in motor nuclei of the medulla, pons, and spinal cord. Other
secondary connections include commissural fibers, projections to the
cerebellum and to the acousticolateral area, and ascending connections.
Ascending fibers terminate in the optic tectum but pass mainly to the
thalamus in higher vertebrates.

Taste

The medulla of all vertebrates contains a visceral sensory column of
descending fibers and neurons. The fasciculus and nucleus solitarius are
the lower portion of this column, particularly those parts caudal to the
entrance of the vagus. They subserve general visceral sensibility and are
relatively small in aquatic lower vertebrates, but become progressively
larger in terrestrial vertebrates. The specialized rostral part of the visceral sensory column is the primary gustatory nucleus, serving the special visceral sense of taste. It is large in teleostean fishes and causes a
prominent bulge on the surface of the medulla at the entrance of the
facial, glossopharyngeal, and vagal nerves.

The perceptions of ionized chemical substances and of taste are not
identical, but at times may overlap. Chemical sensibility is transmitted
by general somatic afferent fibers of the trigeminal nerve or dorsal spinal
nerves. It may initiate reflexes of avoidance, but not of attraction. Taste
is perceived by specialized receptors, taste buds, and is conducted by
special visceral afferent fibers of the facial, glossopharyngeal, and vagal
nerves. Taste may initiate reflexes attracting the animal to a source of
food. Some substances, such as acids, stimulate free somatic nerve end-

ings and are perceived as pain, and also taste buds to be recognized as a sour taste.

Taste buds are lacking in amphioxus. They are sparsely distributed on the surface of the head and on the mucous membranes in the mouth of cyclostomes. The buds become more numerous in higher fishes. Teleosts have the most taste buds of any vertebrates. In fishes, the buds are distributed not only in the mouth, but are widespread on the surface of the body. They are less numerous in amphibians, and fewer still in reptiles and birds. Olfaction, a related sense in many respects, also degenerates in birds. The number of taste buds increases in mammals, but the sensation of taste is not as well developed as in teleosts.

The increase in number and distribution of taste buds in teleosts is associated with enlargement of the visceral sensory root of the facial nerve. This root transmits all impulses from taste buds on the skin and in the anterior (ectodermal) part of the mouth. In mammals, the facial nerve conducts taste from the anterior two-thirds of the tongue, but the number of taste buds in that area is small, as is true of the number of facial nerve fibers carrying taste. Glossopharyngeal and vagal fibers innervate taste buds in the posterior (endodermal) part of the mouth in all vertebrates.

The gustatory nucleus of teleosts is larger and more highly differentiated than in other vertebrates, indicating the importance of the sense of taste in fishes. In some species of teleosts, the gustatory nucleus is laminated.

Secondary gustatory nuclei lie rostral to the primary nucleus in fishes. The inferior secondary gustatory nucleus (lateral funicular nucleus) receives not only fibers related to taste, but also secondary fibers of the descending trigeminal nucleus for correlation with tactile stimuli. These secondary gustatory centers are less differentiated in amphibians and a few reptiles, and are absent in higher vertebrates. In reptiles and mammals, other secondary gustatory nuclei develop in a location different from that of fishes. They are the nucleus intercalatus (of Staderini) and the nucleus prepositus, lying in close relation to the motor nucleus of the hypoglossal nerve in the dorsal part of the medulla. The absence of these perihypoglossal nuclei in teleosts may be related to the absence of a true tongue in fishes. In addition, the most important nerve transmitting taste is the facial nerve in fishes, but the glossopharyngeal nerve in mammals. The prepositus and intercalatus nuclei may also serve as secondary generally visceral centers or possibly as proprioceptive centers for the tongue (DuBois, 1929). The function of the nucleus of Roller, another perihypoglossal nucleus, in mammals is uncertain.

Secondary gustatory fibers decussate and then descend or ascend. Descending fibers synapse in motor nuclei of the medulla to establish reflexive pathways for chewing and for movements of the tongue. Many fibers ascend to the hypothalamus to correlate gustatory and olfactory impulses. In mammals, these fibers are in the dorsal longitudinal fasciculus. Correlation of taste and smell is important to identify food. Most persons experiencing temporary impairment of olfaction because of nasal congestion testify to the bland taste of food. Olfactory discrimination is more highly developed than that of taste in mammals. In higher vertebrates, gustatory impulses also ascend to the thalamus.

The early phylogenetic development of gustatory sense is reflected ontogenetically. Human newborns often reject water or sugar-water feedings but avidly take milk. Even young infants usually prefer sweet fruits to vegetables and may have individual food preferences.

General visceral sensibility

Lower vertebrates have fewer sensory fibers from the viscera than do higher animals. The posterior part of the fasciculus solitarius is correspondingly small in lower species. In all vertebrates, fibers partially decussate at the caudal end of the fasciculus solitarius. This decussation is the commissura infima. The nucleus solitarius of each side meets in the midline at the decussation and becomes the nucleus of the commissura infima. These neurons are particularly associated with vagal impulses from the lungs in terrestrial vertebrates in whom the nucleus of the commissura infima greatly enlarges. Most fibers of the fasciculus solitarius terminate in the nucleus solitarius and in the nucleus of the commissura infima, but some descend to the upper part of the cervical cord.

Secondary visceral fibers from the nucleus solitarius descend to the spinal cord to synapse with motor neurons of respiratory muscles, especially those of the mammalian diaphragm. Descending fibers also synapse with preganglionic sympathetic neurons innervating smooth muscle of the bronchi; similar fibers synapse in the parasympathetic motor nucleus of the vagus. In mammals, neurons of the nucleus solitarius surround the fasciculus solitarius. The small portion of the nucleus lying laterally (nucleus parasolitarius) has many connections with the lateral reticular formation. It helps regulate respiration. Those neurons of the nucleus solitarius and adjacent reticular formation concerned with respiration are termed the "respiratory center" by neurophysiologists. The homologous region in fishes is also a respiratory center, regulating the rhythmic movements of the mouth and gill covers for pumping water through the gills (von Baumbarten and Salmoiraghi, 1962). Russell (1955) proposed that the locus coeruleus of mammals, a derivative of the superior reticular nucleus in lower vertebrates, is the "pneumotaxic center." This nucleus is discussed in Chapter 11.

Ascending fibers from the nucleus solitarius terminate in the optic tectum, hypothalamus, and thalamus.

Motor components of branchial nerves

Motor fibers are associated with each of the branchial nerves of the medulla. They are of two types: those innervating smooth muscle of the viscera and glands and comprising preganglionic parasympathetic fibers, and those innervating striated muscle of the branchial arches, which become the muscles of the jaw, face, pharynx, larynx, and some muscles of the neck.

In accordance with the functional organization of the medulla, all vertebrates have distinct motor nuclei in the form of rostrocaudal columns of neurons similar to the sensory nuclei of the medulla.

The motor components of the branchial nerves are discussed in Chapter 7.

Terminalis nerve

The terminalis nerve is probably the most rostral branchial nerve, although the associated cleft is absent even in amphioxus. A pair of terminalis nerves enters the ventral surface of the diencephalon or telencephalon of all vertebrates. The close anatomic relation of the course of the terminalis nerve, vomeronasal nerve, and olfactory bulb and tract has led to some misunderstanding.

In amphioxus, the terminalis is a sensory nerve to the skin over the rostrum. This nerve retains some sensory function throughout phylogeny, although the area of distribution is small. In man, this area is limited to a portion of the mucosa of the nasal septum. The terminalis nerve has no known olfactory function.

Large ganglion cells occur along the course of the terminalis nerve in all vertebrates. These neurons are scattered or organized into one or more ganglia, and the postganglionic fibers innervate small vessels in the mucosa of the nasal septum. The terminalis is regarded as a branchial nerve because of the combination of autonomic and somatic sensory components.

The terminalis nerve does not emerge dorsally from the brain, as do other branchial nerves and dorsal spinal nerves, because the sulcus limitans extends forward only as far as the preoptic recess; the forebrain rostral to that point is derived from the alar plate. Within the central nervous system, the terminalis nerve has been traced to the preoptic area and hypothalamus in urodeles (McKibben, 1911), but further details and secondary connections are not known.

5
Lateral line, vestibular, and acoustic systems; tactile vibratory perception

An important factor enabling passive filter-feeding protochordates to become active and mobile predators was the evolution of organs of orientation in space. Centers in the central nervous system developed concurrently to receive and interpret appropriate information and translate it into motor responses. Organs of equilibrium and receptors for sense of motion, therefore, were early developments in vertebrate evolution. Although they are not identified in amphioxus, they occur in all presently living true vertebrates, as well as in many invertebrates. Even some plants have static organs in their rootlets for orientation with reference to gravity.

The vestibulospinal tract was the first motor tract from the brain to exercise control over the motor neurons of the spinal cord, reflecting the importance of information about motion and spatial orientation. Its importance as a major pathway for postural control even in man often is underestimated, although the reliance on vestibular control is diminished by vision and other senses of orientation in space.

The development of hearing was an adaptation of existing mechanisms of vibratory perception developed so successfully in the lateral line organs and labyrinth. Hearing ability provided vertebrates with still another means of tracking prey and avoiding enemies, thereby enhancing survival. Later developments enabled animals, particularly birds
· and mammals, to use this ability as a means of communication.

It is instructive to review the phylogenetic development of the special receptor organs before discussing the evolution of those centers and pathways in the central nervous system concerned with spatial orientation and vibratory perception.

Lateral line organs

All aquatic vertebrates from cyclostomes through amphibians possess aggregates of specialized neuroepithelial cells, each having a hair-like projection into the surrounding media and often covered with a gelatinous secretion. These cells are generally arranged in aggregates (neuromasts) along lines on the lateral surfaces of the head and trunk (Fig. 5-1). Primitively, as in cyclostomes, the neuromasts lie in open pits or grooves in the epidermis. As fishes evolved further, a canal system of lateral line organs became buried in the skin beneath the scales. In some higher fishes, these canals no longer communicate openly with the surrounding sea water. They become closed fluid systems, although the membrane over the openings of the canals is thin enough to transmit vibrations from the surrounding water (Kappers et al., 1936). Among aquatic amphibians, the lateral line organs are more primitive than in higher fishes and do not form complex canals. The lateral line system is well developed in the tadpole or larval stage of frogs, but degenerates at the time of metamorphosis and does not return. This system was lost in the evolution of the earliest reptiles and has not reappeared in aquatic reptiles, birds, or mammals.

Figure 5-1   Lateral line system in the head of a shark.

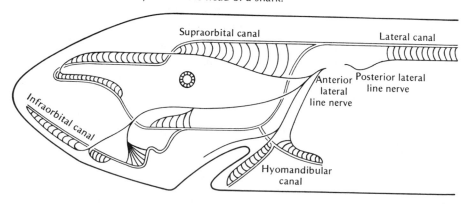

Lateral line organs perceive both water currents and displacements of water near solid objects. Blind predatory fish may find their prey with these organs. Lateral line organs are stimulated by vibrations of low frequency, but they are not sensitive to pressure waves, and therefore do not perceive sound (Dijkgraaf, 1963a, b; van Bergeijk, 1966). In fishes, experimental denervation or destruction of lateral line organs results in collisions with the wall of the aquarium and other solid objects in the environment and decreased movement of the fish. It has no effect, however, on coordination of swimming, or on spatial orientation of the body (Cahn, 1967). Impulses recorded from lateral line nerves are continuous, but they increase transiently in response to ripples in the water, body movement, and sudden changes in pressure or temperature (Cahn, 1967).

Because man has nothing comparable to the lateral line system, it is difficult to appreciate how valuable this special sense is to aquatic vertebrates. Its importance to man is in the pathways of the central nervous system which develop to accommodate it. These tracts eventually become the auditory system of the cochlea, first appearing in advanced amphibians.

Labyrinth

A vestibular organ is not found in amphioxus. The embryogenesis and the nature of its sensory endings in the labyrinth suggest that this structure arose from a further specialization of the lateral line system of the head. It developed as a part of the organ detecting motion of external fluid. This organ then was isolated from outside disturbances and thereby became capable of detecting movements of the body of the animal. The labyrinth of modern vertebrates is a series of canals and sacs in the otic region on either side of the braincase. Aggregates of neuroepithelial sensory cells with hair-like projections comparable to neuromasts of lateral line organs occupy an ampulla at one end of each canal and on the wall or the floor of the sacs. In myxinoids, the labyrinth has a single canal and ampulla, and a common sac. Petromyzonts have two canals, forming a semicircle in the vertical plane in an anteroposterior direction. An ampulla is present at either end and also a peculiar series of sacs. Elasmobranchs possess three canals, each with an ampulla, the characteristic arrangement in all jawed vertebrates. Although it is sometimes suggested that the simple labyrinths of cyclostomes are retrogressive rather than primitive, it is unlikely that these structures would degenerate in actively swimming animals, yet retain their complexity in sedentary teleostean fishes (van Bergeijk, 1966). The floor of the utriculus has a macula (neuromast) lying in the horizontal plane. The sacculus has a macula in the vertical plane. Cyclostomes and elasmobranchs still have an open communication through the top of the head, the lymphatic duct, situated between the labyrinth and the outside. In all higher vertebrates, however, the labyrinth becomes a completely closed, fluid-filled system. The evolution of the labyrinth exemplifies increasing precision in the development of a biologic measuring device.

A blind endolymphatic sac continuous with the labyrinth occurs in many teleostean fishes, amphibians, and reptiles. It contains calcareous matter and may be large; the sacs of the two sides may connect above or below the brain in some amphibians, and in many frogs it even extends the length of the spinal canal (Dempster, 1930). This spinal extension of the endolymphatic sac in frogs may be a vestige of an auditory conducting system similar to the dorsal sail of the extinct pelycosaur (Tumarkin, 1965). A perilymphatic space lies outside the system of semicircular canals and endolymphatic sacs, between the membranous and bony labyrinths. The basic arrangement of three semicircular canals each in a plane at right angles to the other two, and two sacs, all freely communicating, is a constant pattern repeated throughout phylogeny.

The anatomic orientation of the semicircular canals as well as physiologic studies reveal that their function is to perceive and report changes in spatial orientation and motion (linear acceleration) of the animal. The mechanism is similar to that of the lateral line organs.

The function of the utriculus and sacculus is probably related to perception of gravity, but may additionally serve as a detector of low frequency vibrations.

Lagena, basilar papilla, and cochlea

The lagena is an outpocketing of the posterior part of the sacculus and contains a lagenar macula, similar to the macula of the sacculus and utriculus. A second sensory area of the lagena, the basilar papilla, develops in some urodelan and anuran amphibians. The lagena precedes the development of the primordial cochlea. In reptiles and higher vertebrates, the lagena and its associated basilar papilla lengthen to form the cochlea, a relatively straight structure in reptiles, birds, monotremes, and marsupials, but coiled in all placental mammals. The sensory membrane of the basilar papilla becomes the organ of Corti. The lagena has a perilymphatic space forming the scala vestibulae and the scala tympani of the cochlea. The lagenar macula disappears as the cochlea enlarges.

Four different mechanisms are identified for the stimulation of hair cells in the cochlea of terrestrial vertebrates (Wever, 1971). Each involves relative motion between the ciliary tuft and the body of the hair cell. Variation among lizards in the design of the middle ear may be related to these different mechanisms.

Lateral line and acoustic nerves

In all aquatic vertebrates possessing lateral line organs, the peripheral fibers of these organs gather into two main trunks, the anterior and posterior lateral line nerves, serving the head and trunk respectively before entering the medulla. These lateral line nerves do not combine with other components of the facial, glossopharyngeal, or vagal nerves from which they are derived (Chapter 4). The nerve of the anterior lateral line is distributed peripherally with the sensory branches of the trigeminus, and the posterior lateral line nerve with those of the vagus (Kappers et al., 1936). A small ganglion on each nerve contains the bipolar neurons giving origin to the lateral line nerves. The nerves synapse with the hair cells of the neuromasts.

The acoustic nerve contains both coarse and fine fibers. It enters the medulla as two roots in all vertebrates, although a few fibers separate to form a third small root in some reptiles. Of the two main acoustic nerve roots entering the medulla, the more anterior (and ventral in all vertebrates except higher mammals) contains fibers from the anterior and lateral (horizontal) semicircular canals and the utriculus. Its associated ganglion outside the neuraxis is the utricular ganglion, although this structure is usually referred to in higher vertebrates, including man, as the vestibular or Scarpa's ganglion. The cells of origin of the vestibular nerve are within this ganglion. The dendrites of these cells synapse with the hair cells of the labyrinth. The posterior root (dorsal in all vertebrates except higher mammals) is composed of fibers from the posterior semicircular canal, sacculus, lagena, and also the cochlea, in animals possessing this latter structure. This pattern remains fairly constant throughout the phylogenetic series including monotremes and marsupials, but in placental mammals, fibers from the sacculus and posterior semicircular canal gradually shift to the anterior root, as the cochlear fibers of the posterior root increase in number. In man, therefore, vestibular (anterior) and auditory (posterior) roots are separate. The vestibular fibers of the posterior root in animals with this arrangement have central connections appropriate to vestibular function, and are not related to cochlear centers. A saccular ganglion or the spiral ganglion in higher vertebrates is present on the posterior root of the acoustic nerve. The lagena and cochlea in birds may have individual ganglia (Boord, 1969). Dendrites of auditory fibers synapse on hair cells of the organ of Corti (basilar papilla). Until the development of a large contribution of auditory fibers from the cochlea, the posterior root is the smaller of the two, but in man it is the larger.

In various amphibians, the fibers from the sacculus differ: they form part of the anterior root in some species, but in others are in the posterior root, or, some fibers are both roots. In crocodiles and turtles, the fibers from the sacculus form a separate small root between the two main roots and enter the skull through a separate foramen (Larsell, 1967).

Central connections of lateral line and acoustic nerves

The central connections of the lateral line and acoustic nerves in lower vertebrates were extensively studied by investigators in the late nineteenth and early twentieth centuries. They are reviewed by Kappers et al. (1936), Kappers (1947), and Larsell (1967). Later investigation centered on mammals and birds. Little knowledge of this subject in lower vertebrates has been added, with the exception of Herrick's (1948) treatise on the salamander brain.

Within the dorsolateral area of the medulla of an early ancestral vertebrate, a group of neurons was derived from the sensory column of the branchial nerves in the region including the developing sensory nuclei of the facial, glossopharyngeal, and vagal nerves. In myxinoids, this region remains a relatively undifferentiated mass of gray matter. It contains small and large neurons. The larger cells resemble those of the dorsal horn of the spinal cord or the descending root of the trigeminal nerve. This region is known as the acousticolateral area (area acusticolateralis, tuberculum acusticum, area statica) and receives fibers of both lateral line nerves and both roots of the acoustic nerve. Many fibers of these nerves bifurcate into ascending and descending branches within the acousticolateral area. Some join the descending trigeminal root, others enter the primordial cerebellum, but most terminate in relation to neurons of the acousticolateral area.

In petromyzonts, the acousticolateral area is differentiated into three longitudinal columns of cells, the dorsal, middle, and ventral nuclei. Fibers of the anterior lateral line nerve end mainly in the dorsal nucleus, but a few thin fibers pass into the middle and ventral nuclei, and some end in the cerebellum. Almost all fibers of the posterior lateral line nerve terminate within the middle nucleus and cerebellum. Vestibular fibers of both roots of the acoustic nerve terminate predominantly in the ventral nucleus; a few end in the dorsal and middle nuclei as well, and some fibers also pass into the cerebellum. Many fibers terminating in the primordial cerebellum are collaterals or ascending branches of bifurcated lateral line and acoustic nerve fibers; the other branches end in the nuclei of the acousticolateral area (Larsell, 1967). It is certain that the terminations of lateral line and vestibular fibers greatly overlap, and impulses are correlated both in the acousticolateral area and in the cerebellum. General somatic sensory afferents of the other branchial nerves (trigeminal, facial, glossopharyngeal, and vagal) also are correlated through collaterals of these nerves to the acousticolateral area.

This area in elasmobranchs is larger and more highly differentiated than in petromyzonts, reflecting the greater complexity of the lateral line system, the larger number of fibers in the lateral line nerves, and the development of a labyrinth with three canals. The dorsal nucleus is more dorsomedial because of its large size and the parallel development of the crest of the cerebellum. This nucleus is also termed the lobe of the anterior lateral line nerve, and the middle nucleus, the lobe of the posterior lateral line nerve; the latter, however, receives fibers from the anterior lateral line nerve as well, and both lateral line lobes receive vestibular fibers.

The pattern of secondary connections of the acousticolateral area is generally constant throughout phylogeny. It is evident even in myxinoids, but is more clearly defined in petromyzonts and elasmobranchs. The five principal connections are (1) an acousticolateral commissure decussating anteriorly to interconnect the corresponding acousticolateral areas of the two sides; (2) fibers to the ipsilateral medullary reticular formation; (3) fibers to the cerebellum; (4) internal arcuate fibers coursing ventromedially to enter the medial longitudinal fasciculus of both sides. Some fibers descend to lower medullary and spinal cord levels (octavospinal and vestibulospinal tracts). Others ascend to terminate in more rostral motor nuclei; (5) ventral internal arcuate fibers decussate and turn rostrally in the lateral medulla of the opposite side, then ascend to the midbrain as a bundle called the lateral bulbar lemniscus (acousticolateral lemniscus, lateral longitudinal fasciculus).

The lateral bulbar lemniscus also contains many nondecussated fibers from the acousticolateral area of the same side. At least some fibers of this bundle are the homolog of the lateral lemniscus of mammals, although they have not yet acquired an auditory function, and many fibers are added after the development of the cochlea in amphibians. The lateral bulbar lemniscus terminates in the torus semicircularis (primordial inferior colliculus of mammals), nucleus isthmi, primordial medial geniculate body, nucleus of the posterior commissure, and a few fibers pass to the optic tectum. The major portion of the lateral bulbar lemniscus arises from the dorsal and middle nuclei, the centers of termination of lateral line nerves. This feature is important because these nuclei are destined to become the cochlear nuclei of terrestrial vertebrates, and the lateral bulbar lemniscus, the principal auditory pathway.

Collections of large motor cells with coarse axons lie within the acousticolateral area of petromyzonts and elasmobranchs. These masses are sometimes designated the anterior and posterior octavomotor nuclei. The anterior octavomotor nucleus contributes ascending fascicles to the opposite medial longitudinal fasciculus. Fibers of the posterior octavomotor nucleus contribute to the internal arcuate fibers which give rise to the ipsilateral vestibulospinal tract, although vestibulospinal fibers arise also from the smaller granular cells of the acousticolateral area. Those cells giving rise to internal arcuate fibers and the uncrossed vestibulospinal tract are the homologous forerunners of the mammalian lateral vestibular nucleus of Deiters, although they are not yet arranged into a compact nucleus.

The cerebellar crest (Chapter 6) is predominantly a layer of fibers in the primordial cerebellum continuous with the middle nucleus. It covers the entire acousticolateral area in lower vertebrates (Larsell, 1967). Numerous reciprocal connections with the acousticolateral area are present; axons and collaterals of many root fibers of the lateral line and acoustic nerves enter the cerebellar crest. An intimate relation between the cerebellum (archicerebellum of mammals) and the vestibular centers thus exists from the earliest stages of these structures.

Teleosts have the same general pattern of development and connections of the acousticolateral area. The arrangements differ considerably among the various families. A general enlargement in the dorsal and middle nuclei (lateral line lobes) reflects the increased complexity of the lateral line system and is associated with an increase in the size of the lateral bulbar lemniscus. The acousticolateral commissure is a ventral decussation in elasmobranchs but is dorsal in teleosts. This feature illustrates that anatomic position alone is not an adequate criterion of homology of structure.

The vestibulospinal tract in teleosts courses on the same side in the medial longitudinal fasciculus. The cells of origin are organized into a well-defined nucleus, the nucleus of Deiters; the afferent innervation is mainly by vestibular fibers. A tangential nucleus is lacking in elasmobranchs but is differentiated in teleosts and lies ventral to the nucleus of Deiters. It receives root fibers of the acoustic nerve; the axons descend bilaterally in the medial longitudinal fasciculus. The tangential nucleus remains prominent in amphibians, reptiles, and birds, but regresses in mammals, although vestiges may be found even in man. The nucleus of Deiters and the tangential nucleus also project to the giant cells of Mauthner (Chapter 7), allowing even more rapid conduction of vestibular impulses for reflexive tail movements than can be provided by the direct vestibulospinal tract. Most incoming fibers of the acoustic nerve in teleosts terminate in the nucleus of Deiters and in the tangential nucleus.

Elasmobranchs have some fibers that originate in the acousticolateral area, ascend in the opposite lateral bulbar lemniscus, and terminate in the optic tectum. In teleosts, fibers of the acousticolateral area do not project directly to the optic tectum, but have intermediate synapses in the torus semicircularis (inferior colliculus). The correlation of optic and vestibular impulses is therefore by tertiary vestibular fibers in teleosts and most higher vertebrates.

Groups of cells constituting the torus semicircularis (nucleus profundus mesencephali, area posticum, inferior colliculus) are scattered in the ventral part of the midbrain of elasmobranchs. The torus increases in mass proportionate to the development of the lateral line system in teleosts. The lateral bulbar lemniscus terminates mainly in the medial part of this area, but the lateral portion receives fibers of the descending trigeminal nucleus, carrying information on touch, pain, and temperature. Connections between the medial and lateral parts of this midbrain area provide for correlation of lateral line, vestibular, and tactile information.

The gap between fishes and reptiles is not bridged by presently living amphibians. Urodeles have either lagged or regressed, and anurans have extremes of specialization. Study of these modern species, however, provides a basis for speculation on the development of the nervous system of extinct ancestral amphibians. This consideration is important because the move from aquatic to terrestrial life required extreme changes in lateral line and acoustic systems and brought adaptive changes in the related centers of the central nervous system.

The regression of the acousticolateral area in urodelan amphibians is consistent with the dedifferentiation generally in the nervous system of these animals. The acousticolateral area of the urodeles is therefore comparable to that of the most primitive vertebrates having barely distinguishable dorsal, middle, and ventral nuclei (Herrick, 1948).

The acousticolateral area of larval anurans such as the frog tadpole is similar to that of fishes. At the time of metamorphosis, the lateral line fibers degenerate and disappear, leaving the neurons of the dorsal and middle nuclei (lobes of the lateral line nerves) under the influence of the newly developing cochlear fibers. The vestibular fibers that terminated in these nuclei also degenerate, and the entire vestibular innervation is directed to the ventral nuclei, including the well-differentiated nucleus of Deiters. The secondary vestibular connections persist unchanged. The secondary connections of the dorsal and middle nuclei do not degenerate, but they are enhanced by the development of new fibers and by the growth of primary peripheral cochlear fibers. The middle nucleus of the tadpole is the dorsal magnocellular nucleus in the adult frog. This nucleus formerly received afferent fibers from the anterior and posterior lateral line nerves, as in all lower aquatic vertebrates. Secondary fibers pass medially from this nucleus in the frog; some decussate in either of two bundles, one near the ventricular floor, and another, more ventrally situated, and known as the trapezoid body. A new aggregate of cells appears in the lateral region of the trapezoid body. This aggregate, the superior olivary nucleus, has no known primordium in lower vertebrates. Some fibers of the trapezoid body synapse on its cells. After decussation, the dorsal bundle and the trapezoid body join and turn rostrally, accompanied by superior olivary fibers and many uncrossed secondary auditory fibers. The combined bundle of fibers is the lateral lemniscus (lateral bulbar lemniscus). It terminates in the torus semicircularis (inferior colliculus). The two sides of the torus are fused posteriorly to form the cerebral aqueduct (aqueduct of Sylvius, iter), but are still primitively separate anteriorly, allowing formation of the optic ventricles (Chapter 2).

Unlike the condition in teleosts, some fibers of the lateral lemniscus pass directly to the optic tectum, which is continuous with the torus semicircularis. The torus of the frog, in addition to contributions from the lateral lemniscus, also receives fibers of the spino- and bulbo-mesencephalic tracts (Chapter 3), and from the contralateral nucleus isthmi. The torus serves as one correlation center for auditory and tactile (? vibratory) impulses.

The dorsal nucleus of tadpoles is less easily distinguished after metamorphosis and is intermingled with the dorsal and anterior portion of the former middle nucleus, the dorsal magnocellular nucleus (Larsell, 1934, 1967). It emerges once again in reptiles as a distinct morphologic entity, the angular nucleus.

The fate of the acousticolateral area of the frog illustrates a successful experiment by nature in the use of existing anatomic structures and pathways as the basis for functional adaptation to new environmental requirements. This phenomenon not only occurred in evolution over millennia but is repeated in the metamorphosis of each animal, allowing direct observation and serving as an experimental model for modification of the process.

Reptiles have extreme contrasts in the relative development of axial and appendicular muscles, as illustrated by turtles and snakes. Agility also varies greatly, exemplified by the differences between lizards and alligators (Chapter 1). These contrasts are accompanied by alterations in the vestibular nuclei and are representative of adaptive changes for motor needs.

The vestibular nuclei of reptiles have five subdivisions: (1) the tangential nucleus is similar to that of teleosts. It lies ventral to the lateral vestibular nucleus of Deiters, is best developed in lizards and snakes, but is smallest in turtles; (2) the lateral vestibular nucleus of Deiters (ventrolateral vestibular nucleus) has larger but fewer neurons, and more collaterals in snakes than in other reptiles. It gives rise mainly to the ipsilateral direct vestibulospinal tract; (3) the inferior or descending vestibular nucleus is a caudal continuation of the smaller neurons of the lateral vestibular nucleus. It also gives rise to fibers of the vestibulospinal tract. Most spinovestibular fibers terminate in this nucleus; (4)

the superior vestibular nucleus (dorsolateral vestibular nucleus, anterior vestibular nucleus) receives vestibular fibers of fine caliber from
the cristae of the ampullae and maculae of the sacculus and of the cerebellum; (5) the ventromedial vestibular nucleus is small and is the
homologous primordium of the mammalian medial vestibular nucleus
(Kappers, 1947). An even smaller superior group occurs only in turtles.

The rapid trunk and tail movements allowing crocodiles to be good
swimmers are mediated by fibers of the tangential nucleus that reach
the cord by the medial longitudinal fasciculus, and also by the direct
vestibulospinal tract from the lateral and descending vestibular nuclei.
Their clumsy movements on land are partly related to a slower multisynaptic vestibulo-reticulo-spinal pathway to those ventral horn cells innervating muscles of the limbs. Lizards, in contrast, run quickly on land,
and have a unique second direct vestibulospinal tract to the cervical and
lumbar regions of the cord. Running is a coordinated sequence of reflexive activity partly accomplished by the spinal cord alone, but is initiated and reinforced by suprasegmental mechanisms. In submammalian
forms, the vestibulospinal tracts are the major motor pathways to the
cord; both the coordinating function of the cerebellum and postural control are expressed through vestibulospinal pathways. The function of the
efficient vestibulospinal tracts of lizards is analogous to that of the corticospinal tracts, the most important motor pathway in man.

Reptiles have two cochlear nuclei. The angular nucleus is larger and
contains more neurons than in the frog. The dorsal magnocellular nucleus is closely related to the laminar nucleus, a row of cells not receiving direct fibers from the cochlea, but rather secondary fibers of the
dorsal magnocellular nucleus of both sides. It then contributes internal
arcuate fibers to the superior olive and lateral lemniscus, and also sends
fibers to the cerebellum. The lateral lemniscus terminates in the torus
semicircularis, a structure similar in anatomy and connections to that in
anuran amphibians. Other terminations include the nucleus isthmi for
intermediate synapse in passage to the optic tectum, and a scattered nucleus of the lateral lemniscus which may be formed by displaced cells
of the superior olivary nucleus. The nucleus of the lateral lemniscus is
found also in birds and mammals.

A complex vestibular system is required for animals with the ability
to fly in constantly changing winds and to navigate rapidly and accurately around branches of trees and other small obstructions. In many
ways, the differentiation and connections of the vestibular nuclei of

birds is more complex than those of mammals, including man. Birds have inherited the basic reptilian vestibular system and have elaborated upon it with enlarged and subdivided nuclei, particularly the superior vestibular nucleus (dorsolateral vestibular nucleus).

The cochlear nuclei of birds are comparable to those of reptiles, but they are also more highly differentiated. The connections are similar (Boord, 1969). Cochlear fibers terminate in a somatotopic fashion in the angular nucleus and the dorsal magnocellular nucleus. Lagenar fibers also terminate in a unique receptive area of the cochlear nuclei and, in addition, disseminate in the vestibular and cerebellar nuclei. The torus semicircularis (inferior colliculus) of birds remains nonlaminated and can be subdivided by neuronal characteristics and by afferent connections. The lateral portion receives the lateral lemniscus and projects to thalamic centers, mainly on the same side. Impulses then are relayed to a specially differentiated region of the corpus striatum (Chapter 12). Portions of the torus semicircularis receive fibers associated with tactile sensation. This midbrain center correlates auditory and tactile impulses, thus relating hearing by bone conduction, transmitted through the birds' legs after alighting, with the well-developed hearing by air conduction.

Nucleus isthmi

The nucleus isthmi is a rostral continuation of the acousticolateral area in the dorsal and posterior part of the midbrain near the trochlear nucleus. Afferent fibers are mainly from the adjacent lateral bulbar lemniscus and torus semicircularis and perhaps from the secondary ascending trigeminal tract. It has many reciprocal connections with the optic tectum. The nucleus is thus thought to be a correlative center between the vestibular and auditory systems, and the visual system in lower vertebrates.

The nucleus isthmi is present in almost all vertebrates except cyclostomes. In some reptiles it is prominent, and different portions contain large or small neurons. The dorsal part of the nucleus isthmi in birds has unique afferent fibers from the optic tract and efferent connections with the oculomotor and trochlear nuclei. The homology of the nucleus isthmi in mammals is uncertain, but it may become the mammalian nucleus of the lateral lemniscus, or perhaps even contribute to the formation of the medial geniculate body (Kappers et al., 1936).

Acousticolateral area of mammals

The structure and connections of the vestibular nuclei in mammals are fairly constant. Five vestibular nuclei are identified: (1) the tangential nucleus has scattered neurons among the intramedullary vestibular fibers and is much smaller than its homolog in lower vertebrates; (2) the lateral vestibular nucleus of Deiters has both large and small neurons; (3) the inferior or descending vestibular nucleus is a caudal continuation of the small neurons of the lateral vestibular nucleus; (4) the superior vestibular nucleus (of von Bechterew) lies anterior to the lateral vestibular nucleus; (5) the medial vestibular nucleus (of Schwalbe) is not clearly identified in submammals, although it differentiates in reptiles and birds. It lies near the floor of the anterior part of the fourth ventricle, just medial to the lateral vestibular nucleus, is triangular in shape, and extends in man from the abducens nucleus to the rostral end of the hypoglossal. Because of its great extent, it has been called the "principal" vestibular nucleus in man, but in view of the evolution of the acousticolateral area and the connections of the vestibular nuclei in mammals this name is not entirely appropriate. The physiologic importance of each of the vestibular nuclei in man is still conjectured. The lateral vestibular nucleus, however, is the source of the direct lateral vestibulospinal tract and the earliest to differentiate phylogenetically. It may be the most important for reasons to be discussed.

Primary vestibular fibers from the labyrinth project to some areas within each of the main vestibular nuclei, afferents from nonvestibular sources supplying those areas of the vestibular nuclei devoid of vestibular afferents (Brodal and Pompeiano, 1957; Walberg et al., 1958). Primary vestibular fibers also pass to the cerebellum.

Among the afferent fibers to the vestibular nuclei, those from the cerebellum are most numerous. They exceed even the number of acoustic nerve fibers from the labyrinth (Brodal and Pompeiano, 1957). Direct fibers of cells of Purkinje from the flocculus and nodulus (archicerebellum) project to all the vestibular nuclei, but mainly to the medial and superior vestibular nuclei (Brodal and Pompeiano, 1957). The fastigial nucleus also receives afferents of cells of Purkinje from the flocculus and nodulus, and projects upon all major vestibular nuclei, but mainly on the lateral vestibular nucleus of Deiters (Carpenter et al., 1958). Fibers from the cells of Purkinje in the anterior and posterior parts of the vermis (paleocerebellum) subserve axial muscles. These fibers project to the lateral and inferior vestibular nuclei and are somatotopically organized (Brodal and Pompeiano, 1957). There are no reciprocal fibers from the lateral vestibular nucleus to the cerebellum (Carpenter, 1960). The vestibular nuclei are the only site of termination of axons of Purkinje's cells other than the deep cerebellar nuclei.

An uncrossed lateral vestibulospinal tract originates from both large and small neurons of the lateral vestibular nucleus of Deiters and extends as far as the sacral cord. It has somatotopic organization (Pompeiano and Brodal, 1957a; Nyberg-Hansen and Mascitti, 1964). In man, neurons of the lateral vestibular nucleus also are topographically arranged (Loken and Brodal, 1970). The superior and inferior vestibular nuclei send fibers to the brainstem and cerebellum, but not to the spinal cord (Carpenter, 1960). Vestibulospinal fibers from the medial vestibular nucleus course in the medial longitudinal fasciculus, mostly ipsilaterally, as far as the upper part of the thoracic cord (Nyberg-Hansen, 1964). This vestibular component of the medial longitudinal fasciculus in the spinal cord is the medial vestibulospinal tract. It originates exclusively from the medial vestibular nucleus (Carpenter, 1960; Carpenter et al., 1960; Nyberg-Hansen, 1964). Fibers of both vestibulospinal tracts terminate in the laminated gray matter of the ventral horns, but not directly on lower motor neurons, cells of the column of Clarke, or the intermediolateral cell column (Nyberg-Hansen and Mascitti, 1964). Direct spinovestibular fibers are sparse. They have been traced only to that part of the lateral vestibular nucleus subserving the hindlimbs (Pompeiano and Brodal, 1957b). Collaterals of fibers from the dorsal spinocerebellar tract enter the lateral vestibular nucleus, however, and these may be a feedback from the spinal cord. Cerebellovestibular fibers contribute to another circuit.

Vestibular contributions to the medial longitudinal fasciculus originate in the lateral, medial, and superior vestibular nuclei to innervate motor nuclei of the brainstem, especially those related to extraocular muscles. Fibers do not ascend from the inferior vestibular nucleus (Carpenter, 1960). The lateral vestibular nucleus of Deiters gives rise to ascending fibers in the medial longitudinal fasciculus, most of which cross, then enter the abducens, trochlear, and oculomotor nuclei, and also the nuclei of Cajal, of Darkschewitch, and of the posterior commissure (Carpenter, 1960). All fibers from the superior vestibular nucleus ascend; the abducens nucleus does not receive any (Szentágothai, 1964b).

Commissural fibers (acousticolateral commissure) traverse the midline of the brainstem to interconnect the inferior, lateral, superior, and medial vestibular nuclei with the corresponding nuclei of the other side (Carpenter, 1960). Interconnections between the various vestibular nuclei of the same side are also present. All vestibular nuclei connect extensively with the ipsilateral pontine and medullary reticular formations.

A few efferent vestibular fibers of small caliber arise from the lateral vestibular nucleus and course with the vestibular nerve through its ganglion without synapsing, to end in the neuroepithelium of the inner ear (Rasmussen and Gacek, 1958; Rasmussen, 1960; Carpenter, 1960; Ross, 1969).

The vestibular nuclei in man are usually thought to relate to primitive reflexive movements of eye and head, and to gross postural reflexes. It was demonstrated by Martin (1967) that labyrinthine function is not essential for static posture or righting reactions in man. Proprioception and visual compensation are not sufficient, however, when the supporting base is unsteady, if the surface on which the person walks is uneven, or if he is in water. The vestibulospinal pathways, particularly the lateral, remain in man among the most important long descending motor tracts of the brain. Their importance lies not so much in postural adjustments to motion perceived by the labyrinth, but rather as the principal mediator of cerebellar influence on the spinal cord for the maintence of proper postural tone and coordinated changes in posture.

The vestibular fibers that ascend and descend in the medial longitudinal fasciculus in mammals are largely pathways of reflexive movements of eyes and head. Some of these secondary vestibular fibers to extraocular motor nuclei lie in the reticular formation, just lateral to the medial longitudinal fasciculus (Szentágothai, 1964b). Ocular movements in the cat have a characteristic and reproducible pattern when the nerves from each of the semicircular canals are stimulated individually and in combination (Cohen et al., 1964). The details of the individual projections of each of the vestibular nuclei of the monkey to the abducens, trochlear, and oculomotor nuclei have been described by Carpenter (1966).

The dorsal magnocellular nucleus lies dorsal to the angular nucleus in reptiles, birds, and some lower mammals. It tends to migrate laterally and ventrally in the phylogeny of mammals, however, to become the ventral cochlear nucleus in most higher mammals, including man. It has intermediate positions in various mammals. In some widely divergent families, as bats and whales, it occupies a position even more ventral than that of man. The ventral cochlear nucleus is also larger in mammals than in lower forms. The angular nucleus of lower terrestrial vertebrates becomes the dorsal cochlear nucleus in most mammals. It is better developed in the rabbit, pig, and cat than in man or other primates. Various synaptic terminations of auditory nerve fibers within the cochlear nuclei, and cytoarchitectural differences within these nuclei have been found in the rat (Harrison and Warr, 1962; Harrison and Irving, 1966; Feldman and Harrison, 1969).

The secondary central connections of the cochlear nuclei in mammals have the basic reptilian pattern but with minor differences. The laminar nucleus migrates toward the superior olivary nucleus and becomes the superior accessory olivary nucleus. In higher mammals, the trapezoid body originates largely from the ventral cochlear nucleus (dorsal magnocellular nucleus of reptiles). It becomes larger than the dorsal decussation. This finding correlates well with the decreased size of the dorsal cochlear nucleus in primates. The dorsal bundle courses near the floor of the fourth ventricle to the midline under but not in the stria medullaris where it decussates (commissure of Held) ventral to the medial longitudinal fasciculus, and swings ventrolaterally to the superior olivary complex and the lateral lemniscus. A few fibers of the superior olivary nuclei and of the nuclei of the lateral lemniscus decussate (commissure of Probst) to ascend in the opposite lateral lemniscus. Crossed olivo-cochlear fibers have been demonstrated in the cat. They act on the hair cells of the organ of Corti to inhibit activity in primary auditory neurons (Fex, 1968). Variations of the central auditory system among primates were described by Moskowitz (1969).

One important feature of the central auditory system is constant throughout phylogeny: the secondary fibers of the nuclei related to the lateral line nerves and later the cochlea ascend bilaterally, each lateral lemniscus containing fibers from both sides.

Conclusive evidence is lacking that fibers of the vestibular system pass to the inferior colliculus by the lateral lemniscus in mammals, although the phylogenesis of the lateral lemniscus suggests that such connections may be present (Kappers et al., 1936). At present, only the cochlear centers, which are concerned with discriminatory reactions, are known to have highly developed thalamic and cortical connections, although clinical evidence is accumulating of vestibular projections to the postero-ventro-lateral nucleus of the thalamus and then to the para-acoustic area of the superior temporal gyrus in man (Behrman and Wyke, 1959; Cantor, 1971). Vertiginous seizures may be related to involvement of this temporal neocortex.

Secondary connections from the cochlear nuclei to the facial nerve nucleus probably mediate reflexive auditory control of the stapedius muscle, which acts as a variable attenuator of sonic intensity. The stapedius is well developed in bats, who localize objects by the use of ultrasonic echoes (Pye, 1968). A similar mechanism is used under water by dolphins.

Ontogenetic development of the mammalian acousticolateral area was studied in the early pig embryo by Shaner (1934).

Auditory centers in thalamus and cerebral cortex

Auditory projections from the inferior colliculus or torus semicircularis to the dorsal thalamus (Chapter 8) probably occur in all vertebrates but have not been studied extensively in submammalian species. The medial geniculate body is a thalamic nucleus receiving auditory fibers, but is clearly differentiated only in mammals. In lower species of mammals, including the marsupial phalanger (Rockel et al., 1972) and the hedgehog (Schroeder et al., 1970; Jane and Schroeder, 1971; Ebbesson et al., 1972), the thalamic auditory center also receives many fibers from the dorsal column system via the medial lemniscus and secondary ascending projections from the trigeminal nucleus (Fig. 5-2). This overlap is anatomic evidence in support of the hypothesis that sound perception is a refinement of tactile vibratory sense, and is reminiscent of the phylogenetic origin of the auditory nerve from somatic sensory components of branchial nerves. The greater overlap in such generalized mammals as the hedgehog, but not in higher mammals, is also related to the development of specificity of function in the thalamus (Chapter 8).

Auditory fibers from the inferior colliculus and lateral mesencephalic nucleus ascend to thalamic nuclei in birds (Karten, 1969) and probably also in reptiles. These thalamic centers are the nucleus ovoidalis and reuniens, and may be homologous with the medial geniculate body of mammals.

Auditory radiations from the thalamus of mammals are confined to a specialized area of neocortex, with less overlap than is found between the somatic sensory and motor systems, even in primitive mammals. Auditory and visual radiations overlap slightly, however, in the cortex of

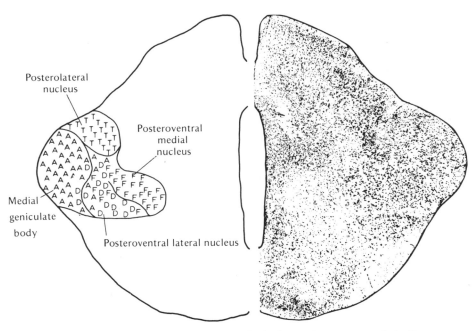

Figure 5-2   Coronal section of diencephalon of hedgehog, a lower mammal. Auditory projections (A) terminate mainly in the medial geniculate body; fibers from the dorsal column nuclei (D) and trigeminal nucleus (F) terminate respectively in the posteroventral lateral and posteroventral medial nuclei. These thalamic nuclei are contiguous, however, and the auditory and tactile projections overlap considerably. The similarity of hearing to distal vibratory sense in man is related to the phylogenetic origin of the auditory system from branchial nerves. Optic tectal projections (T). Right hemisection stained with cresyl violet. (Ebbesson et al., 1972).

marsupials and in lower placental mammals (Lende, 1969). In man and other primates, the specialized area of neocortex subserving audition is in the superior temporal gyrus.

Evolution of hearing

"Do fish hear?" is a question debated for centuries by both philosophers and scientists. We now know that fish can indeed hear, but their process of audition is different from that of mammals. Mechanisms of hearing among vertebrates in general exemplify convergent analogy; evolving lines of vertebrates independently develop a similar function but use different means.

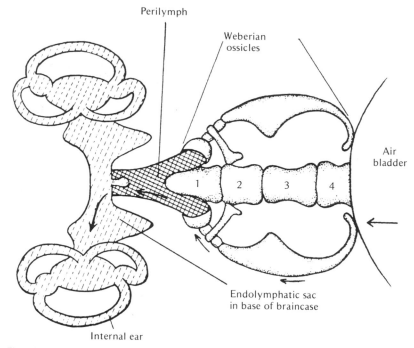

Figure 5-3   Diagrammatic horizontal section of Weberian ossicles and labyrinth of a teleostean fish. Arrows indicate the course of transmission of vibrations from the swim (air) bladder to the endolymphatic sac. Numerals indicate the vertebrae of the cervical spine from which the Weberian ossicles are derived (Romer, 1970, after Chvanilov, 1929).

It was long thought that elasmobranchs could not hear (Kappers et al., 1936) and that the low frequency vibrations detected by the lateral line organs were not heard. It was later found that the labyrinth of the dogfish shark could detect tones of 180 cps (Dijkgraaf, 1963a) and others have reported on hearing by sharks (Enger, 1968; Nelson and Johnson, 1972). Although the difference in acoustic properties between water and cartilage may be sufficient for the detection of low frequency sound by elasmobranchs (Enger, 1968), specialized structures for the detection, conduction or amplification of sound do not exist in these fishes (Romer, 1970).

Teleosts have a hydrostatic organ called the swim-bladder, a structure lacking in elasmobranchs. They have secondarily used this air-filled internal cavity formed by an outpouching of the gut as an effective transducer of sound, analogous to the tympanic membrane of man. The swim bladder is a trapped bubble of air. It changes volume when pressure is altered and follows variations in pressure over a broad range of frequencies (van Bergeijk, 1966). All reports on sound perception in teleosts support the concept that an air bubble within the animal greatly improves hearing (Enger, 1968). Some teleosts, such as the catfish, have an elaborate series of small, articulating bones. These Weberian ossicles are detached transverse processes of the first four cervical vertebrae (Fig. 5-3). The Weberian ossicles transmit the vibrations from the anterior part of the swim bladder to a perilymphatic sac, which then conducts the vibrations to an endolymphatic sac continuous with the labyrinth (Romer, 1970). The fish thus hears with the vestibular apparatus and uses vestibular nuclei and pathways in the central nervous system. Another family of teleosts with an acute sense of hearing, the Clupeidae, has a thin diverticulum leading from the swim-bladder rostrally and expanding into bullae adjacent to the sensory epithelium of the utriculus. Other teleosts have various modifications of the principle of using endolymphatic vibrations to perceive sound. It has long been suggested that the sacculus of fishes is sensitive to vibrations that can be perceived as sound, and that fishes thus hear with the sacculus, particularly because the cochlea of terrestrial vertebrates arises from the lagena of the sacculus. The enormous otoliths of most teleosts would make the sacculus a poor acoustic organ, however.

Fishes are said to have well-developed discrimination of pitch (Enger, 1968), although they do not have a frequency analyzer, such as a cochlea. The system illustrated in Figure 5-3 has a single resonating membrane (swim-bladder) transmitting sound equally to both inner ears. This arrangement could not permit localization of sound as with separate tympanic membranes in each ear. Although it is simplest to postulate that fishes localize sound by tracking the source according to changes in intensity, kinociliary localization is probably equally important (Tumarkin, 1972). Initial orientation in a field of sound results from modulation of the angle of turning in response to variations in pressure (Kleerekoper and Malar, 1968). The lateral line organ, in contrast, is capable of accurately locating the source of near-field motion (Dijkgraaf, 1963b). The two crucial factors for such localization are the distribution of the lateral line system over the body, and the orientation of sensory hairs of receptor cells in the neuromasts (Erulkar, 1972).

The evolutionary change, still taking place, from reliance upon dis-

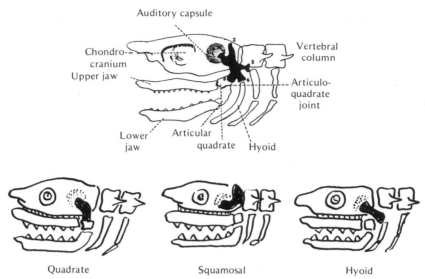

Figure 5-4 Evolution of the hyomandibular bone with multiple processes in fishes (above) to produce three different bone-conducting mechanisms of hearing in different vertebrates: vestibuloquadrate, vestibulosquamosal, and vestibulohyoid. The hyomandibular bone becomes the stapes in mammals (Tumarkin, 1968).

placement receptors (lateral line organs) to reliance upon pressure receptors (resonating membrane and labyrinth) has important consequences for localization of sound (Erulkar, 1972). Acoustic information perceived by pressure receptors is processed mainly in the central nervous system rather than peripherally. Also, two ears on the sides of the head, rather than sensory receptors distributed over the entire body, establish two fixed relations for time, intensity, and phase difference that can be compared. Thresholds for different frequencies differ at the two ears, dependent on the direction of the sound, because of blocking of high frequencies by surrounding tissues. Different mechanisms of localization of sound among animals have been reviewed by Erulkar (1972).

The mechanisms of auditory conduction in fishes were useless on land. The emerging amphibians of the Devonian period therefore developed new hearing mechanisms. The earliest terrestrial vertebrates spent much time in water and went on land only when the lagoons evaporated. They were prostrate on land, the head and body remaining in contact with the ground at all times. They evolved detectors of substrate vibrations by using bone conduction. The hyomandibular bone later evolved into the stapes and was an articular structure important in the support of the upper jaw in fishes. It had internal attachments to the auditory capsule as well as external processes articulating with the squamosal, quadrate, and hyoid bones. Each articulation was used for hearing by bone conduction in various amphibians and reptiles (Fig. 5-4), and each is found today in their modern counterparts. In both urodelan and anuran amphibians, an additional vestibuloscapular ossicle, not derived from the hyomandibular bone, has developed. This ossicle permits hearing by bone conduction through the forelimbs and allows the head to be raised from the ground without sacrificing auditory perception (Fig. 5-5).

Bone conduction can be accomplished directly by vibrations carried from the stapes to the inner ear. A reverse route may also be used, vibrations being conducted to the inner ear through the body and the cerebrospinal fluid, to emerge via the stapes. As animals assumed a more erect posture and used the limbs to lift their entire body from the ground, and even assumed bipedal posture, the reverse route of hearing

Figure 5-5 The vestibuloscapular mechanism, found in all modern amphibians, enabled primitive amphibians to detect vibrations of the substrate even when the head was raised off the ground (Tumarkin, 1968).

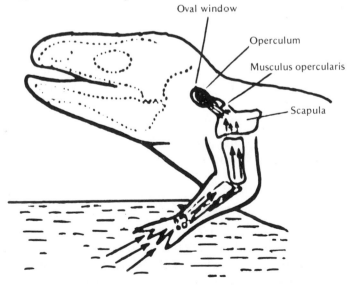

Oval window

Operculum

Musculus opercularis

Scapula

by bone conduction became increasingly important. The mass of the stapes therefore increased, and culminated in enormous stapes in the earliest mammals, the therapsids. Bone conduction of substrate vibrations was limited, however, in animals with erect posture, as well as in large animals for whom ground vibrations were more remote, and in flying reptiles and birds. Incoming sound was also masked by movements of the animal. Finally, bone conduction could not readily be adapted to the use of sound for communication.

The use of the vertebral column to transmit vibrations to the cerebrospinal or endolymphatic fluid is another possible mechanism of hearing in some animals. The greatly enlarged endolymphatic sac of frogs extends down the spinal canal and serves to transmit such vibrations more readily. Tumarkin (1965, 1968) suggested that the tremendously enlarged spinous processes of the extinct, mammal-like, pelycosaur reptile *Dimetrodon* carried an enormous "tympanic membrane" to transmit vibrations to the cerebrospinal fluid. This structure would have been the Earth's first "ear" to perceive sound by air conduction! The spinal extension of the endolymphatic sac in frogs may be a vestige of such a mechanism.

The need for an ear using air conduction was satisfied by several more practical adaptations. The vestibulohyoid ear of some early amphibians was best adapted for air conduction. It used the soft tissues of the floor of the mouth as a crude tympanic membrane. The spiracle, a branchial pouch or pharyngeal diverticulum (Chapter 4), would have been capable of immediately functioning as a middle ear filled with air in a Devonian vertebrate making the transition from water to land. The air bubbles rested against the labyrinth without an intervening chain of ossicles. The presence of a receptor of sound on each side allowed the directional hearing not possible with a single swim-bladder.

The archosaurs refined the principle of the vestibulohyoid ear. The hyomandibular bone became a fine and delicate stapes to conduct airborne sound in these dinosaurs, and in their modern descendants, the birds.

The vestibuloquadrate conductor was not adapted as easily to air conduction as the vestibulohyoid. Modern snakes and many lizards have inherited this type of ear but they have remained largely prostrate and continue to hear by bone conduction of substrate vibrations.

Modern urodelan amphibians possess both vestibulosquamosal and vestibuloscapular connections, but both conduct sound by bone. The anurans, the modern frogs, in addition to retaining their vestibuloscapu-lar bone conductor, also have a vestibulotympanic mechanism for air conduction. The anuran columella is probably a new creation not homo-logous with the hyoid bone that became the stapes of reptiles, birds, and mammals. The origin of the tympanic membrane among vertebrates is still uncertain (Romer, 1970). All tympanic membranes may not be homologous or derived from the spiracle of fishes, as once thought.

A persistent hyocolumellar ligament in the ear of the bird reveals its origin from the primordial vestibulohyoid arrangement of some reptiles. *Sphenodon,* a primitive reptile which has survived, illustrates the transi-tional stage from the bone-conducting vestibulohyoid ear to the air-conducting type of some modern reptiles, birds, and mammals.

The ear of birds is well developed and conducts sound through air. Birds also have well-developed sense organs of vibration (Herbst cor-puscles) on the tibia. They have a sensitivity of about 40 decibels, more than that of the human fingertip. They comprise a bone-conducting mechanism of hearing substrate vibrations except in flight (Schwartzkopff, 1968).

The therapsids were the earliest mammals, although they retained many reptilian features. They had a vestibuloquadrate ear and a mas-sive stapes well suited to bone conduction. They appeared in the early Mesozoic era, when dinosaurs proliferated. The dinosaurs had perfected a far superior air-conducting vestibulotympanic ear with a thin and deli-cate stapes, despite the immensity of these creatures. The poorer hearing of the larger therapsids may have been a factor in their eventual extinc-tion. The stapes of the therapsids could not be transformed into a ves-tibulotympanic ear by reduction in size and by contact with a tympanic membrane as in lizards. The bone was unable to reach the surface of the head because of the development of the mammalian jaw, and corre-sponding hypertrophy of the overlying masticatory muscles. As the mammalian jaw developed, the articular and quadrate bones were no longer needed to suspend the mandible. They atrophied and articulated with the stapes to form the triple ossicles unique to the middle ear of modern mammals. Not all mammals possess a tympanic membrane, how-ever. In the whale, the entire massive petrous bone has become de-tached; it hangs from the base of the skull by a single ligamentous pedicle and is surrounded by air space. It thus is isolated from tissue vibrations except those reaching it by the ossicular chain; the whale is a biologic seismograph (Tumarkin, 1965).

This scheme of evolution of hearing in terrestrial vertebrates by the independent development of four different bone-conducting mechanisms, and the later evolution of tympanovestibular air-conduction mechanisms, was proposed by Tumarkin (1965, 1968, 1972) and is based upon functional adaptations. It is a departure from the more traditional explanation (Romer, 1970) of the immediate development of an air-conducting ear in the emerging amphibians by deriving a tympanic membrane from the spiracle, or of the evolution of the tympanic membrane and stapes in ancestral fishes in whom it allegedly functioned under water as well as in air (van Bergeijk, 1966). In the usual theory, transitional bone-conduction mechanisms in many presently living amphibians and reptiles are dismissed as "degenerate." Tumarkin (1965, 1968) points out the limitations and inconsistencies of the traditional theory.

Relation of hearing and distal vibratory sense in man

Calne and Pallis (1966) reviewed the literature regarding vibratory sense in man and concluded that it is not a distinct "modality" as are proprioception, temperature, pinprick, or pressure. They regarded vibratory sense as a temporal modulation of tactile sense, analogous to the relation between flicker and vision. They also concluded that the impulses ascended in both the dorsal and lateral columns of the spinal cord. It is still unresolved whether the specificity of a modality arises in the peripheral end-organ receptor or in its central nervous system connections (Sinclair, 1967); the nervous system has the ability to distinguish repetitive stimulation and also to summate impulses at a critical frequency. This ability is exploited in visual and auditory as well as tactile perception. In this sense it can be argued that vibratory sensibility is indeed a distinct modality in its own right.

What is the relation of hearing and of bone conduction of vibration transmitted through the extremities or spine in man? The evolution of hearing in terrestrial vertebrates clearly illustrates the use of distal bone conduction for hearing. In terms of specific neurologic structures, distal vibratory impulses are relayed by the dorsal roots, from which the acoustic nerve is phylogenetically derived (Chapter 4). It is therefore understandable that dorsal spinal root nerves and the acoustic nerve should have retained some common qualities, such as the ability to relay rapid successive tactile impulses or "vibration." This ability is retained by both the more highly specialized primary sensory neurons of the dorsal columns and those synapsing in the dorsal gray matter of the cord to relay impulses via the spinothalamic tracts of the lateral columns in man.

In lower vertebrates, many collateral fibers from the descending nucleus of the trigeminal and other branchial nerves end in the acousticolateral area to correlate tactile (? vibratory) and specialized vibratory impulses transmitted by the lateral line and acoustic nerves. In mammals, the external or accessory cuneate nucleus (of von Monakow) lies close to the posterior end of the inferior vestibular nucleus. Collaterals of external cuneate fibers ascending into the cerebellum may pass into the inferior vestibular nucleus and allow further correlation of proprioceptive impulses from the upper part of the body with vestibular impulses. Tactile and acoustic impulses also are correlated in the torus semicircularis and the mesencephalic tegmentum of lower vertebrates. Auditory and tactile projections extensively overlap in the dorsal thalamus of reptiles and of relatively unspecialized species of mammals, such as the tree shrew and hedgehog (Fig. 5-2; Chapter 8). Correlation in the cerebral cortex of man is also probable.

The important point, however, is that it is not necessary for vibratory sense by distal bone conduction to be perceived by the acoustic nerve, the cochlear nuclei, or any part of the central nervous system associated with hearing by air conduction. Vibratory perception is a crude, non-specific type of "hearing" relayed by all general somatic sensory nerves. Bone conduction does not have the discriminatory properties characterizing the specialized cochlear and central auditory mechanism, but nonetheless many forms of vertebrates hear in this manner; distal vibratory sensibility remains one form of "hearing," even in man. In spite of the critical discrimination by the cochlea and higher cerebral structures associated with the interpretation of sound in man, vibrations of equal frequency transmitted by the fibula is basically not different in quality than that transmitted by the stapes. It is understandable that the frequency range of appreciation of distal bone-conducted vibrations in man is well within the range of auditory frequency.

Objection could be raised that the definition of "hearing" should be limited to perception through the cochlea and auditory nerves. Not only would that definition fail to emphasize that the auditory nerve has the same capability of all somatic sensory nerves to transmit vibration, but it would exclude as "deaf" all animals lacking a cochlea and those using bone conduction of substrate vibrations arriving through the extremities or trunk. Finally, hearing by bone-conduction through the human skull is relayed, in part, by the trigeminal nerve, as evidenced by the ability of patients with bilateral auditory nerve deafness to perceive tuning fork vibrations on the head, mandible, and teeth.

Hearing, in the most general sense, may be defined as the perception and appreciation of vibration; more limited definitions fail to relate audition in man to the evolution of hearing.

6
Cerebellar system

The elucidation of the organization of the nervous system by studies of comparative anatomy has been most successful in the study of the cerebellum and related structures. The phenomenon of selective involvement of phylogenetically recent structures in some neurologic disorders of man is well illustrated by the panorama of developmental, retrogressive, and metabolic disease affecting the cerebellar system. Cerebellar evolution is thus relevant to clinical neurology. Because of the precisely defined uniform architecture of the cerebellar cortex, its anatomy has been extensively studied in more species of vertebrates than any other part of the brain. Significant contributions and reviews include those of Bolk (1906), Cajal (1909-1911), Larsell (1967, 1970), Jansen and Brodal (1954), Larsell and Jansen (1972), Fox (1962), Nieuwenhuys (1967), Llinás and Hillman (1969), Schnitzlein and Faucette (1969), Larramendi (1969), and others.

The cerebellar system as used here includes the cerebellar cortex and nuclei, spinocerebellar nuclei, red nucleus, inferior olivary nuclei, pontine and arcuate nuclei, and all pathways interconnecting these structures.

Origin and evolution of cerebellum

A cerebellum is lacking in amphioxus. This finding is consistent with the absence of a vestibular system and of suprasegmental motor centers in a primitive creature. A primordial cerebellum in myxinoids consists of a medial cellular extension of the acousticolateral area toward the fourth ventricle (Larsell, 1947a, 1967). In petromyzonts, the primordial cerebellum extends dorsally from the medial part of the acousticolateral area as a small ridge on the rostral margin of the fourth ventricle on either side. This ridge constitutes the lateral lobes or auricles of the cerebellum, structures homologous with the flocculi of higher vertebrates. The region where the auricles meet in the midline at the anterior margin of the fourth ventricle is a primordial nodulus and corpus, indistinguishable from each other.

Elasmobranchs and bony fishes have a common pattern of cerebellar development, although species differ considerably (Schnitzlein and Faucette, 1969). Auricles are present, as in petromyzonts. The lateral recess of the fourth ventricle sometimes divides the auricles into dorsal and ventral leaves. The dorsal leaves meet in the midline above the fourth ventricle. The ventral leaves are continuous with the acousticolateral area. A transverse fissure demarcates the auricles from a large, dorsal, midline structure, the corpus of the cerebellum.

The corpus is homologous with the vermis of higher vertebrates. Its development in fishes is associated with the appearance of truncal musculature and spinocerebellar tracts. Sagittal and transverse fissures of the corpus differ among species and sometimes even divide the cerebellum asymmetrically. A deep transverse fissure is common and may be the primordium of the primary fissure of mammals. In many fishes, a tonguelike structure, the valvula, extends anteriorly from the corpus of the cerebellum to protrude beneath the optic tectum. The cerebellar ventricle is a dorsal diverticulum of the fourth ventricle into the corpus of the cerebellum. It extends anteriorly into the valvula.

In one group of teleosts, the mormyrids, an enormous and complexly folded valvula extends above the optic tectum and covers the entire brain (Nieuwenhuys and Nicholson, 1969). This fish possesses a pair of electric organs in its tail, and the lateral line organs have become electroreceptors. Speculation that the cerebellar hyperplasia of this fish is related to the electric system is not yet experimentally confirmed; other fishes with electric organs lack this modification of the cerebellum.

Coelacanths and lungfishes have cerebella typical of fishes. Urodelan amphibians have only paired flocculi (auricles) and a nodulus (Larsell, 1967), but frogs have a corpus in addition. The corpus lies anterior and dorsal to the fourth ventricle and extends into it as a large midline structure continuous with the flocculi. The valvula of fishes is absent in all terrestrial vertebrates. The flocculi decrease in size in terrestrial vertebrates, associated with disappearance of the lateral line system; the increase in somatic afferents from muscles is accompanied by enlargement of the vermis.

In reptiles, the corpus of the cerebellum has medial and lateral portions. The medial part and the nodulus correspond to the vermis of the mammalian cerebellum. The lateral portion of the corpus is largest in those reptiles with legs. It is the primordium of the paravermal (medial) part of the cerebellar hemispheres, although it lacks convolutions in reptiles and birds (Brodal et al., 1950). The cerebellum of birds is similar to that of reptiles; new structures do not develop, although the cerebellum is larger and has more convolutions or folia. The lateral portion of the cerebellar hemispheres appears in mammals. The most lateral part is associated with fine coordination of the fingers. It is present only in primates, and it is best developed in man.

The lateral hemispheres of the mammalian cerebellum are called the neocerebellum because of their recent development. They are connected with other phylogenetically recent structures, principally the cerebral cortex and ventrolateral nucleus of the thalamus. The neocerebellar hemispheres are not masses separated from the vermis, but are continuous, lateral expansions of the vermal lobules, a relation seen most clearly in small mammals and in embryos of larger species (Jansen, 1969). Functionally, the neocerebellum is related to the muscles of the extremities, particularly distal groups. The vermis, except the nodulus, is the paleocerebellum, and deals mainly with axial muscles of the trunk. The large corpus of the cerebellum in fishes makes possible the well-coordinated truncal movements in swimming, particularly when changing direction and compensating for shifting water currents. The flocculi and nodulus, the archicerebellum, are the phylogenetically oldest portions and are intimately related to the vestibular nuclei.

Many subdivisions of the cerebellum have been described, but the major fissures are the one separating the flocculus and nodulus from the remainder of the cerebellum, and the primary fissure (preclival fissure), which divides the vermis and hemispheres into anterior and posterior lobes. This division is anatomic and does not correspond to the somatotopic arrangement of the cerebellar cortex. The anterior lobe is associated with coordination of the lower extremities and caudal part of the trunk, and the posterior lobe with the rostral part of the body (Snider and Eldred, 1952; Hampson et al., 1952). These findings explain why degenerative changes involving predominantly the anterior lobe of the human cerebellum in chronic alcoholism are characterized clinically by ataxic gait and less involvement of the upper extremities.

Comparative development of cerebellar cortex

The cerebellar cortex is a constant feature of the brain, except in the most primitive species. The organization is similar in all classes of vertebrates (Fig. 6-1). The progressive increase in the area of the cerebellar cortex in phylogeny is facilitated by the development of small convolutions, the folia, in higher vertebrates; transverse fissures occur in the cerebellar cortex, even in fishes. New cerebellar structures, such as the lateral hemisphere of mammals, are characterized microscopically by repetition of the architecture of the phylogenetically oldest parts of the cerebellar cortex.

The primordial cerebellar neurons extending from the medial side of the acousticolateral area in myxinoids are poorly differentiated granular cells. These cells form large aggregates in fishes, and are a distinct layer in most terrestrial vertebrates. Dendritic claws of granular cells synapse with afferent mossy fibers in reptiles, birds, and mammals. Parallel fibers are axons of granular cells even in anuran amphibians (Crosby, 1969). A superficial molecular layer composed largely of parallel fibers is present in all vertebrates except cyclostomes and urodeles.

An external granular layer is found in all young reptiles, birds, and mammals. Granular cells are not normally found as the most superficial layer of the cerebellar cortex of adult vertebrates of any class. The granular cells that extend to the surface in some regions of the cerebellum of adult fishes are associated with focal absence of the molecular layer in those regions. In parts of the valvula the layers may be reversed, with the granular cells superficial to the molecular zone.

The external granular layer would seem to be an exception to the rule that ontogeny recapitulates phylogeny; in addition the traditional explanation that this layer is composed of neuroepithelial cells that have migrated away from the subependymal zone while retaining the bipotentiality of neurogenesis and gliogenesis signifies a unique condition in the ontogenesis of the central nervous system. Woodard (1960) refuted this theory and demonstrated that the external granular layer in human embryos is formed by adhesion of the roof plate of the medulla to the

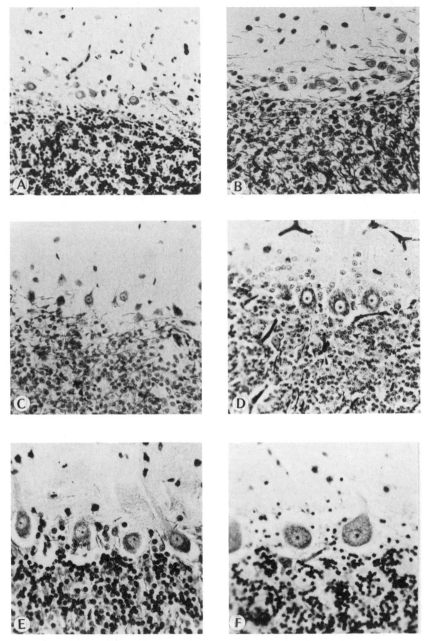

Figure 6-1　Representative sections of cerebellar cortex in (A) goldfish; (B) frog; (C) alligator; (D) pigeon; (E) opossum; and (F) man. Laminar arrangement of granular cells, Purkinje's cells, and molecular zone is common to all vertebrates, except the most primitive or retrogressive species of cyclostomes and urodeles. Luxol fast blue and cresyl violet, X 200.

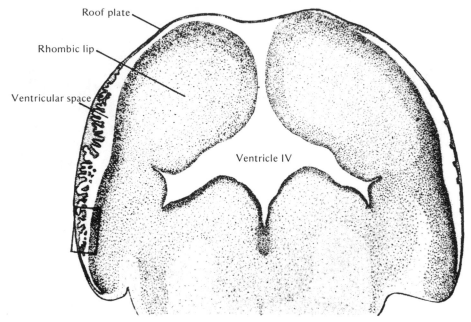

Figure 6-2 Section of medulla of 10-week human embryo (40 mm crown-rump length). Developing cerebellum is an intraventricular structure. External granular cell layer is formed by adhesion of the roof plate of the medulla to the intraventricular cerebellar surface rather than by the migration of primitive neuroepithelial cells. (Woodard, 1960).

intraventricular cerebellar surface with obliteration of this intraventricular space; the cerebellum is an intraventricular structure until 10 weeks gestational age in man (Fig. 6-2). This condition is reminiscent of intraventricular portions of the cerebella of many fishes.

Primitive cells of Purkinje in petromyzonts are large neurons with widely branching dendrites; they are randomly scattered among granular cells. In fishes, Purkinje's cells are loosely arranged into a layer at the junction of the granular cells and the molecular zone. Although cells of Purkinje are frequent among the granular cells, the layer of Purkinje's cells may be thicker than one cell in places, and these neurons are unevenly distributed in the cerebellar cortex. They are particularly sparse in the valvula. The dendrites of Purkinje's cells are oriented in a plane perpendicular to the long horizontal fibers of the molecular layer in higher teleosts, anurans, reptiles, birds, and mammals.

A few basket cells occur in fishes, but they are more numerous in reptiles, birds, and mammals. Golgi's cells can be identified only in higher vertebrates, suggesting that inhibitory pathways in the cerebellar cortex may be well developed only in advanced vertebrates.

The cerebellar crest (crista cerebellaris) is a continuation of the molecular layer of the cerebellum in fishes. It overlies the acousticolateral area of the dorsal part of the medulla and is associated with the development of the lateral line system (Chapter 5). Terminal climbing fibers of lateral line and acoustic (vestibular) nerves synapse with dendrites of the primitive cells of Purkinje in the cerebellar crest.

Afferent fibers arising outside the cerebellum enter the cerebellar cortex as either climbing or mossy fibers. Climbing fibers synapse with dendrites of cells of Purkinje in the molecular layer. Mossy fibers end in the granular layer where they branch extensively and synapse with terminal dendritic claws of granular cells. Climbing fibers are found even in petromyzonts and change little in evolution; the mossy fiber-granular cell system has, in contrast, undergone many changes of increasing complexity with phylogenetic development (Llinás and Hillman, 1969). Simple mossy fibers are found in teleosts. Pontine and inferior olivary nuclei give origin to both types of fibers in the cat, and reticular centers project mainly climbing fibers (Murphy et al., 1973).

Short association fibers occur between adjacent folia, and long fibers connect distant parts of the cerebellar cortex, including connections between the hemispheres and vermis (Jansen, 1933).

Electron microscopy of the cerebellar cortex in various vertebrates, particularly with regard to synapses, has been performed by Fox et al. (1967), Kaiserman-Abramof and Palay (1969), Sotelo (1969), Mugnaini (1969), Uchizono (1969), Meller and Glees (1969), and Larramendi (1969).

Cerebellar nuclei

The cerebellar nuclei are aggregates of neurons within the deep white matter of higher vertebrates. Most afferent projections to these nuclei are axons of Purkinje's cells, but the nuclei also receive fibers originating in the brainstem and spinal cord, such as the vestibulocerebellar and spinocerebellar tracts. Fibers arise from the cerebellar nuclei to form the principal efferent pathways from the cerebellum. Fishes and urodelan amphibians lack cerebellar nuclei. Purkinje's cells then project to the mesencephalic tegmentum without intermediate synapse. The reticular neurons receiving axons of Purkinje's cells in fishes thus serve as cerebellar nuclei and may be primordial homologs of these nuclei. In advanced animals, the only destination of the axons of Purkinje's cells other than to the cerebellar nuclei or opposite cerebellar cortex is to the vestibular nuclei. These fibers arise in the flocculus, nodulus, and probably in some regions of the vermis.

The size and differentiation of the cerebellar nuclei generally parallel that of the cerebellar cortex. In reptiles, the medial and lateral cerebellar nuclei are homologous with the fastigial and part of the interpositus nuclei, respectively, of mammals. The nuclei are continuous with the vestibular area and are variably demarcated from each other. In most birds, especially the strong fliers, the cerebellar nuclei are a single, well-developed, greatly convoluted mass of neurons, also homologous with the fastigial and interpositus nuclei of mammals. Most mammals, including marsupials, have three cerebellar nuclei. The most medial, the fastigius, is related to the flocculi and nodulus. An intermediate nucleus interpositus is associated with the vermis. The lateral nucleus, the dentate, receives projections predominantly from the lateral hemisphere of the cerebellum. In higher primates, including man, the nucleus interpositus is subdivided into globose and emboliform nuclei. The dentate nucleus is a convoluted semicircle of neurons with a dorsomedially directed hilus. It is somatotopically organized in harmony with the cerebellar cortex of the same hemisphere (Korneliussen, 1967, 1968) and with the contralateral chief nucleus of the inferior olive (Lapresle and Ben Hamida, 1970). The medial parts of the dentate nucleus are older and are related to the paravermal part of the hemisphere.

Spinocerebellar nuclei and tracts

Spinocerebellar tracts convey both proprioceptive and tactile information. These tracts may be lacking in cyclostomes. The size of the pathway is proportionate to that of the cerebellum. The dorsal spinocerebellar tract in mammals enters the cerebellum through the inferior cerebellar peduncle, and the ventral tract enters by hooking back through the superior cerebellar peduncle. Because of this difference, a distinction is sometimes made between dorsal and ventral tracts in lower vertebrates, based on whether the entrance of spinocerebellar fibers is rostral or caudal to the trigeminal nerve root. By this criterion, most vertebrates have both tracts, although the two intermingle as they ascend in the spinal cord. If, however, the two tracts are more properly distinguished on the basis of origin and destination, the dorsal spinocerebellar tract is phylogenetically newer.

The ventral spinocerebellar tract in mammals originates from cells in the periphery of the anterior horn (nucleus pericornualis anterior; nucleus anteromarginalis). The fibers decussate near their origin and ascend in the opposite lateral funiculus of the spinal cord. A homologous tract is found in fishes, amphibians, reptiles, and birds, but few details of the spinal cells of origin in lower species are available. The fibers terminate in the cerebellar cortex and in the fastigial nucleus. In fishes and amphibians, they also synapse with reticular cells of the medulla.

Anuran amphibians have unique cells in the dorsal root ganglia of the cervical and lumbar regions. Fibers extend peripherally into the extremities and also project centrally to the cerebellum without intermediate synapse. They ascend in the dorsal funiculus of the same side of the spinal cord (Joseph and Whitlock, 1968a). Similar neurons have not been found in fishes, perhaps related to the absence of extremities. Direct ipsilateral connections from the periphery to the cerebellum are also lacking in higher vertebrates, but the basic pathway is retained by the addition of an intermediate synapse.

The dorsal nucleus or column of Clarke in reptiles, birds, and mammals progressively differentiates on the medial side of the dorsal horn of the spinal cord in the lower cervical, thoracic, and upper lumbar regions. This nucleus receives fibers from the dorsal root ganglia. The fibers from lower lumbar and sacral regions ascend within the spinal cord before terminating, but even in the thoracic region, they generally end a few segments rostral to the level of entry. Fibers from the dorsal root ganglia of the cervical region ascend and terminate in the paracuneate nucleus (posterior external arcuate nucleus) of the medulla, comparable to the dorsal nucleus of the spinal cord. From the column of Clarke, secondary fibers ascend in the dorsolateral part of the spinal cord without decussating, and they are joined by secondary fibers of the paracuneate nucleus as they pass to the cerebellum through the restiform body (inferior cerebellar peduncle). These ascending fibers compose the dorsal spinocerebellar tract. A similar monosynaptic ascending system, also limited to one side of the spinal cord and brain, parallels the dorsal spinocerebellar tract in mammals and carries similar proprioceptive information to the thalamus. These impulses travel in the dorsal funiculus of the spinal cord. Secondary fibers form the medial lemniscus (Chapter 8).

Termination of the spinocerebellar tracts within the cerebellum is in a somatotopic pattern. The ventral spinocerebellar tract projects to the vermis after a partial decussation in the cerebellum, thus effectively making an ipsilateral system of part of the ventral spinocerebellar tract. Fibers of the dorsal spinocerebellar tract, also an ipsilateral system, project to the paravermal and lateral hemisphere of the cerebellar cortex.

Cerebellospinal fibers in reptiles, birds, and most mammals complete a reciprocal feedback loop with the spinocerebellar tracts. Cerebellospinal fibers originate in the fastigial nucleus, decussate in the cerebellum, hook around the branchium conjunctivum in the uncinate fasciculus or hook bundle, and emerge through the restiform body. They then send collateral fibers to the vestibular nucleus of Deiters, and descend in the ventral funiculus of the spinal cord to be distributed to motor neurons in the cervical region of mammals. These fibers go to multiple levels of the spinal cord in birds, in whom this tract is particularly well developed. The uncinate fasciculus also contains crossed fastigial fibers extending to the other vestibular nuclei, and to the pontine and medullary reticular formations.

Other fiber connections of cerebellum

The cerebellar commissure is composed of axons of Purkinje's cells interconnecting the cerebellar cortex of the two sides in all vertebrates. In some species, dorsal and ventral commissures are present, but only the ventral is found in man.

Afferent fibers originating outside the cerebellum arise in the vestibular system, spinal cord, reticular formation, optic tectum, and trigeminal nuclei in all vertebrates except possibly myxinoids and urodeles, which lack almost all but vestibular connections. Higher vertebrates have additional connections from the inferior olivary nucleus, and mammals have a large cortico-ponto-cerebellar tract from an extensive region of cerebral cortex. Birds may have a direct afferent cerebellar tract from the highly developed corpus striatum (Craigie, 1928; Huber and Crosby, 1929), but this tract is lacking in mammals. Projection of the various afferent fiber systems upon the cerebellar cortex is somatotopic, and distribution is limited to certain regions of the cerebellar cortex. In mammals, the vestibular nuclei project to the flocculus and nodulus (archicerebellum); spinal cord centers supplying axial muscles project to the vermis (paleocerebellum); spinal cord centers subserving distal muscles project to the lateral hemispheres (neocerebellum); the cerebral cortex projects to both the vermis and lateral hemispheres, after intermediate synapses.

Axons of Purkinje's cells constitute the cerebellar fibers projecting to the vestibular nuclei and reticular centers of the brainstem in fishes. In higher vertebrates, these axons terminate almost exclusively in well differentiated cerebellar nuclei that then give rise to efferent fibers projecting outside the cerebellum. Axons of Purkinje's cells still enter the vestibular nuclei in all vertebrates, however. The vestibular nucleus of Deiters is particularly important, even in man, as a pathway of cerebellar influence upon motor centers of the spinal cord, and is associated with tonic posture (Chapter 5). In terrestrial vertebrates, the cerebellar nuclei discharge to the red nucleus and reticular formation of the midbrain, as do the cells of Purkinje in fishes. Other cerebellar fibers in fishes enter the hypothalamus. A reciprocal hypothalamocerebellar projection (lobocerebellar tract) arises mainly in the inferior lobes of the hypothalamus in fishes and is probably related to hydrostatic mechanisms of depth control (Chapter 9).

In mammals, the predominant projection of the cerebellar nuclei is to the ventrolateral nucleus of the opposite thalamus. This large cerebellothalamic pathway, arising mainly from the dentate nucleus, constitutes most fibers of the brachium conjunctivum, although a decussated efferent cerebellar pathway ascends even in fishes and terminates in the tegmentum of the midbrain. Evidence is incomplete that all vertebrates have direct connections from the cerebellum to motor nuclei of the brainstem, including the nuclei subserving the extraocular muscles. A few dentato-oculomotor fibers were found in the monkey (Carpenter and Strominger, 1964).

The comparative phylogenesis of cerebellar pathways is summarized in Table 6-1. The basic cerebellar pathways throughout phylogeny are remarkably constant.

Red nucleus

Efferent cerebellar fibers directed rostrally synapse with large reticular cells (superior reticular nucleus) in the tegmentum of the midbrain in fishes and amphibians, but the red nucleus is well organized only in rep-

Fiber Connections	Petromyzonts	Fishes	Urodelan amphibians	Anuran amphibians	Reptiles	Birds	Mammals
Vestibular root to cerebellum	━	━	━	━	━	━	━
Vestibulocerebellar and cerebellovestibular	━	━	━	━	━	━	━
Lateral line root and secondary fibers to cerebellum	━	━					
Trigeminal root to cerebellum		━	━	━	━	━	▪▪
Secondary trigeminocerebellar fibers	━	━	━	━	━	━	━
Reticulocerebellar and cerebelloreticular	━	━	━	━	━	━	━
Ventral spinocerebellar	▪						
Dorsal spinocerebellar					━	━	━
Tectocerebellar	▪						
Olivocerebellar		▪▪	▪	▪ ▪	▪▪▪▪▪▪	━	━
Hypothalamocerebellar	━	━	━	━	━	━	━
Striatocerebellar						━	
Pontocerebellar					▪ ▪ ▪	▪▪▪▪▪▪	━
Cerebellotegmental	━	━	━	━	━	━	━
Cerebellospinal					━	━	━
Cerebellorubral				━	━	━	━
Dentato-olivary							━
Dentatorubrothalamic							━
Dentatothalamic							━

Table 6-1. Phylogenetic distribution of cerebellar fiber connections. Broken lines indicate inconstant pathway, absent in some species, or incompletely documented (modified from Crosby, 1969).

tiles, birds, and mammals. Neurons of the red nucleus are also derived from the primitive entopeduncular nuclei, clusters of neurons lying along the posterior course of the ventral (descending) peduncle of the lateral forebrain bundle (Crosby et al., 1962). This tract is the precursor of the ansa lenticularis and fasciculus lenticularis, the principal discharge pathways of the corpus striatum in higher vertebrates. Cells of the entopeduncular nuclei also differentiate into part of the substantia nigra, deep tegmental nuclei of the midbrain, subthalamic nucleus, and a few smaller nuclei (Chapter 12).

In reptiles and birds, the red nucleus is composed of large, multipolar neurons. This type of cell is also found in mammals (pars magnocellularis of the red nucleus), but a second, smaller neuron also develops in the rostral part of the red nucleus (pars parvocellularis). The number of large neurons decreases as the small cells of the red nucleus reciprocally increase in the phylogeny of mammals. In primates, large cells are few and small neurons are numerous. The red nucleus is anatomically distinct in the rostral part of the midbrain of birds and mammals because the nucleus is surrounded by heavily myelinated fibers of the brachium conjunctivum.

The principal afferent connections of the phylogenetically old magnocellular part of the red nucleus are those from the contralateral dentate and interpositus nuclei of the cerebellum, the ipsilateral globus pallidus, the superior colliculi of both sides, and the frontal lobe of the cerebral cortex; the latter projection terminates topographically in the cat (Kuypers and Lawrence, 1967). The efferent pathways are crossed rubrobulbar and rubrospinal tracts to the motor nuclei of the brain stem and spinal cord, particularly of the cervical region. The somatotopic distribution and termination of rubrospinal fibers in the cat was described by Pompeiano and Brodal (1957c) and Nyberg-Hansen and Brodal (1964). The reduced number of large neurons of the red nucleus in advanced mammals is accompanied by a lesser size of the rubrospinal tract. In man, this tract is small, its distribution is uncertain, and it is probably of minimal functional significance.

Axons of the newer parvocellular part of the red nucleus, accompanied by a few fibers from the large neurons, ascend to the ventrolateral nucleus of the ipsilateral thalamus. Other fibers descend to the medulla in the central tegmental tract to terminate in the inferior olivary and facial nuclei on the same side (Courville, 1966).

Reciprocal rubrodentate and rubro-interpositus fibers are few.

Inferior olivary nuclei

The phylogenetic development of the inferior olivary nuclei is intimately associated with that of the cerebellum. A few neurons of a primordial olive are found, even in petromyzonts (Kooy, 1916). Elasmobranchs have a large elongated nucleus in the caudal half of the medulla; a bundle of fibers emanates from the concave medial side, or hilus. These fibers decussate and ascend along the upper border of the medulla to terminate in the corpus of the cerebellum, but probably not in the auricles (Crosby, 1969). Although the inferior olive is less compact in most teleosts, the connections are similar. Afferent fibers originate in the dorsal horn of the spinal cord, in the optic tectum, and in reticular cells of the midbrain, probably of the primordial red nucleus. The inferior olivary nucleus of fishes is homologous with the medial accessory olivary nucleus of mammals.

An inferior olivary nucleus cannot be recognized in amphibians or in some reptiles. This lack of differentiation is associated with the relatively poor development of the cerebellar vermis. An incompletely differentiated inferior olive is recognized in other reptiles.

Birds have a well-developed cerebellar vermis; a highly differentiated inferior olivary nucleus in the medulla consists of two parallel laminae. The larger medial lamina is homologous with the inferior olive of fishes; the lateral part is a new development. The dorsal portion of the lateral lamina becomes the dorsal accessory olive in mammals. The ventral portion of the lateral lamina of birds is homologous with the chief inferior olivary nucleus of mammals. It is least well developed in primitive birds, such as the ostrich, and is largest in advanced birds that fly well.

The inferior olivary nucleus of mammals has three portions: the medial and the dorsal accessory olivary nuclei, projecting to the cerebellar vermis, and the chief inferior olivary nucleus, related mainly to the lateral hemisphere of the cerebellum, and also projecting to the spinal cord. The accessory olives predominate in lower mammals and change little in mammalian phylogeny, although the medial accessory olive is large in aquatic mammals, such as whales, who have well-developed muscles in tail and trunk. The chief inferior olivary nucleus progressively enlarges in advanced mammals (Fig. 6-3). As it expands, greater surface area is achieved by the development of the convolutions similar to those of the dentate nucleus. The medial and rostral part of the chief olivary nucleus is the older portion, already present in birds. Anatomic continuity between the chief and accessory olivary nuclei is found in lower mammals, but is lost in higher species.

The medial accessory olivary nucleus projects to the contralateral flocculus, nodulus, and posterior vermis, as well as to the fastigial nucleus in

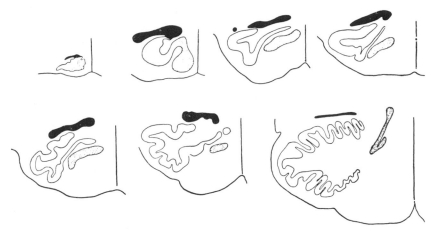

Figure 6-3 Comparative development of the inferior olivary nuclei in several mammals. Top row, left to right: opossum, anteater, carnivore, lower primate; bottom row: two lower primates and an anthropoid ape. Black, dorsal accessory olive; stippled, medial accessory olive; white, chief olivary nucleus (Kooy, 1916).

mammals. It is of interest that the homologous olivary nucleus of fishes projects predominantly to the corpus, rather than to the auricles (flocculi). The dorsal accessory nucleus sends fibers to the vermis and to the lateral part of the anterior lobe of the cerebellum in mammals.

The phylogenetically newer portions of the chief olivary nucleus in mammals are related to the neocerebellar hemisphere, and relate to the extremities rather than the trunk. Proprioceptive spino-olivary fibers from the spinal cord partially decussate in the medulla and end mainly in the accessory olivary nuclei. They are supplemented by fibers from the gracile and cuneate nuclei, terminating in the chief inferior olive.

Fibers from the cerebellar nuclei, both primary (Lapresle and Ben Hamida, 1970) and after intermediate synapse in the red nucleus, descend in the central tegmental tract. They are accompanied by a few phylogenetically old fibers from the superior colliculus, and fibers from the periaqueductal gray matter of the midbrain. The idea that the central tegmental tract contains thalamo-olivary fibers has not been verified. Fibers from the corpus striatum are also doubtful. Short fibers from specific parts of the reticular formation enter the chief olivary nucleus (Brodal, 1953). Cortico-olivary fibers from a wide area of cerebral cortex ac-

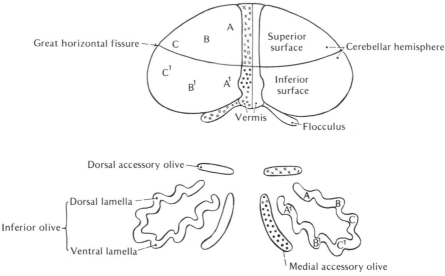

Figure 6-4   Pattern of topographic distribution of crossed olivocerebellar fibers in man (Crosby, Humphrey, and Lauer, 1962).

company the corticospinal tract. Interolivary fibers connect the chief olivary nuclei of the two sides.

Most efferent olivary fibers emerge from the hilus of the chief olivary nucleus and pass to the contralateral cortex of the cerebellum, forming the largest component of the restiform body. The somatotopic distribution of these fibers is illustrated in Figure 6-4. Some fibers decussate and turn caudally to descend in the spinal cord as the olivospinal tract, terminating in ventral horns at cervical levels and probably more caudally.

Connections of the olive with the vestibular and lateral line nuclei have not been found in any vertebrates.

Pontine and arcuate nuclei

Pontine and arcuate nuclei are not found in most reptiles or lower vertebrates. Primordial pontine nuclei and paired accumulations of neurons along the base of the medulla occur in a few reptiles and in most birds (Brodal et al., 1950). Pontine and arcuate nuclei are a constant feature of the mammalian brain, and progressively enlarge in mammalian phylogeny.

The rhombic lip of the mammalian embryo gives origin to the cerebellum and also to other neurons intimately connected with the cerebellum in the adult brain. Those neurons migrating ventrally and caudally in the medulla become the inferior olivary and arcuate nuclei (Ellenberger et al., 1969); other neurons, perhaps influenced by the developing corticopontine tract, migrate ventrally and rostrally from the rhombic lip to become the pontine nuclei. The presence of these neurons and their fibers distinguishes the pons from the medulla in mammals.

Corticopontine fibers arise from a widespread area of cerebral cortex, including the posterior frontal lobe (frontopontine tract or Arnold's bundle), the caudal part of the second and third temporal gyri (temporopontine tract or bundle of Tuerck), and the anterior occipital lobe occipitopontine tract). The number of corticopontine fibers and the proportion of those fibers to other components of the internal capsule progressively increase in the phylogeny of mammals. Synapses are made with pontine neurons. Axons of the latter cross the midline to form the

Figure 6-5 Projections from precentral and postcentral cerebral gyri to cerebellar cortex of monkey (Snider and Eldred, 1952).

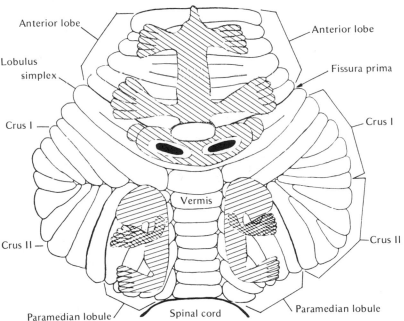

brachium pontis (middle cerebellar peduncle) and enter the cerebellum to terminate in a topographic pattern (Fig. 6-5).

The arcuate nuclei are similar to the pontine nuclei in origin and in connections. Afferent fibers enter from the nearby medullary pyramids (corticospinal tracts). Efferent fibers course to the cerebellum in two bundles, around the lateral surface of the medulla and dorsally near the median raphé. They then turn laterally in the floor of the fourth ventricle, where they compose the stria medullaris to enter the cerebellum through the restiform body. The reason is not known for the more caudal migration of the arcuate nuclei than that of the pontine nuclei.

Functional evolution of cerebellar system

The analogy of the human brain to a computer has been suggested. The cerebellum is a part of the brain for which this analogy may be appropriate. The repetitious architecture of the cerebellar cortex is even more highly organized than is evident on cursory examination. In man, for example, each basket cell of the molecular layer synapses with all cells of Purkinje within a length of about 20 of these neurons and a width of 12 cells. Overlap of distribution of adjacent basket cells allows a precise pattern of convergence and divergence (Fox, 1962). The dendritic branches of Purkinje's cells arranged perpendicular to the long parallel fibers of the molecular layer allows these neurons to be stimulated in temporal succession, as shown physiologically (Freeman, 1969). The concept of the cerebellum as a timing device, achieving motor coordination by the temporal sequencing of contraction of muscle fibers, the reciprocal relaxation of antagonistic muscles and the damping of oscillations, is discussed by Eccles et al. (1967) and Freeman (1969). The similarity of fundamental cerebellar function in all vertebrates including man is further supported by evidence of similar disorders of synergy, motor coordination, and muscle tone in all classes of vertebrates with comparable lesions of the cerebellum.

The need for coordination in contractions of muscle was satisfied early in evolution by the development of the cerebellum, the basic plan of which changed little throughout phylogeny. Creatures with small or poorly developed cerebella, such as urodelan amphibians, rely on sequential spinal cord reflexes and vestibular control to achieve coordination in running; these animals are limited in their ability to use the extremities for other purposes. In running, the rhythmic movements of the trunk and appendages of urodeles and many reptiles are similar to the undulations of the trunk used by fishes in propulsion through water. Swimming, however, requires more coordination because of the greater external forces, such as water currents, and because vertical movements and depth control are additional factors.

Another important feature related to the increased need for an organ of motor coordination in some vertebrates is the development of the forebrain. Other cerebral structures associated with more motor responses to stimuli and to volitional motor activity are the correlative centers of the midbrain and diencephalon. Fishes, particularly teleosts, have evolved a more highly differentiated and complex brain than urodeles. The advanced development of the cerebellum in fishes and relative lack of the cerebellum in urodeles is partly dependent upon the complexity of the anterior part of the brain; fishes are correspondingly capable of more intricate activities than are salamanders. The evolution of neocerebellar hemispheres is correlated with the need for such structures by animals with fine motor control of the distal extremities. This development was limited in lower vertebrates by the degree of differentiation of the extremities themselves, and by the meager growth of the cerebral cortex and other forebrain structures. Further evidence of the dependence of the lateral cerebellar hemispheres upon enlargement of the cerebral cortex is found in examining the brains of whales. These mammals have atrophic extremities but a highly developed cerebral cortex and relatively large cerebellar hemispheres (Jansen, 1969).

Destruction of the cerebellum in man and other advanced mammals usually results in permanent ataxia. Simpler animals are able to compensate for loss of this structure, however. Murphy and O'Leary (1973) showed that cerebellectomy does not appear to affect the sloth, a primitive mammal. Racoons, of a higher phylogenetic order, exhibit signs of cerebellar deficit after this operation, but they compensate rapidly and within a week are again able to climb. Cats compensate poorly for loss of the cerebellum. Even, in man, however, cerebellar hemiatrophy may occur early in life and not be accompanied by clinical deficits (Fig. 6-6). The ability of lower animals to compensate for loss of cerebral structures is found also in other systems; destruction of occipital neocortex thus does not cause blindness in lower mammals (Chapter 8).

The inferior olivary nuclei gather proprioceptive information from the spinal cord, from primitive correlative centers in the midbrain, such as the optic tectum and red nucleus, additional information from the cere-

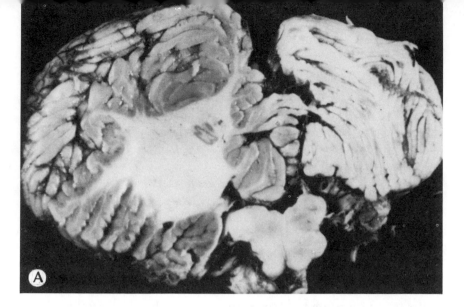

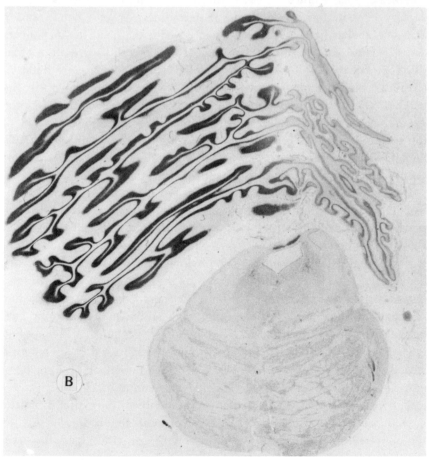

Figure 6-6 Hemiatrophy of cerebellum, contralateral pontine nuclei and inferior olive. This finding was unexpected in a 67-year-old woman in whom a neurologist found no evidence of cerebellar deficit during life. (A) Gross section of medulla and cerebellum. (B) Stained section of pons and cerebellum. Nissl's method.

bellum, and, in mammals, from the cerebral cortex. The information is returned to the cerebellum, where it is integrated with unmodified proprioceptive information from the spinocerebellar tracts, and appropriate adjustments are made in muscular tone.

The red nucleus correlates impulses from the cerebellum and globus pallidus and relays this correlation back to the cerebellum through the inferior olivary nuclei. It also directly influences ventral horn cells of the spinal cord by way of the rubrospinal tract. In higher vertebrates, this function of correlating cerebellar and striatal impulses is largely supplanted by the ventrolateral nucleus of the thalamus. The red nucleus actually becomes incorporated into the thalamic system in mammals by the growth of the parvocellular portion of the red nucleus, relaying rubral impulses directly to the ventrolateral thalamic nucleus. In addition, fewer large rubral neurons act directly upon the ventral horns of the spinal cord; the rubrospinal tract is consequently reduced in size.

From the earliest phylogenesis of vertebrates, from cylostomes through man, the discharge of the cerebellum to the midbrain is to areas also receiving efferent fibers from the corpus striatum. Direct connections between cerebellum and corpus striatum, two important systems regulating muscle tone, failed to develop except in birds. The need for harmony between cerebellum and corpus striatum underscores the importance of the red nucleus in lower vertebrates and of the ventrolateral nucleus of the thalamus in mammals. In birds, the corpus striatum is highly developed and serves many functions performed by the cerebral cortex of mammals, but it probably incorporates the homologous neocortical primordium (Chapter 12). The development of a direct striatocerebellar pathway in birds is perhaps analogous, therefore, to the great development of the cortico-ponto-cerebellar pathway in mammals. Both tracts similarly activate the cerebellum to coordinate muscle contractions in voluntary motor acts. Evidence is lacking that the cerebellum alone is capable of initiating motor activity in vertebrates.

Because of its function, the cerebellum requires not only continuous monitoring of information from the spinal cord, but also continuous feedback from other cerebral centers with which it is integrated. The most important of these feedback loops are: (1) the vestibulocerebellar and cerebellovestibular connections, involving mainly the flocculi and nodulus, but also other parts of the vermis; (2) the spinocerebellar and cerebellospinal pathways, including the indirect cerebellar influence on the spinal cord of the vestibulospinal, reticulospinal, and corticospinal tracts; (3) the cerebello-rubro-olivo-cerebellar loop, or the Guillain-Mollaret triangle. Lesions in the inferior olivary nuclei may result in palatal myoclonus and other rhythmic motor disturbances of the eyes and extremities (Tahmoushi et al., 1972); (4) the cerebello-thalamo-cortical pathway, which allows cerebellar modification of corticospinal tract impulses, and the reciprocal cortico-ponto-cerebellar, cortico-olivo-cerebellar pathways. The feedback loops involving the cerebral cortex are features only of the mammalian brain.

The somatotopic organization of the cerebellar cortex is such that each hemisphere serves the ipsilateral side of the body, although some projections are bilateral (Snider and Eldridge, 1952), in contrast to the predominantly contralateral projections of the cerebral cortex and corpus striatum.

The cerebellar hemispheres evolve by lateral expansion; more cerebellar cortex is added in mammals with progressive development of the cerebral cortex. This phylogenetic growth pattern of the cerebellar cortex results in the functional development of longitudinal zones. The most lateral zone in man is related to the finest distal coordination (Dow and Moruzzi, 1958).

Clinical implications of cerebellar evolution

A group of diseases in man, of unknown origin, are collectively termed the "spinocerebellar degenerations." Pathologic features include demyelination of some tracts and degeneration of neurons of specific nuclei. Structures are affected in various combinations. Some disorders such as Friedreich's ataxia, are predominantly spinal; others involve predominantly the cerebellum and the brainstem. The pathologic classification of these disorders is discussed by Greenfield (1954), Dow and Muruzzi (1958), Netsky (1968), and others.

The spinocerebellar degenerations have several components suggesting they are variants of one process. One common feature is that these diseases affect the cerebellar system, but often not exclusively. Another feature of the spinocerebellar degenerations is the selective involvement of phylogenetically recent structures and relative sparing of older structures (Winkler, 1923). For example, in olivo-ponto-cerebellar atrophy, the pontine and arcuate nuclei degenerate, as well as the chief inferior olivary nucleus and the cortex of the cerebellar hemispheres. The phylogenetically older accessory inferior olivary nuclei and vermis of the

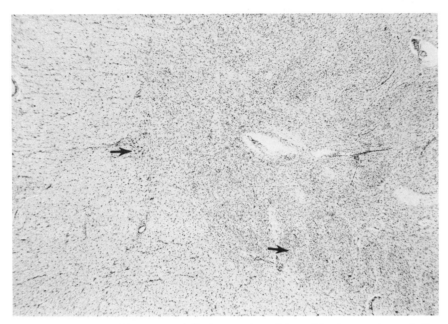

Figure 6-7   Section of human medulla from patient dying with olivo-ponto-cerebellar atrophy. The chief inferior olivary nucleus (lower arrow) is gliotic, and only a few scattered neurons remain; the phylogenetically older medial accessory olive (upper arrow) is intact, however. Cresyl violet, X 32.

cerebellum, however, may remain normal and contrast sharply with degenerated adjacent structures (Fig. 6-7).

In Freidreich's ataxia, the nucleus of Clarke degenerates, as well as the dorsal spinocerebellar tract, gracile and cuneate fasciculi, and anterior and lateral corticospinal tracts, but the older ascending sensory pathways of the lateral funiculus of the spinal cord, including the ventral spinocerebellar tract, are little affected. The older parts of the cerebellar system may be mildly affected in the spinocerebellar degenerations, so that the phylogenetic alteration is not absolute. Because of the striking pattern of involvement, however, the spinocerebellar degenerations may be regarded as examples of diseases in man related to phylogeny.

Several disturbing features complicate the hypothesis that selective involvement of phylogenetically new structures in the spinocerebellar degenerations is related to differences in metabolism that developed during evolution. Involvement of all phylogenetically new structures within the cerebellar system does not occur in any known disease. Even in olivo-ponto-cerebellar atrophy, the dentate nucleus, almost exclusively a mammalian structure, is not involved. Significant metabolic differences may exist between different regions of cerebellar cortex that are uniform in structure and function. The evolutionary history of the cerebellum is largely one of increase in size of a cerebellar cortex that is thus far indistinguishable in structure and function. Subcellular differences need not necessarily be reflected in morphologic appearance, however, and further investigation of metabolic changes in phylogeny may eventually resolve these questions. Comparative neurochemical studies of submammalian vertebrates and mammals may be rewarded by the discovery of specific metabolic mechanisms of the spinocerebellar degenerations. The hereditary nature of most of these diseases further suggests that an enzyme system appearing late in evolution may be deficient, as occurs in some of the lipidoses and leukodystrophies.

Phylogenetic implications of developmental disorders involving the cerebellum, such as the malformations of Arnold-Chiari and of Dandy-Walker, and cerebellar hypoplasia are discussed in Chapter 1. Disorders of migration of the inferior olivary nuclei implicate phylogeny only as the latter is reflected in embryonic development of the human brain. They may be associated with disorders of embryonic neuronal migration in the forebrain, such as lissencephaly and pachygria, or with other developmental anomalies, such as the Dandy-Walker malformation (Hanaway and Netsky, 1971).

7

Motor system of brainstem

The motor cranial nerves evolved from ventral spinal roots at the upper end of the neural tube in a manner analogous to the development of branchial nerves from dorsal spinal nerves in protochordates (Chapter 4).

Hypoglossal nerve

Fishes lack a true tongue; oral manipulation of food is relatively easy for animals living in water. During the evolution of terrestrial vertebrates, the somatic muscles associated with gills were no longer needed for respiration. They became a mobile, muscular tongue, anchored at the base by hyoid bones derived from modified gill bars (Romer, 1970). Although some amphibians still lack tongues, most frogs have an elongated, sticky tongue to catch insects. In animals such as lizards, snakes, woodpeckers, and anteaters, the tongue specializes for various purposes.

The hypoglossal nerve innervates the muscles of the tongue. It is homologous with the numerous spino-occipital nerves of cyclostomes and elasmobranchs. These emerge outside the primitive cranium. In many advanced teleosts, the occipital and first spinal nerve roots have disappeared. In the frog, a single occipital nerve on each side joins the second spinal root to form the hypoglossal nerve; the first spinal root is absent. The hypoglossal nerve still emerges between the second and third vertebrae in frogs (Kamali and Braitenberg, 1969), although the neurons of origin of these fibers form a dorsal column in the caudal part of the medulla.

In phylogenesis, motor neurons of the spino-occipital nerves migrate from the ventral horns of the cervical cord to a more rostral and dorsal position in the floor of the fourth ventricle. These neurons form a column of cells, the hypoglossal nucleus. The dorsal and medial migration of this nucleus brings it near the medial longitudinal fasciculus as well as near the visceral, tactile, and gustatory centers of the medulla that influence movements of the tongue. The hypoglossal rootlets also emerge more rostrally, from the ventral aspect of the medulla.

In many teleosts, the lower ends of the gill bars slant forward into the floor of the mouth, and they are beneath and between the jaws. In cyclostomes, similar structures form an extrusible rasp with sharp, irregular edges to tear the flesh of fishes upon which these creatures prey. The structures are sometimes called "tongues," but are not homologous with the muscular tongues of tetrapods. The visceral muscles associated with them are innervated by the vagal nerve, as with other corresponding branchial arches.

Spinal accessory nerve

The spinal accessory nerve supplies the trapezius and sternocleidomastoid muscles in mammals. The primordia of these branchial muscles are associated with the gills of fishes, although even in sharks, slips of these muscles run above the gills to attach to the shoulder girdle (Romer, 1970). In spite of the branchial origin, it is not surprising that the nucleus supplying these muscles in mammals retains a location within the spinal cord. It lies near the motor neurons supplying other muscles of the neck and shoulder girdle. In man, the spinal accessory column extends caudally as far as the sixth or seventh cervical segment. A homologous nucleus in amphibians and reptiles has not been definitively identified, probably because the trapezius and sternocleidomastoid muscles are well developed only in mammals.

The cranial portion of the accessory nerve arises from the nucleus ambiguus. In the rat, some fibers of the dorsal motor nucleus may accompany the accessory nerve (Zeman and Innes, 1963). Herrick (1948) regarded the most caudal rootlets of the vagus as a primordium of the accessory nerve in the salamander, but this separation is arbitrary.

Motor components of branchial nerves

As with the sensory system of the medulla (Chapter 4), the visceral efferent neurons of the branchial nerves are organized in columns of functionally similar cells, without regard to the peripheral cranial nerves in
which their axons travel. Motor components of the accessory, vagal,
glossopharyngeal, facial, and trigeminal nerves arise from one of two
columns in the medulla. The general visceral efferent column serves the
glands and viscera and is the parasympathetic portion of the autonomic
nervous system (Chapter 10). Neurons of the special visceral efferent
column innervate the striated muscles derived from the visceral muscles
of the branchial arches (Chapter 4).

The general visceral motor column is the dorsal motor nucleus of the
vagus. It contains preganglionic parasympathetic neurons innervating
thoracic and abdominal viscera. Axons are in the glossopharyngeal
and accessory nerves but they are mainly in the vagal nerve. The dorsal
motor nucleus of the vagus is present in all vertebrates but enlarges in
phylogeny as the distribution of those autonomic fibers increases (Chapter 10). The inferior (glossopharyngeal) and superior (facial) salivatory
nuclei are interrupted rostral continuations of the general visceral motor
column in mammals. They innervate the salivary glands after synapsing
in the otic or submandibular ganglia (Chapter 10). The Edinger-
Westphal nucleus of the oculomotor nerve is also included in this category of general visceral efferent or autonomic nuclei.

The special visceral motor column is composed of discontinuous aggregates of motor neurons, usually more ventrally situated than the general visceral efferent column but variable in position. The phylogenetic
development of the nucleus ambiguus parallels the differentiation of
pharyngeal and laryngeal muscles which it innervates. The fibers are
distributed in the vagal and glossopharyngeal nerves. The facial nerve
mainly supplies the muscles of the face, but even in man it continues to
innervate several small submandibular muscles, and the tiny but important stapedius of the middle ear. Facial muscles are best developed in
mammals, in whom they afford additional protection for the facial ori-
fices by allowing tight closure of eyes, lips, and also the nostrils in some
species. In primates, facial muscles also serve as a means of communicating feeling and emotion. The motor nucleus of the trigeminal nerve
supplies the muscles of mastication and is well developed in all vertebrates except the jawless cyclostomes. The only striated muscle still in-

nervated by the glossopharyngeal nerve in man is the small stylopharyngeus.

The relative position of the various motor nuclei of the branchial nerves in the medulla differs in various species, particularly in submammalian vertebrates. The general visceral efferent column usually is dorsal; the fibers emerge from the lateral surface of the medulla as multiple rootlets. The special visceral motor nuclei are more variable in position and probably are determined by those fiber systems conducting the most stimuli to them (Kappers et al., 1936). The principles of the debated theory of neurobiotaxis (Chapter 1) are exemplified by the migrations of the motor nuclei of the medulla (Kappers, 1919).

The facial motor nucleus in various vertebrates may be ventral or dorsal, a single mass or several subnuclei, independent or continuous with the nucleus ambiguus or trigeminal motor nucleus. It tends to be near the gustatory nucleus in animals with an acute sense of taste, and is more rostral in cyclostomes and birds in whom this sense is poor. The position of the facial motor nucleus is probably influenced to an even greater extent by the descending sensory nucleus of the trigeminal nerve. The shift in position of the facial motor nucleus during human embryogenesis results in a loop of fibers in the brainstem coursing around the more dorsal abducens nucleus before the facial nerve emerges from the brain. This condition is also found in some reptiles and most other animals. It exemplifies the ability of groups of similar neurons to migrate together.

The trigeminal motor nucleus may also be divided into two or even three nuclear groups in many teleosts, reptiles, and birds. It is variable in position in different species.

The origin of parasympathetic fibers for the striated muscle of the heart is uncertain (Crosby et al., 1962). Some authors contend that the neurons of origin lie in the dorsal motor nucleus of the vagus; others maintain that they are in the nucleus ambiguus.

In birds, the caudal part of the nucleus ambiguus forms a special center in association with the hypoglossal nucleus. This center, the intermediate nucleus, gives origin to fibers innervating the syrinx, a specialized bronchial derivative most prominent in songbirds.

Abducens nerve

The abducens nerve innervates the lateral rectus muscle of the eye and is present in all vertebrates except some cyclostomes. In elasmobranchs, the abducens nucleus is loosely arranged. It consists of large motor neurons scattered along the medial longitudinal fasciculus. In many fishes, amphibians, and reptiles, two or more nuclei of the abducens nerve may occur on each side. The position of this nucleus differs in submammalian vertebrates; the root fibers may emerge rostral or caudal to those of the glossopharyngeal nerve. The abducens therefore is the sixth cranial nerve only in some vertebrates, mainly birds and mammals, in whom the position of the nucleus is fairly constant. The fibers of the abducens nerve are uncrossed in all species.

In most reptiles and birds, and in some mammals, a transparent, retractable fold of skin lying beneath the eyelids protects the eye when drawn over the cornea. This nictitating membrane prevents damage to the eye by wind and dust, without losing vision. It is vestigial in man, but present in most other primates (Arao and Perkins, 1968). Retraction of the nictitating membrane is mediated by an accessory abducens nucleus with fibers accompanying the abducens nerve.

Trochlear nerve

The trochlear nucleus lies dorsally in all vertebrates. Primitively, it is far caudal to the oculomotor nucleus, but in advanced species, it approaches this nucleus, or is in direct continuity with it.

Fibers of the trochlear nerve decussate in the anterior medullary velum before supplying the superior oblique muscle of the eye. The crossing of trochlear roots is incomplete in the adult lamprey, however, and the roots emerge without crossing in the larval forms of this primitive creature (Larsell, 1947b). The decussation of the trochlear roots in higher vertebrates is the result of migration of neurons across the midline during embryogenesis. Decussation and dorsal emergence of fibers are features unlike any somatic motor nerve, but are similar to the visceral motor components of some branchial nerves, such as the vagus. Hoffman (1894) found that in elasmobranchs, the superior oblique muscle separated from the muscles innervated by the trigeminal nerve during embryogenesis. In the chick, visceral efferent roots develop 20 to 24 hours before somatic motor roots; the trochlear nerve develops with the visceral efferent system, considerably earlier than the oculomotor nerve (Bok, 1915). It is therefore probable that the trochlear nerve is not a true somatic motor nerve as are the other nerves supplying ocular muscles but rather is a detached special visceral motor component of the trigeminal nerve. That the trigeminal nerve itself is derived from two branchial nerves (Chapter 4) makes this hypothesis even more tenable.

Oculomotor complex

Amphioxus lacks eyeballs and associated neural structures. Myxinoids have retrogressive eyes (Chapter 8) and have lost the extraocular muscles, nuclei, and nerves supplying these muscles which probably existed in their ancestors. Petromyzonts have less retrogressive eyes than myxinoids, and poorly differentiated ocular muscles persist. A few motor neurons of the small oculomotor nucleus of petromyzonts have already migrated dorsally from the primitive ventral position in the midbrain near the emergence of the oculomotor root. In almost all other vertebrates except some amphibians, the oculomotor nucleus is dorsal, in close relation to the medial longitudinal fasciculus. In some teleosts, however, part of this nucleus returns almost to the base of the midbrain. This secondary shift probably is influenced by the ventrally placed tectobulbar tracts in fishes.

The six extraocular muscles in man are also present in most other vertebrates. The cells of origin of nerves to the four muscles supplied by the oculomotor nerve come together and form subnuclei of the oculomotor complex. In most fishes and amphibians, only dorsolateral and ventromedial groups can be distinguished, but in some reptiles, and in birds and mammals, the oculomotor nuclear complex is well organized and subdivided according to muscles innervated.

In almost all vertebrates, some fibers of the oculomotor nerve originate from the contralateral oculomotor nucleus. Whether these decussated fibers are associated with specific extraocular muscles is still uncertain in most species, but the pattern in mammals is well defined. In both the cat (Szentágothai, 1942) and the monkey (Warwick, 1953, 1964), and probably in man, fibers to the superior rectus muscle originate from neurons in the contralateral oculomotor nucleus and decussate near the origin. Fibers to the medial and inferior recti and inferior oblique muscles arise from the same side of the brain.

The "central nucleus of Perlia" lies in the midline between the two oculomotor nuclei. It was long regarded as a nucleus of convergence. These neurons are now known to be cells of origin of fibers to the superior rectus muscle, rather than to the medial rectus (Warwick, 1953, 1964). During embryogenesis, the neurons incompletely migrate across the midline. In addition, this midline aggregate is small in monkeys and man and largest in some mammals lacking binocular vision such as the tree shrew and squirrel (Warwick, 1964). Another nucleus in the midline of the oculomotor complexes of the two sides gives origin to fibers innervating the levator palpebrae muscle of mammals (Warwick, 1964).

Petromyzonts lack intrinsic eye muscles, ciliary ganglia, and an Edinger-Westphal nucleus. In most other vertebrates, a nucleus within the oculomotor complex gives origin to parasympathetic fibers to the intrinsic ocular muscles. In elasmobranchs and teleosts, these fibers innervate the dilator muscle of the iris, but in terrestrial vertebrates, corresponding fibers innervate the pupillary constrictor (Chapter 10). The Edinger-Westphal nucleus is best developed in birds and mammals.

Reticular motor system of brainstem

Amphioxus lacks direct descending pathways from the primordial brain to the spinal cord, and relies entirely on multisynaptic pathways through the poorly differentiated reticular formation. The adaptability of this primitive pathway to the conduction of a variety of impulses explains its persistence throughout phylogeny, even in man. Synaptic delays in conduction, however, limit its usefulness in mediating quick reflexive responses.

As with living cyclostomes, the earliest vertebrates lacked fins and the muscles of the trunk were weak, leaving only the tail as an organ of locomotion and as a means of maintaining equilibrium. With the evolution of organs of special sense and integrative centers at the upper end of the neural tube, a faster means was needed to conduct impulses from the brain to caudal segments of the spinal cord controlling movements of the tail. This need was satisfied by the development of several long descending motor tracts originating in the midbrain and medulla. The most important of these pathways are the vestibulospinal (Chapter 5) and reticulospinal tracts, the latter undergoing some unique modifications in different classes of vertebrates. Other motor pathways, lacking in the lowest vertebrates, include the olivospinal, rubrospinal, and tectospinal. The corticospinal tract is the only direct descending pathway from the forebrain to the spinal cord and is found only in mammals (Chapter 12).

Large multipolar neurons, with axons coursing caudally in or near the medial longitudinal fasciculus, occur in the medulla and midbrain of all vertebrates. Primitively, these reticular motor neurons are close to the motor roots of the cranial nerves, but in advanced species, they shift in position toward the midline and may lie in the median raphé. They send dendrites in several directions and are a final common pathway for stimuli from several sources. These neurons form several aggregates, comprising the motor nuclei of the reticular formation of the midbrain and medulla. The axons synapse with lower motor neurons.

The reticular motor nuclei in petromyzonts contain only a few neurons, but these cells are highly specialized and enormous in size, with long, thick axons. The giant cells of Mueller in petromyzonts are reminiscent of the specialized giant neurons of some invertebrates, such as the squid. Another primitive type of overgrown motor neuron, the collosal cell of Rohde, is found in the spinal cord of amphioxus and sends axons to more caudal segments of the opposite side (Chapter 3). The giant cell of Mueller in petromyzonts originates both in the medulla and in the midbrain, but only six to eight occur on each side. The large axons decussate and descend in the medial longitudinal fasciculus and synapse with motor neurons in the most caudal segments of the opposite side of the spinal cord. Dendrites of interstitial and motor neurons along the course of the large fibers come into intimate relation with them, but the fibers of Mueller do not branch. Cyclostomes thus rely entirely on these few giant neurons to mediate locomotion and equilibrium by use of the tail.

Cyclostomes and many teleosts have a pair of giant cells of Mauthner. They also occur in amphibians, but the dendritic arborizations are most complex in teleostean fishes. The bodies of these neurons are near the floor of the fourth ventricle on each side; the dendrites extend laterally and ventrally, almost to the periphery of the medulla. Impulses are gathered by the cell of Mauthner by synapses with the lateral line and vestibular nuclei, optic tectum, sensory trigeminal nuclei, reticular formation, and cerebellum. Vestibular root fibers make synaptic contact with the dendrites and body of the ipsilateral cell of Mauthner, and with the axon hillock of the contralateral neuron; stimulation of these root fibers on one side excites the cell of Mauthner on the same side of the medulla and simultaneously inhibits discharge of its contralateral counterpart (Retzlaff, 1957). This arrangement results in strong movement of the tail, and hence the animal, away from the side of stimulation because of decussation of the large descending axon of Mauthner's cell near its origin (Stefanelli, 1951; Retzlaff, 1957). The axon then extends to caudal segments of the spinal cord. The cell of Mauthner is an example of cephalization of the decussating interneuron in evolution (Chapter 3).

Piatt (1947) found that when the developing vestibular roots of larval lampreys were experimentally removed, the cells of Mauthner failed to develop. These results suggest that the relation of the cell of Mauthner and the vestibular centers is not only one of anatomic proximity but also of dependence for development. Resorption of the tail of tadpoles during metamorphosis was reported to be associated with atrophy of the cells of Mauthner, in spite of persistence of the lateral line organs and nerves in a species of aquatic frog (Stefanelli, 1951). Other investigators found only cytologic changes during metamorphosis, but preservation of the cell of Mauthner in adult frogs (Moulton et al., 1968). In lungfishes, the axons of four or five cells of Mauthner on each side become surrounded by a single, common myelin sheath.

Other terrestrial vertebrates have lost all giant upper motor neurons of their ancestors. A rapid conductive pathway to the caudal part of the spinal cord is still needed, however, not only to initiate running, but also because the tail remains an important mechanical organ of balance in most reptiles, and in many mammals. The use of the tail in this fashion is easily imagined in the strides of the enormous bipedal dinosaurs with heavy, muscular tails, or in the delicate balancing movements of a cat walking on a fence. Birds use the tail as a stabilizing rudder in flight. The vestibulospinal tracts serve these functions in part, but they are aided in these functions by other descending motor pathways that have developed further. Among the most important of these is the direct reticulospinal tract from the reticular motor nuclei near the midline of the brainstem. This tract is best developed in mammals, but reptiles and birds have similar fibers that descend into the spinal cord in the medial longitudinal fasciculus.

The tectospinal tract is prominent in anuran amphibians and reptiles. The cells of origin of these fibers may be homologous with some of the giant reticular motor neurons, in the midbrain of an ancestral fish, that became secondarily incorporated into the optic tectum.

The interstitial nucleus of Cajal lies in the midbrain of reptiles, birds, and mammals. It is derived from part of the mesencephalic reticular motor nucleus of lower vertebrates. This nucleus may mediate some vertical eye movements. It gives rise to fibers projecting bilaterally to the oculomotor and trochlear nuclei; some fibers cross in the posterior commissure.

Fibers of the interstitial nucleus also descend in the medial longitudinal fasciculus to synapse with cells of the medial vestibular, perihypoglossal, and paramedian reticular nuclei of the medulla; others continue caudally to reach the lumbar region of the spinal cord (Carpenter, 1971).

The deep lateral reticular nucleus (nucleus lateralis profundus) is a motor center, lateral to, and associated with the red nucleus. Fibers descend in the central tegmental tract to terminate in the facial nucleus of the same side, in the cat (Courville, 1966). Some cells of the red nucleus itself may also be derived from the reticular motor nucleus of the midbrain.

The reticular motor nuclei of the brainstem differ from other nuclei in which descending fibers originate, such as the vestibular nucleus of Deiters and the red nucleus, because the reticular coordinating centers remain independent of domination by any one system. They continue to receive stimuli from several relatively unrelated sources and provide a final common pathway. When a reticular group becomes dominated by a single system, it assumes more structured nuclear organization and usually migrates toward the source of its main stimulation (Kappers et al., 1936).

The reticular formation in mammals mediates transmission of cerebral cortical impulses to motor nuclei of the brainstem. Corticobulbar fibers terminate among reticular neurons in the rat and cat (Walberg, 1957; Kuypers, 1958a; Zimmerman et al., 1964); these cells then relay impulses to both motor and sensory nuclei of pons and medulla (Scheibel and Scheibel, 1958). Only in man and other primates is this phylogenetically old, indirect pathway supplemented by a few direct corticobulbar fibers that terminate upon neurons of the trigeminal, facial, and hypoglossal nuclei (Kuypers, 1958b). Analogous terminations of corticospinal fibers upon interneurons rather than motor neurons is also the condition in the spinal cord.

Medial longitudinal fasciculus

The medial longitudinal fasciculus is the oldest and most constant longitudinal fiber tract in the central nervous system. It is large in all vertebrates and relatively greater in size in lower species, except in the most primitive. The medial longitudinal fasciculus extends on each side from the midbrain to the most caudal segments of the spinal cord, although it is smaller in the caudal part of the medulla and in the spinal cord. Few

if any individual fibers extend the entire length. In man, the spinal continuation of the medial longitudinal fasciculus is the medial vestibulospinal tract (Chapter 5).

The position of the medial longitudinal fasciculus near the midline in
the tegmentum of the midbrain and beneath the floor of the fourth ventricle in the medulla and pons is constant in all vertebrates, although
shifts in position of many nuclei toward this tract may be related to neurobiotactic influence.

The medial longitudinal fasciculus contains a mixture of ascending
and descending fibers connecting many parts of the brainstem. The most
important fascicles are those related to the vestibular nuclei and to the
nuclei innervating ocular muscles. Other prominent internuclear components include connections between the oculomotor and facial nuclei to
coordinate the opening and closing of the eyes, connections between the
motor trigeminal and facial nuclei, and the contralateral nucleus ambiguus and hypoglossal nucleus to harmonize chewing, swallowing, and
speech (Crosby et al., 1962).

Among the debated issues in clinical neurology is the mechanism of
coordinated eye movement in man, and the pathogenesis of the syndrome of internuclear ophthalmoplegia. Voluntary gaze is initiated in
the neocortex (Chapter 8). The cortical pathways from various cerebral
areas converge toward the midbrain. They decussate near the oculomotor and trochlear nuclei to continue caudally in the paramedian zone of
the pontine tegmentum in the monkey (Bender and Shanzer, 1964). The
presence of synapses of these descending cortical fibers with neurons innervating the medial rectus muscle is uncertain, but the fibers probably
end in or near the abducens nucleus. From this region, secondary projections ascend in the opposite medial longitudinal fasciculus to the oculomotor neurons serving the medial rectus. This arrangement allows simultaneous abduction of one eye and adduction of the other. Internuclear
ophthalmoplegia may result from the effects of a lesion in the medial
longitudinal fasciculus, which blocks ascending impulses from the abducens nucleus to the opposite oculomotor nucleus. This focal lesion is
usually related to demyelination, as in multiple sclerosis, or less often to
a small infarct. In a patient with internuclear ophthalmoplegia on the
right side, voluntary gaze to the left results in abduction of the left
eye and failure of the right eye to adduct. Anterior and posterior syndromes of internuclear ophthalmoplegia are sometimes distinguished on
the basis of preservation or loss of accommodation.

A coordinating mechanism of conjugate eye movement is of little importance in mammals lacking stereoscopic vision such as the horse, but even in these animals, the eyes move synchronously. In many submammalian vertebrates, however, movement of one eye is independent of the other. A mechanism to link the nuclei supplying the ocular muscles of the two eyes probably is lacking in reptiles such as the chameleon. Reciprocal inhibition of antagonistic muscles of the same eye during deviations from the primary position of gaze is still needed, however; the fibers associated with this function probably are in the medial longitudinal fasciculus.

Posterior commissure

At the junction of the optic tectum and thalamus, some fibers of the medial longitudinal fasciculus decussate and join other crossing fibers to form the posterior commissure. This structure is present in all vertebrates including cyclostomes, but is smaller in primates than in most mammals. It contains various components, including fibers from the habenula, pretectal area, optic tectum, Edinger-Westphal nucleus, interstitial nucleus of Cajal, nucleus of Darkschewitch, ascending connections from the vestibular nuclei, and other less well documented connections from more caudal areas of the brain and possibly even the spinal cord (Crosby, 1962). This commissure does not contain fibers from the forebrain, however, in any vertebrate. Neurons among fibers of the posterior commissure form the nucleus of the posterior commissure.

8
Visual system and dorsal thalamus

Variations of the eye among vertebrates

Amphioxus has a group of pigmented cells within the spinal cord. Whether these spots are photoreceptors is speculative. Eyes as well as other organs of special sense are lacking. Photoreceptive processes of cells lining the cerebral vesicle (third ventricle) of amphioxus were described by Eakin (1962), however, and would favor the theory of evolution of the visual system described in this chapter.

Paired eyes occur in almost all vertebrates. In cyclostomes, particularly myxinoids, the eyes are small and degenerate. A similar retrogression of the visual system has occurred in the evolution of animals living in darkness, such as cave amphibians, moles, and other burrowing animals. In these species, the central neural structures of vision are also small. Well-developed orbits and canals for the optic nerves are found even in the fossilized skulls of ancient ostracoderms (Polyak, 1957).

Other structures of the eye, including the lens, ciliary body, choroid, sclera, and cornea are derived from mesenchyme and cutaneous ectoderm. Most intrinsic muscles of the eye originate in ectoderm rather than mesoderm. The comparative anatomy of the eye was reviewed by Walls (1942), Polyak (1957), and Romer (1970). The eye is fundamentally similar in all vertebrates, and it has specialized features in each class and in many species.

The lens in fishes is a firm sphere giving the highest possible magnification. It is situated forward in the eye to afford the maximum distance to converge rays of light on the retina. In terrestrial vertebrates, however, light rays are strongly refracted by the cornea to achieve most of the focusing performed by the lens in fishes. The lens of land animals is therefore flatter, farther back in the eye, and may be freely distorted to adjust focus finely.

Accommodation is accomplished in lower vertebrates by moving the entire rigid lens. In petromyzonts and in teleosts, the lens is normally forward for near vision and retracts to bring distant objects into focus. In elasmobranchs and in amphibians, the opposite condition exists; the lens rests behind for far vision and is moved forward to accommodate for near objects. Reptiles, birds, and mammals have a pliable lens, the shape of which can be controlled. The resting shape is flattened when focused for distant vision. The lens is expanded to a more spherical shape for near objects.

The mechanism of movement of the lens evolved independently and differently in each class of vertebrate. Even the modification of the shape of the lens is accomplished differently in mammals than in reptiles and birds. Some mammals, including the rat and cow, have poorly developed ciliary musculature and lack the ability to accommodate, resulting in permanent far-sightedness in those animals.

The choroid is pigmented in most vertebrates and absorbs most of the light reaching it through the overlying retina. The choroid of many vertebrates has a surface that also reflects light. This phenomenon is lacking in man, but is well developed in cats, nocturnal animals, and in fishes living deep in the sea. Sparse rays of light are conserved by returning them to the retina. The reflection is accomplished by the tapetum lucidum. This structure is either a sheet of glistening connective tissue or an epithelium filled with crystals of guanine. Some teleosts lack a tapetum lucidum but develop a mirror of guanine crystals in the pigmented layer of the retina.

The iris outlines the pupil and is the anterior segment of the choroid and retina that has lost the characteristic functions of both parent structures, that is, vascular supply and photoreception. An iris is present in all vertebrates and is almost universally pigmented. The size is fixed in some teleosts, and the pupil is distended by the forward position of the lens. In most vertebrates, however, muscle alters the size of the pupil in response to light. Amphibians and mammals have smooth muscle in the iris, but most reptiles and birds have striated muscle; crocodilians have both. The muscle is arranged in circular and radial patterns, but the autonomic innervation of these sphincters and dilators of the pupil is reversed between fishes and terrestrial vertebrates (Chapter 10). In primitive species, the muscle of the iris may respond directly to light rather than to neural impulses, a feature reminiscent of the derivation of the iris from the margin of the retina.

Congenital clefts or colobomas of the eye are rare developmental defects in man. They variably involve the inferior part of the iris, optic disk, choroid, and sclera. This normally results from defective closure of the embryonic choroidal fissure of the eye. It is the normal condition in teleostean fishes. An elongated vascular structure, the falciform process, protrudes through the cleft in these fishes to serve a nutritive function for the interior of the eye.

A similar vascular structure, the pecten, projects into the eye of reptiles and is especially well developed in birds. The comb-like shape of the pecten may be a visual aid. The shadows of the parallel ridges fall on the retina as a grilled ruling. Small or distant moving objects are more readily detected as the images pass from one area to the next on the grill. This phenomenon accounts for the high visual acuity at great distances of birds such as eagles (Romer, 1970).

Differences in phylogenetic development of the retina

The two embryonic layers of the optic cup fuse to form the adult retina in all vertebrates. The outer layer has pigmented cells but lacks neurons; the complex neural structure of the retina develops from the inner layer alone. The various theories to explain the phylogenetic origin of the retina are discussed by Walls (1942).

The retina is similar in most vertebrates, consisting of a series of three neurons arranged in laminae alternating with layers of synapses (Cajal, 1909-1911; Polyak, 1957). The light receptors are the rods and cones. They are processes of the first neurons and are in contact with the pigmented epithelium of the outer layer of the retina. Because the rods and cones are oriented away from the source of light, the rays must pass through the retina to be perceived. The reason for this arrangement common to all vertebrates is illustrated in Figure 8-1 and it is discussed later in this chapter. Only in a few invertebrates are the photoreceptors nearest the source of light. In man, rods are receptors of crude light, but cones are the receptors of detail and color. These cell processes are histologically distinct in mammals; in many classes of vertebrates, however, the shape of rods and cones is similar, hence may be difficult to distinguish. Color vision is widespread among vertebrates, but only advanced primates and man have exceptional sensitivity to color. Retinas with rods alone occur in some fishes and a few terrestrial vertebrates, including even a primate, the tarsier (Polyak, 1957). The central retina of some sharks contains one cone per fifty rods (Stell, 1972). The presence of even a few cones may be decisively advantageous to such predatory species of sharks; other elasmobranchs that dwell on the bottom of the sea and rely more on olfaction than vision to locate their crustacean prey have retinas with only rods (Stell, 1972). Cones predominate in the retinas of most reptiles and birds.

The tips of the rods in terrestrial vertebrates and most marine fishes contain rhodopsin or visual purple, a derivative of vitamin A. Light catalyzes the breakdown of this substance and the stimulation of neurons; in the absence of light, rhodopsin is reconstituted. A simpler chemical, porphyropsin or visual red is formed by an analog of vitamin A in the rods of petromyzonts, fresh-water fishes, and larval amphibians. Cones have the visual pigments iodopsin and cyanopsin, of violet and blue tints, similar respectively to the substances in the rods (Romer, 1970).

A second, bipolar neuron relays the impulses from the photoreceptor cell to a third ganglion cell. From these latter neurons arise the fibers that converge to form the optic nerve. A fourth type of neuron, the amacrine cell, is also present in the vertebrate retina (Cajal, 1909-1911, 1972). It is probably involved only with intraretinal relations.

The bipolar cells are associated with either rods or cones exclusively, and converge upon a smaller number of ganglion cells. Some of these neurons are a final common pathway for closed systems of impulses perceived by either rods alone or only by cones. Bipolar cells synapsing with rods, and others with cones, together converge on other ganglion cells, suggesting that some retinal neurons conduct two kinds of impulses to the brain; simple brightness and color (Cajal, 1909-1911, 1972).

Animals with good vision have a central area of the retina of greatest visual acuity. This region is the macula. It contains predominantly cones and a few rods in man. In the center of the macula of some animals is a depression in which the inner layers of cells and vessels are pushed aside. The most acute perception of detail occurs in this central macular depression, the fovea centralis. A central macula without a fovea occurs in many species of fishes, reptiles, birds, and mammals, but many other animals have a larger fovea than does man (Polyak, 1957). Amphibians lack a macula altogether, rendering such animals unable to fixate for tracking moving targets in the same way that mammals follow objects in the visual field (see Visual tracking and cerebral control of gaze, page 184).

Many birds and some lizards have two maculae in each eye. One macula is situated centrally as in mammals; the other is in the lateral part of the retina. Because the eye of the bird is usually on the side of the head, the central macula perceives the lateral visual field, and the lateral macula allows the bird to have good forward visual acuity in flight. The macula is not developed in amphibians or in fishes with poor vision. Other teleosts, including most marine species, have maculae and foveas with different degrees of development (Polyak, 1957). Animals lacking both macula and fovea cannot fixate and cannot track in the same fashion as do vertebrates with more differentiated retinas. The development of the fovea is greatest in species capable of extensive movements of the eye (Polyak, 1957).

The detailed histologic structure of the retina in the phylogenetic series of vertebrates was described by Cajal (1909-1911, 1972), whose observations remain as valid today as when first published, although his techniques did not permit him to appreciate the complexities of the synapse.

Parietal eye

Some lower vertebrates have a third eye medially situated on the forehead and directed upward. This eye may lie within the integument, beneath a depigmented area of the skin, or in a depression in the roof of the skull. Ostracoderms had a socket on the dorsal surface of the skull, similar to but smaller than that of the paired lateral eyes. This median or parietal eye was also present in placoderms, in all major groups of bony fish of the Devonian period, and in ancestral amphibians and reptiles. By the Triassic period, however, many fishes, amphibians, and reptiles lacked the parietal eye (Romer, 1970). Among living vertebrates, it is still found in some fishes, anuran amphibians, and lizards and it is best developed in the primitive reptile *Sphenodon* of New Zealand. The "frontal organ" of frogs is a poorly differentiated parietal eye (van de Kamer, 1965).

Embryologically, the parietal eye develops from the distal end of the pineal or parapineal evagination of the epithalamic ependyma. It becomes separated from this primary evagination and continues to develop similar to the fashion of the paired lateral eyes, forming a retina, lens, and cornea. Nerve fibers from the retina of the parietal eye grow into the habenula (Ortman, 1960; Kappers, 1965); further investigation may demonstrate a projection to the optic tectum. The parietal eye has been extensively studied by electron microscopists (Eakin, 1962; Eakin and Westphal, 1959, 1960; Oksche and von Harnack, 1963; Steyne, 1960a, b; Hendrickson and Kelly, 1971).

In petromyzonts, both pineal and parapineal bodies develop ocular structures. This observation raises the speculation that a remote ancestral vertebrate had paired dorsal eyes as well as the persistent lateral eyes.

The cyclopian eye found in human monsters with defects of cleavage of the forebrain and face is the result of fusion of the paired eyes of man and is not homologous with the parietal eye of lower vertebrates.

Optic nerve, chiasm, and tract

The optic nerve is composed of axons of retinal ganglion cells. It is a fiber tract of the central nervous system rather than a peripheral nerve. In lower vertebrates, thin fibers with sparse myelin predominate, but in advanced teleosts and terrestrial vertebrates, most fibers are heavily myelinated. The convergence of nerve fibers before emerging behind the eye forms the optic disk or papilla in all animals; this retinal structure is a blind spot in the visual field.

The optic nerves form the chiasm by decussating below the floor of the diencephalon. In all submammalian vertebrates and in some lower mammals, the decussation is complete or almost complete. A few fibers project ipsilaterally in the frog (Scalia et al., 1968), in lizards and snakes (Armstrong, 1951; Ebbesson, 1970), and in the duck (Bons, 1969). In advanced mammals, however, and particularly in primates, the decussation is partial. Only those fibers from the nasal side of the retina cross; those from the temporal side remain ipsilateral. The optic chiasm does not contain neurons or synapses. The need for decussation of optic nerves associated with image reversal in the chambered eyes of all vertebrates is illustrated in Figure 8-3.

The optic tract is the continuation of the optic nerves posterior to the chiasm. Because of the partial decussation in advanced mammals, the optic tract contains some fibers from both optic nerves in these species. In man, as in other primates, the optic tract has an almost equal number of fibers from each eye. An intermediate condition occurs in other mammals; fibers from the contralateral eye still predominate in each optic tract. In the rat, 90 per cent of the optic nerve fibers decussate in the chiasm (Zeman and Innes, 1963).

In submammalian vertebrates, most fibers of the optic tract terminate in the tectum without further decussation. A few fibers or collaterals pass to the thalamus. In mammals, by contrast, almost all fibers end in the thalamus, although even in man some fibers still terminate in the superior colliculus.

The basal optic root is a small bundle of thin fibers that separates from the optic tract in terrestrial vertebrates, passes around the cerebral peduncle in mammals, and terminates in the basal optic nucleus (ectomammillary body), associated with the medial part of the substantia nigra. A few fibers of the basal optic root end in the lateral reticular formation of the tegmentum of the midbrain and in the oculomotor nucleus (Zeman and Innes, 1963). The basal optic root arises in the contralateral eye.

A few optic nerve fibers project to the hypothalamus in some submammalian species (Chapter 9).

Degenerative diseases of the nervous system in man sometimes involve the optic nerves. An example is Leber's hereditary optic atrophy, occurring as an isolated process or associated with Friedreich's ataxia (Woodworth et al., 1959). This involvement is not inconsistent with the pattern of sparing of phylogenetically old structures in such diseases. Although optic nerves are found in all vertebrates with eyes, the fibers terminating in the optic tectum of lower animals are not homologous with those projecting to the lateral geniculate body in mammals. Both types of fibers actually co-exist in most vertebrates, but the latter predominate in mammals. Opticogeniculate fibers of lower vertebrates may be collateral branches of opticotectal fibers, rather than separate axons.

A theory of origin of retina, optic tectum, and dorsal thalamus

The proposal is made in many modern textbooks of embryology that the retinas originate as paired outgrowths of the embryonic neural tube, and that the optic stalk becomes the optic nerve. This concept is derived from the appearance of sections of embryos at a particular stage of development. This interpretation does not consider the entire dynamic

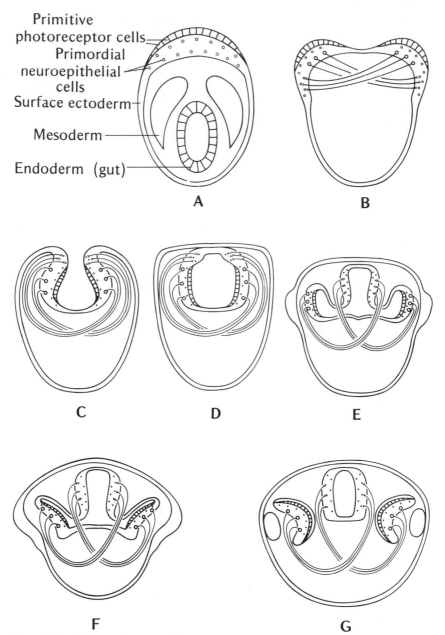

Figure 8-1   A theory of origin of the visual system. See text for explanation.

process. It fails to explain how the photoreceptor cells and ganglion cells become reversed in position in the adult retina, nor does it explain the formation of the optic chiasm ventral to rather than within the brain.

The primordial retina is more properly considered as the wall of the diencephalic portion of the neural tube and differentiates earlier than most other parts of the brain. The eye is not a secondarily derived appendage of the brain that grows outward to reach the integument; rather, the medullary plate and subsequent neural tube are formed from surface ectoderm. The optic vesicles originate when the neural ectoderm is at the surface and remain peripheral while the rest of the brain becomes a deeper structure because of the growth of mesodermal tissue between it and skin. Invagination of the optic vesicle forms the optic cup and eventually the retina.

A theory to explain the arrangement of the retina with photoreceptor cells facing away from the source of light was first proposed by Balfour in 1881 (quoted by Walls, 1942) and elaborated by Polyak (1957). This theory can be further expanded to explain the derivation of the entire optic system, as illustrated in Figure 8-1: (A) An early ancestor had only surface ectoderm, part of which differentiated into neuroectoderm, similar to the open neural plate stage of human embryonic development. The most superficial cells of the primordial neuroectoderm had photoreceptive properties permitting crude differentiation of intensity of light. Similar photosensory cells are found in the integument of the earthworm and some other invertebrates.

(B) With the evolution of bilateral symmetry as the basic feature of the vertebrate body, an incipient median invagination concentrated the photoreceptive epithelium into paired placodes. This arrangement, still seen in the open neural groove stage of embryonic amphibians, resulted in more precise localization of sources of light and shadow. Neuroectodermal cells underlying the photoreceptor cells developed processes as they differentiated into neurons. Some neurons became bipolar; the dendritic processes established intimate associations with the photoreceptor cells and the axons synapsed with other neurons. These latter neurons, the ganglion cells, had axons which grew across the midline to innervate motor neurons in the contralateral neuroectoderm of the bilaterally symmetric animal. These crossing axons were the primordial optic nerves. Any change in illumination, either a flash of brightness or a shadow, was interpreted as indicating the presence of a predator. The decussation provided a reflexive pathway for coiling away from the threatened side, the optic nerves thus being similar to the decussating interneurons of the tactile system (Chapter 3). It is unlikely that the earliest optic nerve fibers directly innervated muscles on the opposite side of the body, as suggested by Polyak (1957), because motor neurons do not generally decussate elsewhere in the nervous system. In a few cases, such as the trochlear nerve, the neurons of the nucleus secondarily migrate across the midline during embryonic development.

Crude differentiation of intensity of light in different parts of the receptive field, hence localization without image formation, was the next probable step in the evolution of vision. The actual perception of images did not occur until the optic cup, lens, and other structures of the chambered eye evolved for the focusing of images and until cerebral centers had sufficiently evolved to process such complex information.

The eyes of many invertebrates, such as the snail, are formed at this stage by simple invagination of each of the optic placodes to form optic cups, with photoreceptor cells still facing outward toward the source of light. The optic nerves decussate even in these invertebrates, but a hollow, tubular brain is not formed.

(C) The entire neural plate, including the optic placodes, invaginated.

(D) The closed neural tube is formed. In this scheme, Studnička's (1898) proposal that the retina originated from the ciliated ependyma of the third ventricle is not only plausible but probable. Eakin (1962) found ciliary appendages of cells lining the cerebral vesicle (third ventricle) of amphioxus. He suggested that these processes might be light-sensitive organelles. He also demonstrated that the rods and cones of photoreceptor cells in vertebrates are modified cilia. Amphioxus is small and translucent. Light passes through the animal and could stimulate photoreceptors within the brain; the same principle could have been used by an ancestral pre-vertebrate.

(E) Cerebral tissue proliferated in the dorsal region, allowing the photoreceptor cells to retain proximity to sources of light at the skin. The epidermis overlying the optic vesicles thickened as it formed the lens placode.

(F) and (G) The optic vesicle invaginated and the retina was formed, as in modern embryos. The continuity of the optic vesicle with the ventricular system of the brain was gradually obliterated. The optic nerves continued to decussate ventral to the neural tube. The glial component of the optic nerves was partly derived from the obliterated stalk of the optic vesicle.

That portion of the wall of the neural tube receiving the decussated optic nerve fibers developed into two important and closely related structures. The caudal part became the optic tectum (superior colliculus), and the rostral portion evolved into the dorsal thalamus. Both structures lie dorsal and rostral to the sulcus limitans. Extensive connections between the optic tectum and the thalamus, particularly the ventral nucleus of the lateral geniculate body, are found in almost all vertebrates.

The retina and optic centers of the brain thus were derived from a common neuroectoderm. The optic tectum eventually formed the roof of the midbrain, but in lower vertebrates in whom the cerebral aqueduct is not yet formed, the optic tectum simply extends over the midbrain as a laminated cortex, continuous at its rostral end with the diencephalon and separated from the underlying midbrain by extensions of the third ventricle, the optic ventricles. Thalamic nuclei also extend into the tegmentum of the midbrain in submammalian vertebrates, exemplified by the nucleus rotundus (pulvinar) of reptiles.

Optic nerve fibers terminate chiefly in the optic tectum in submammalian vertebrates, but some fibers also end in the thalamus; the termination of these fibers in mammals is proportionately reversed, the majority ending in the thalamus.

Further evidence of the similar origin and function of the optic tectum and dorsal thalamus is suggested by the ascending fiber projections of nonvisual sensory systems. The optic tectum of submammalian species is a major correlative center of exteroceptive impulses from tactile and vestibulo-auditory centers, receiving crossed, secondary ascending fibers from the spinal cord and trigeminal nucleus and from the acousticolateral areas. Integration of visual and vestibular impulses influences orientation and gaze. Optic reflexes related to feeding, such as the rapid protrusion of the tongue of the frog at an insect flying across the visual field are mediated by the optic tectum. Efferent pathways of the optic tectum to motor nuclei of the brainstem and spinal cord are prominent in lower vertebrates. In mammals, the dorsal thalamus receives most visual, ascending tactile and auditory projections that terminate in the optic tectum of submammalian vertebrates. This anatomic and functional cephalization allows greater cerebral cortical participation in most activities of the central nervous system.

Descending efferent fibers, analogous to the tectospinal and tectobulbar tracts, do not arise in the dorsal thalamus proper but rather in

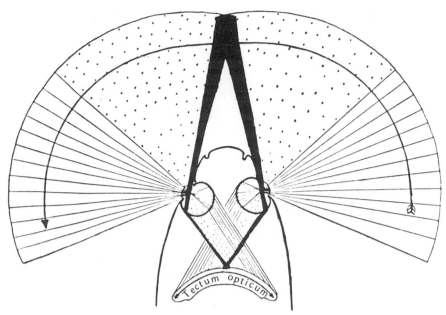

Figure 8-2   Total decussation of the optic nerves in a fish with little more than panoramic vision. Note the convergence in the optic tectum of those fibers carrying impulses from the small portion of the visual fields that overlap. (Kappers, Huber, and
Crosby, 1936).

the telencephalon or cerebral cortex. This latter structure, the volume of
which exceeds that of the entire remainder of the brain in mammals,
may be regarded in part as an efferent extension of the dorsal thalamus
(Chapter 12). The extensive connections between dorsal thalamus and

Figure 8-3   Cajal (1909-1911) theorized that if the optic nerves failed to decussate
and terminated instead in the same side of the brain as the eye, the continuity of
parts of images appearing in the visual fields of both eyes would be retinotopically
projected to the optic tectum in an illogical fashion. This phenomenon would be
caused by the reversal of images projected upon the retina, resulting from the
focusing (crossing) of light rays in the lens of the chambered eye. That hypothetic
condition (A) of total lack of decussation of the optic nerves is not found in any
vertebrate. Complete decussation of the optic nerves (B), the condition of submammalian vertebrates, allows full panoramic vision. Partial decussation of the optic
nerves (C) and (D), the mammalian condition, requires overlap of terminating fibers
in the secondary ascending visual pathway to reconstruct images in a logical retino-
tipic pattern and superimpose corresponding images from the two eyes on the visual
neocortex. In lower mammals, such as the rat (C), most optic nerve fibers still decussate, but in higher species including man (D), nearly half project ipsilaterally.

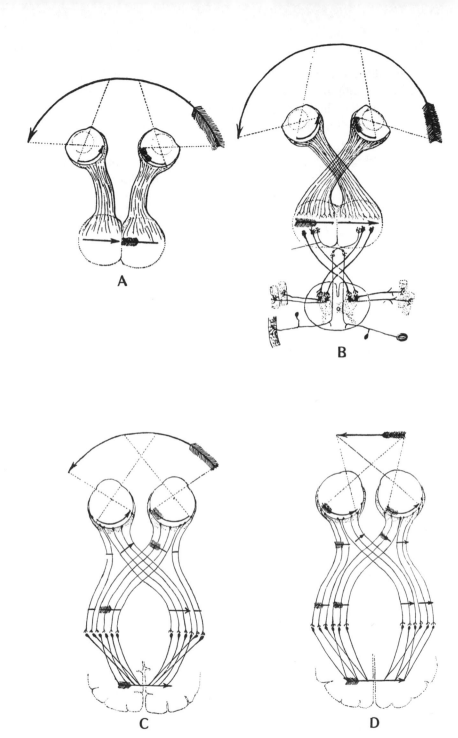

A

B

C

D

telencephalic structures make the entire forebrain and diencephalon a system for integration, correlation, and higher associative activities. The concept that the thalamus is merely a "way-station" for the simple relay of sensory impulses to the cerebral cortex is not in accord with available data.

Whether the optic tectum should therefore be regarded as a diencephalic structure or continue to be assigned to the traditional but arbitrary part of the brain called the mesencephalon is only a semantic difference, if the phylogenetic relationship of these structures and the phenomenon of cephalization of function is understood.

Comparative structure of the optic tectum

The optic tectum, the superior colliculus in mammals, is a laminated structure forming the roof of the midbrain in all vertebrates. It is absent in amphioxus and is poorly differentiated in myxinoids. The optic tectum has relatively the largest size in teleostean fishes.

Although the optic tectum is the primary visual center in all vertebrates except mammals, it has an additional, equally important function in lower vertebrates as the major correlative center of nonoptic exteroceptive impulses. Sensory projections from spinal cord and medulla, particularly from the descending trigeminal nucleus, ascend to the optic tectum on the opposite side in the scattered spinomesencephalic (spinotectal) and bulbomesencephalic tracts. Fibers from the acousticolateral area and torus semicircularis relay vestibular and auditory impulses to the optic tectum (Chapter 5). Information from these sources is integrated with visual information. The descending tectospinal and tectobulbar tracts then modify relations of the body to the environment.

The tectobulbar pathways are largest in the teleosts, are reduced in size in amphibians, and are progressively smaller in reptiles, birds, and mammals. The tectospinal and tectobulbar pathways persist in man, although small and probably of little significance. The optic tectum is regarded by some investigators (Abbie and Adey, 1950) as the highest correlative center of the motor system in the frog and other lower vertebrates. It is, perhaps, partly because of the nonoptic connections that the tectum remains well developed in species with small eyes and poor vision.

Embryologically, the optic tectum differentiates at the posterior end of the third ventricle and cerebral aqueduct from a central zone of gray matter bordered by an acellular zone, as elsewhere in the central nervous system. Neurons migrate peripherally, perhaps under the neurobiotactic influence of incoming fibers, to form layers of cells and fibers. The optic tectum of urodelan amphibians is similar to the early embryologic condition of more advanced vertebrates. It is composed of a central layer of neurons and a superficial layer of fibers, although the latter is stratified with afferent fibers peripheral to the efferent paths (Kappers et al., 1936; Herrick, 1948).

The optic tectum of the lamprey differs from that of other vertebrates in having a superficial layer of ependyma, but the lamination of the optic tectum is particularly well organized relative to other parts of the brain. It has a similar pattern in most other vertebrates: (1) the external white layer (stratum opticum) is composed of afferent fibers of the optic tract and brachium tecti (geniculotectal tract); (2) the intermediate gray and white layer (stratum fibrosum et griseum superficiale; stratum lemnisci) is the main receptive layer for terminal fibers of the optic nerve and the spinotectal and bulbotectal pathways, relaying somatic sensory information for correlation with visual impulses. Reciprocal connections with pars lateralis of the substantia nigra (Chapter 12) also occur. This layer is better differentiated in teleosts and reptiles than in elasmobranchs and anuran amphibians because of the more complete migration of neurons during development. The nonoptic afferent projections are important in lower vertebrates, but in mammals there are fewer of them and they are insignificant; (3) the deep gray layer (stratum griseum centrale or profundum) is a cellular lamina with dendrites extending superficially into the external white layer and intermediate gray and white layer. These cells are the final efferent neurons of the optic tectum, and the axons form the underlying fourth layer; (4) the deep white layer has many commissural fibers connecting the optic tecti of the two sides, as well as other decussating tectal fibers; (5) the superficial neurons of the periaqueductal gray matter have dendrites extending into the optic tectum as far as the external white layer.

Mammals have the same tectal lamination as lower vertebrates. In addition, superficial to the external white layer, they have one more layer of neurons covered by a zonal layer of slightly myelinated and unmyelinated fibers. These superficial white and gray layers in mammals are associated with the development of the visual neocortex. The zonal layer is composed of fibers from the cortical region corresponding to the frontal eye field (Kuypers and Lawrence, 1967) and from the auditory and visual associative neocortex of the temporo-parieto-occipital region (Altman, 1962; Garey et al., 1968). The pathway is called the external corticotectal tract. An internal corticotectal tract from the lateral surface of the occipital lobe (areas 18 and 19 of Brodmann) terminates somato-topically in the intermediate gray and white layer of the tectum in mammals. These heavily myelinated fibers are the largest afferent projection to the optic tectum in man, and the corticotectal paths are larger in man than in any other mammal. Only a few such fibers occur in reptiles. The corticotectal fibers may be related to movements of the eyes in visual tracking, discussed later in this chapter.

The medial tectobulbar and tectospinal tracts emerge from the deep white layer of the optic tectum, curve ventrally around the periaqueductal gray matter, and decussate ventral to the oculomotor nuclei in the dorsal tegmental decussation (dorsal fountain decussation of Meynert), before proceeding caudally, ventral to the medial longitudinal fasciculus. Other tectal efferent fibers project to the large-celled part of the red nucleus and to the reticular formation for relay to the motor nuclei concerned with ocular movement, but direct connection with the oculomotor and trochlear nuclei is probably lacking (Altmann and Carpenter, 1961; Carpenter, 1971). Some tectal efferent fibers pass to pars lateralis of the substantia nigra. A lateral tecto-tegmento-spinal tract contains preganglionic fibers to the superior cervical ganglion; stimulation of the postganglionic neurons causes dilatation of the pupil.

Although fishes have a direct tectocerebellar path, mammals have tectopontine fibers for the relay of visual impulses to the cerebellum via the pontine nuclei. Corticopontine fibers also arise in the primary and associative visual areas of the cerebral cortex in mammals (Brodal, 1972a,b).

Reciprocal connections between the habenulae and optic tectum occur, some fibers crossing in the habenular commissure.

These diverse connections strongly support the hypothesis that the optic tectum is a correlative center capable of initiating or modifying reflexive motor responses, and that the optic tectum and the dorsal thalamus have a similar origin from the same neuroectodermal plate.

Ascending tectal efferent fibers are important in reptiles, birds, and mammals. They are described with the thalamic visual centers in this chapter.

Pretectal area

The pretectal area is primordial in the lamprey and is located at the anterior end of the optic tectum. It is found throughout phylogeny and is well developed in birds, in whom four or more distinct nuclei can be differentiated (Kappers et al., 1936). In several species of lower placental mammals, eight distinct nuclei in the pretectal area can be identified (Scalia, 1972). The pretectal area is regarded by Ebbesson (1972) as one of the six constant diencephalic centers of the visual system in almost all vertebrates.

Homology of the pretectal area in different vertebrates is difficult to determine because the limits of the area are vague, and the term has been applied to several different groups of cells in the same general region of different species. The group of neurons usually designated as the pretectal area is anterior to and continuous with the middle gray layer of the optic tectum. In man, it is incorporated into the superior colliculus, but in some other primates and in many lower mammals it is sometimes regarded as part of the pulvinar of the thalamus. The pretectal area is sometimes confused with the dorsal nucleus of the posterior commissure.

Afferent fibers of the pretectal area are from the optic tract and the lateral geniculate body. The retinopretectal fibers in the mouse, rat, rabbit, and tree shrew are predominantly crossed, although a few fibers also terminate in the pretectal nuclei on the same side as the eye of origin (Scalia, 1972). Other afferent connections from the secondary visual cortex in the monkey have been described. The pretectal area has efferent connections with the optic tectum, lateral geniculate body, nucleus rotundus (pulvinar) of the thalamus, the Edinger-Westphal nucleus, and the tegmental reticular formation of the midbrain. Commissural fibers connect the pretectal areas of the two sides, and other fibers in the posterior commissure relay pretectal impulses to the opposite Edinger-Westphal nucleus. Pretectocerebellar and pretectobulbar fibers occur in fishes.

The pretectal area in man mediates the pupillary light reflex whereby light entering either eye causes ipsi- and contra-lateral (direct and consensual) pupillary constriction. The efferent fibers of the reflex are axons of the Edinger-Westphal nucleus. Occipitopretectal fibers in advanced primates may be important in the pathways mediating vertical eye movements and tracking.

Comparative anatomy of dorsal thalamus

The dorsal thalamus or simply "thalamus" is a large diencephalic structure receiving ascending fiber projections from many systems. It is distinguished from the smaller ventral thalamus that in man includes the subthalamic nucleus (of Luys) and zona incerta.

Within the central nervous system of amphioxus, an optic tectum, acousticolateral area, and olfactory bulbs are lacking. The tissue surrounding the probable homolog of the third ventricle at the rostral end of the neural tube consists of a few scattered neurons. Diencephalic structures cannot be distinguished. All basic sensory systems are present in even the lowest true vertebrates, however, and the optic tectum and dorsal thalamus are readily recognized in all vertebrates.

Four general types of cytoarchitecture are found in the diencephalon of vertebrates (Ebbesson et al., 1972): (A) Primitive periventricular aggregations of neurons are found in cyclostomes, urodelan amphibians, and in mammalian embryos; (B) Neurons migrate outward from the ventricular wall but are still arranged diffusely with minimal differentiation of cell groups, exemplified in the shark and hedgehog; (C) Many neuronal groups are highly differentiated into morphologically distinct nuclei. Not only are nuclei developed, but individual neurons are more highly specialized. This type of organization is characteristic of some teleosts, reptiles, birds, and mammals, including most primates; (D) The nuclei further differentiate or form laminae. Such polar arrangement is not only characteristic of the highest species, but also is found in many primitive mammals. An example is the lamination of the dorsal nucleus of the lateral geniculate body in the tree shrew and in man, but not in most other mammals.

The distinct morphologic pattern of thalamic nuclei in each class of vertebrates, and often between species, precludes the determination of homology from histologic sections of normal brain. The many descriptive names given to thalamic nuclei in different vertebrates are applicable only to particular species or orders because of the inconstancy of the appearance of thalamic nuclei in other species. One feature noted in comparative brain sections is that the caudal limit of the diencephalon is highly variable in submammalian vertebrates. Even in reptiles and birds, some thalamic nuclei, such as the nucleus rotundus, extend well into the midbrain and are clearly seen beneath the optic tectum in coronal sections.

Investigating afferent and efferent connections of thalamic neurons and nuclei is a more rewarding approach to the problem of determining homology, thus elucidating the evolution of the thalamus. Past techniques of study of fibers with degenerating myelin are not generally useful in the thalamus because sparse myelin is associated with the many thin fibers. The application of techniques of impregnation of degenerating axons does not require the presence of myelin. New concepts of thalamic organization have resulted.

Two questions are fundamental in understanding the organization of the thalamus and the phylogenetic development of that organization: (1) Which sensory system was the primary stimulus in the development of the thalamus? (2) What is the extent of overlap of afferent fiber systems upon neurons of the thalamus in primitive and in advanced vertebrates?

A traditional theory expounded by Herrick (1926, 1948) was that the diencephalon and telencephalon of submammalian vertebrates were dominated by olfactory input; the thalamus and forebrain evolved, particularly in mammals, by progressive increase in afferent connections from nonolfactory sensory systems: tactile, auditory, and visual. The restricted distribution of olfactory connections, once thought to be considerably more extensive, is discussed in Chapter 12. Olfactory projections to the dorsal thalamus are sparse or nonexistent, although secondary and tertiary connections have not been fully investigated. Recent studies reveal that the one system dominating the thalamus in all vertebrates by the quantity and distribution of its connections is not the olfactory, but the visual system. It is ironic that the thalamus was named the "optic thalamus" by Galen (Field and Harrison, 1957), but that the adjective was later omitted.

Visual centers in thalamus

The discovery of extensive thalamic participation in visual pathways in lower vertebrates as well as in mammals has only recently allowed the recognition of homology of many thalamic nuclei in different vertebrates. These homologous structures have been summarized by Ebbesson (1972), who also proposed a uniform nomenclature to replace the confusing array of names used in the older literature (Table 8-1). The information about homology of thalamic nuclei is still largely preliminary, however, and not nearly as well understood as are the nuclei of the medulla oblongata.

Table 8-1. Proposal for new nomenclature of thalamic nuclei of the visual system. The advantage of such a classification is in the identification of homologous nuclei by common names in all classes of vertebrates (Ebbesson, 1972).

	Dorsomedial optic nucleus	Dorsolateral optic nucleus	Ventrolateral optic nucleus	Ventromedial optic nucleus	Central optic nucleus
Elasmobranchs	Pretectal area	Lateral geniculate nucleus	Ventrolateral optic nucleus	Unknown	Lateral geniculate nucleus
Teleosts	Dorsomedial pretectal nucleus; dorsolateral thalamic nucleus	Uncertain	Uncertain	Ectomammillary nucleus; nucleus of the posterior accessory optic root	Nucleus rotundus; prethalamic nucleus
Amphibians	Pretectal area	Dorsal thalamus	Visual part of ventral thalamus	Ectomammillary nucleus	Visual part of dorsal thalamus
Reptiles	Posterodorsal nucleus	Dorsolateral geniculate nucleus	Ventral geniculate nucleus	Ectomammillary nucleus	Nucleus rotundus
Birds	Uncertain	Dorsolateral anterior complex	Ventral geniculate nucleus	Ectomammillary nucleus	Nucleus rotundus
Mammals	Pretectal area; posterior pretectal nucleus; olivary pretectal nucleus	Dorsal nucleus of lateral geniculate body	Ventral nucleus of the lateral geniculate body; pregeniculate nucleus	Medial terminal nucleus of basal optic root	Pulvinar; posterior lateral thalamic nucleus

In addition to the importance of the lateral geniculate body in relaying optic impulses to the visual cortex in man and other mammals, this thalamic structure is also well developed in many lower vertebrates lacking a neocortex typical of mammals. The primordium of the lateral geniculate body is found even in the lamprey. It persists, although small, in blind species of fishes (Charlton, 1933; Shanklin, 1935). In many teleosts, a thalamic structure similar to the lateral geniculate body and receiving optic fibers is well developed and even laminated.

The well-developed lateral geniculate body of some lower vertebrates is probably not entirely homologous, however, with the structure in man.

In most vertebrates, the lateral geniculate body consists of ventral and dorsal nuclei. The ventral nucleus is a synaptic center between the optic tectum and the tegmentum of the midbrain, but also receives fibers from the optic tract. This is the nucleus that is so well developed in teleosts. In the phylogenetic series of mammals, the ventral nucleus is large in rodents (Zeman and Innes, 1963) but becomes progressively smaller, and only a few neurons remain in man (LeGros Clark, 1932), as the pregeniculate nucleus. The tectogeniculate pathway is called the brachium tecti and is prominent in teleosts (Shanklin, 1935). The brachium of the superior colliculus persists in man but is mainly an afferent pathway to the optic tectum, rather than efferent. Reciprocal geniculotectal fibers also occur.

The dorsal nucleus of the lateral geniculate body is largest in mammals. It is less well developed but also distinct in reptiles and is probably present throughout phylogeny. Ascending fibers from the dorsal nucleus are found even in elasmobranchs (Ebbesson et al., 1972). Fibers of the optic tract in the monkey synapse with neurons of the dorsal nucleus with a 1 : 1 ratio (Chow et al., 1950). Six laminae of neurons are separated by terminal fibers of the optic tract. Fibers from the ipsilateral eye synapse with neurons in layers 2, 3, and 5; those from the opposite eye end in layers 1, 4, and 6 in monkey and in man. The fibers have a retinotopic distribution. Lamination of the dorsal nucleus of the lateral geniculate body is characteristic in primates, carnivores, and ungulates. This structural feature is not found in all mammals, however, nor in lower vertebrates.

Efferent fibers of the dorsal nucleus of the lateral geniculate body form the optic radiation or geniculocalcarine tract to the primary visual area of neocortex in mammals. Geniculate connections with the forebrain are lacking in teleosts, but anuran amphibians have a few fibers from the posterior part of the lateral geniculate body (the part homologous with the dorsal nucleus of higher vertebrates) to the lateral wall of the cerebral hemisphere (Herrick, 1925).

The lateral geniculate body is large in reptiles and in lower mammals. In reptiles, the ventral nucleus extends the length of the diencephalon. In the opossum, the dorsal nucleus predominates, and forms almost the entire lateral wall of the thalamus. The lateral geniculate body has reciprocal connections with surrounding thalamic nuclei in all mammals, particularly with the overlying pulvinar. This nucleus of

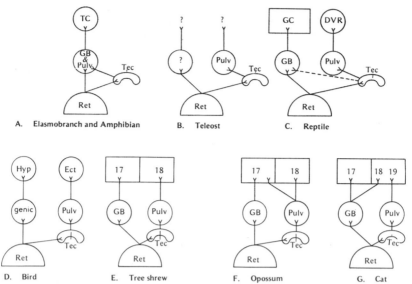

Figure 8-4   Schematic representation of variations in visual pathways among vertebrates, based on studies using Nauta's technique. (A) The shark has a single thalamic
center of the visual system (GB and Pulv) to which both retinal (Ret) and tectal (Tec)
fibers project. This thalamic nucleus discharges to one nonlaminated telencephalic
center (TC). The arrangement in amphibians is similar, although the thalamotelen-
cephalic projection is not well understood. (B) Teleosts have direct retinal connections to a thalamic center different from the center in which tectal fibers terminate
(Pulv). Further ascending pathways to the telencephalon are unknown. (C) Reptiles
have a well-developed geniculate body (GB) of the thalamus that receives retinal and
sparse tectal fibers and projects to the laminated general cortex (GC) of the telencephalon. A second visual pathway ascends from tectum to nucleus rotundus or
pulvinar (Pulv), then to a nonlaminated telencephalic structure of the dorsal ventricular ridge (DVR). (D) Birds have the greatest separation of two ascending visual
systems, terminating in hyperstriatum (Hyp) and ectostriatum (Ect). Both of the latter
structures are of telencephalic origin and are probably homologous with mammalian
neocortex. (E) The tree shrew has the greatest separation of visual systems among
mammals, with no overlap in neocortex. (F) The opossum has two ascending visual
systems with overlap in area 17. (G) The cat has an arrangement similar to the
opossum but with overlap in areas 18 and 19. Area 17 is the primary visual or calcarine cortex, and areas 18 and 19 are associative visual cortex. The extent of the
secondary ascending visual system in man is unknown. (Modified from Ebbesson,
1972).

the posterior part of the thalamus is present in carnivores and ungulates,
but it is well developed only in primates. The nucleus rotundus of submammalian vertebrates is the homologous counterpart of at least part of
the mammalian pulvinar.

In addition to descending projections from the tectum, ascending fibers are prominent in reptiles, birds, and mammals and indeed occur in all vertebrates. Tectogeniculate fibers terminate in both ventral and dorsal nuclei of the lateral geniculate body. The dorsal nucleus projects to the general cortex or primordial neocortex of amphibians and reptiles, and to the calcarine or primary visual cortex of mammals. Such ascending geniculotelencephalic projections have been found even in elasmobranchs (Ebbesson and Schroeder, 1971; Ebbesson et al., 1972).

A second ascending pathway from the optic tectum also occurs in reptiles, birds, and mammals. The diencephalic center of this pathway is the nucleus rotundus, the largest of the reptilian and avian thalamic nuclei and represented in mammals by the portion of the pulvinar receiving only tectal fibers. The nucleus rotundus projects to the telencephalon in turtles (Hall and Ebner, 1969), and to the ectostriatal part of the telencephalon in the pigeon (Karten and Hodos, 1970). Unlike the lateral geniculate body, the nucleus rotundus (pulvinar) does not receive direct retinal fibers of the optic tract. In contrast to the tecto-geniculo-cortical pathway that terminates in the primary visual cortex, the tecto-pulvino-cortical pathway in lower mammals projects to the nonstriate secondary visual neocortex. The two ascending systems partly overlap in some mammals but are separate in the tree shrew (Ebbesson, 1972), although intracortical connections may relate the primary and secondary visual neocortical areas (Diamond et al., 1970). The ascending visual pathways in vertebrates are schematically illustrated in Figure 8-4.

In advanced mammals, the pulvinar receives some tectal fibers as well as short connections from the lateral geniculate body. Fibers ascend from the pulvinar to the secondary visual areas of the occipital lobe in the monkey (LeGros Clark and Northfield, 1937; Truex and Carpenter, 1970). A pulvino-occipital pathway in the cat was suggested also by Talbot (1942). The extent of the secondary ascending visual system in man is uncertain.

It has been postulated that the nucleus rotundus is a remnant of a phylogenetically old thalamic nucleus receiving only tectal fibers, and that the dorsal nucleus of the lateral geniculate body differentiated from it in response to the acquisition of direct retinal input (Snyder and Diamond, 1968; Diamond and Hall, 1969). Ebbesson (1972), however, suggested that the demonstration of direct optic nerve projections to the thalamus in even lower vertebrates indicates that these structures evolved simultaneously rather than sequentially.

Visual centers in telencephalon

The traditional concept that the optic tectum is the principal visual center in submammalian vertebrates, and that its function shifts to the telencephalon (i.e. cerebral cortex) in mammals, is based on the observation that most optic nerve fibers terminate in the tectum of submammalian vertebrates and in the lateral geniculate body of the thalamus in mammals. Cephalization of vision in phylogeny is further suggested by the large size of the optic tectum associated with a relatively small forebrain in lower vertebrates, and the great development of the mammalian cerebral cortex.

This concept of cephalization of visual function may not be entirely correct, however. Extensive tecto-thalamic fiber connections in lower vertebrates are now well documented, and thalamo-telencephalic projections in the visual system also are being discovered in such "primitive" vertebrates as the shark (Ebbesson and Schroeder, 1971). The emerging anatomic evidence of a telencephalic visual center is further supported by behavioral studies demonstrating that sharks are capable of discriminating black from white, and horizontal from vertical stripes, even after bilateral removal of the optic tectum (Graeber and Ebbesson, 1972; Graeber et al., 1973). These data suggest that vision is a telencephalic function that evolved early in at least some lower vertebrates, as well as in mammals, and that if cephalization of vision occurred as an evolutionary change, it did so long before the first primitive mammal appeared on Earth. Sharks evolved almost 200 million years before even the first teleostean fishes, and they have changed little since the Jurassic period (Romer, 1970).

Complete tectal ablation causes permanent blindness in teleosts (Dijkgraaf, 1949; Iwai et al., 1970). These advanced, highly specialized fishes have changed greatly from their early ancestor, in contrast to sharks. Elasmobranchs are not ancestral to teleosts (Chapter 1). One explanation of the difference in the effects of tectal lesions in sharks and teleosts is that the primitive visual system included a telencephalic region as its highest center, and that teleosts departed from this arrangement by developing the tectum as a highly specialized visual structure that incorporated the telencephalic visual functions of other vertebrates. The optic tectum is relatively larger in teleosts than in any other vertebrates. Further anatomic study of telencephalic visual pathways in teleosts, and examination of the visual system of the more primitive, living holos-tean fishes of the same line of evolution that led to teleosts (Chapter 1), will corroborate or deny this theory.

Insufficient evidence is yet available for conclusions regarding visual function in the telencephalon of amphibians and reptiles. The impor-tance of secondary visual pathways through the pulvinar to the neocor-tex of mammals, and perhaps even of man, is not fully known. The optic tectum did not atrophy or disappear with the evolution of higher visual centers in the telencephalon of advanced vertebrates. This fact suggests that these ascending pathways have a specific and probably unique func-tion in the visual system of mammals. In the tree shrew, tectal lesions result in inattention to visual stimuli and impairment of visual identifica-tion of objects (Jane et al., 1972). The cerebral cortex, in contrast, was thought to inhibit incorrect responses to the total visual information re-ceived (Jane et al., 1972). In man, however, inattention or neglect, and visual agnosia are associated with lesions of the neocortical parietal lobe.

A neocortical region for vision is clearly differentiated in the occipital lobe of mammals. In monotremes, the visual neocortex overlaps other regions related to hearing and tactile senses (Chapter 12). The primary visual cortex is relatively isolated from other sensory systems in pla-cental mammals. It lies along the calcarine fissure in the medial wall of the cerebral hemisphere.

In reptiles, and especially in birds, direct retinal projections to the dorsal nucleus of the lateral geniculate body (dorsolateral anterior nu-cleus) occur, in addition to the tectothalamic pathways. Secondary fibers enter the lateral forebrain bundle to be distributed topographically in a dorsal part of the telencephalon in birds, the wulst (Karten and Nauta, 1968; Karten, 1969). This laminated structure, similar to the primary visual neocortex of mammals, is part of the avian hyperstriatum and accessory hyperstriatum. Birds lack neocortex, but the highly differen-tiated, unique structures of the corpus striatum probably incorporate the reptilian primordium of the neocortex and function similarly (Chapter 12). Fibers ending in the wulst synapse with a band of granular cells resembling those in lamina IV of the mammalian visual cortex (Karten, 1969). The highest visual centers in birds thus are in the telencephalon, similar to the condition in mammals. Elasmobranchs and some other lower vertebrates also may have a telencephalic visual system more similar to that of man than was previously recognized.

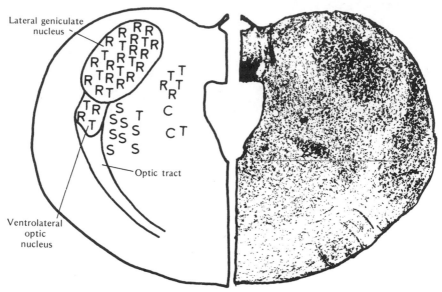

Figure 8-5 Coronal section of forebrain of shark. Overlap of projections from retina (R) and optic tectum (T) occur in the lateral geniculate and ventrolateral optic nuclei. Fibers from spinal cord (S) and cerebellum (C) also ascend to thalamus. The intimate relations of retinal and tectal fibers terminating in common thalamic nuclei supports the concept of a common phylogenetic origin of all neural components of the visual system (Fig. 8-1). Right hemisection stained with cresyl violet. (Ebbesson et al., 1972).

Convergence of sensory pathways in thalamus

Convergence or overlap of thalamic projections to the neocortex occurs to a greater extent in lower mammals than in advanced species (Lende, 1969; Chapter 12). A question raised by this observation is whether afferent projections of sensory systems to the thalamus also overlap to a greater extent in lower than in higher mammals, and whether the isolation of sensory systems within the dorsal thalamus precedes the relative confinement of these systems to restricted regions of neocortex.

Rockel et al. (1972) investigated sensory projections to the thalamus of the phalanger, a marsupial mammal. They found that the overlap between various afferent pathways was no greater in this marsupial than in the cat or monkey. Despite the presence of common sensory and motor regions of the cerebral cortex, the overlap between somatic sensory and cerebellar pathways in the ventral nuclei of the thalamus is probably less in the marsupial phalanger than in higher mammals. Somatic and auditory projections also overlap, but not more extensively than in other mammals (Rockel et al., 1972). Ebbesson et al. (1972) found a broad area of overlap between projections of the dorsal column and trigeminal nuclei and those of the inferior colliculus, in the thalamus of the hedgehog (Fig. 5-2). It should not be surprising that the tactile and auditory

Figure 8-6   Coronal section of diencephalon of the amphibian *Amblystoma*. Fibers from retina (R) and optic tectum (T) overlap extensively in dorsal thalamus and ventral thalamus. Right hemisection stained with cresyl violet. (Ebbesson et al., 1972).

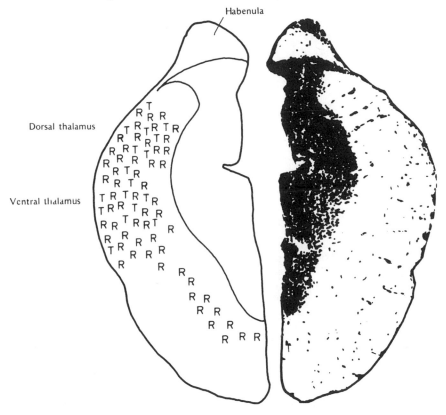

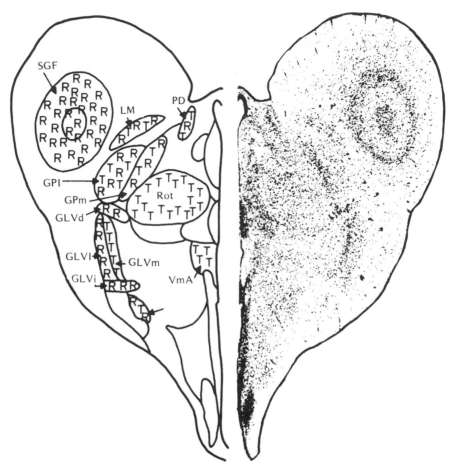

Figure 8-7   Coronal section of brain of lizard at junction of mesencephalon and diencephalon. Specialized thalamic nuclei of the optic system receive either retinal (R) or
tectal (T) projections, although some overlap of projections persists in other thalamic
nuclei. Ventrolateral geniculate nucleus is divided into several parts: dorsal (GLVd),
intermediate (GLVi), lateral (GLVl), medial (GLVm), and ventral (GLVv). Mesencephalic lentiform nucleus (LM), posterodorsal nucleus (PD); nucleus rotundus or pulvinar
(Rot), stratum griseum et fibrosum superficiale of optic tectum (SGF); ventromedial
anterior nucleus (VmA). Right hemisection stained with cresyl violet. (Ebbesson et al.,
1972).

systems overlap in the thalamus: perception of sound is a refinement of
tactile vibratory sense, and the auditory nerve is derived from branchial
nerves (Chapter 5).

The phalanger may not be representative of lower mammals, however, and is certainly not ancestral to primates or to any placental mammal. If the findings of Rockel et al. (1972) are corroborated in lower placental mammals, particularly lower primates, these data would invalidate the theory of Herrick (1929, 1948). His theory is based on the premise that the thalamic nuclei of higher vertebrates differentiate from a single multimodal thalamic nucleus in lower species, the neurons of which receive convergent innervation from all sensory systems. Studies of the responsiveness of single neurons in the thalamus of the hedgehog to multimodal sensory stimulation indicate that sensory impulses from several sources indeed do converge upon individual thalamic neurons in this unspecialized mammal (Erickson et al., 1972). This finding suggests that the specificity characteristic of higher mammals is a result of evolution of thalamic nuclei from a nonspecialized diencephalic mass of gray matter, as originally proposed by Herrick.

Figure 8-8   Coronal section of diencephalon of hedgehog, a lower placental mammal. Very few retinal (R) and optic tectal (T) projections overlap in their thalamic terminations. Ventrolateral nucleus receiving cerebellar projections (C). Right hemisection stained with cresyl violet. (Ebbesson et al., 1972).

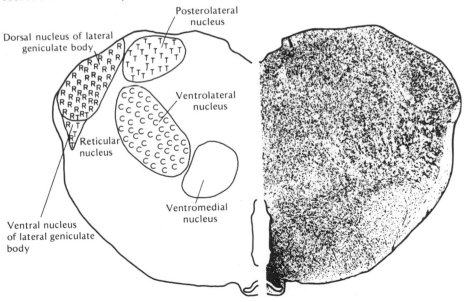

The phalanger is an animal with good vision. Lack of overlap of the visual and other sensory systems in the thalamus of the hedgehog and opossum, mammals with poor vision, was also demonstrated, however (Campbell et al., 1967).

Ebbesson et al. (1972) found that visual projections dominated the thalamus of all classes of vertebrates and that considerable overlap often occurred between projections from the optic tectum and from the retina, but not between the visual and other sensory systems (Figs. 8-5 to 8-8). The extent of convergence of sensory fibers to the thalamus of submammalian vertebrates correlated more with the extent of specialization of individual species than with the hypothetic evolutionary position of those species on the phylogenetic scale. In sharks, almost the entire thalamus is thus dominated by extensive projections from the optic tectum, but only a small amount of overlap with retinal afferents occurs anteriorly, and with spinal afferents posteriorly. Amphibians, both urodelan and anuran, have almost complete overlap of tectal and retinal projections throughout the thalamus, but spinal and medullary projections are limited to a caudal thalamic zone and do not overlap with thalamic regions of the visual system (Ebbesson et al., 1972).

Nonvisual centers of thalamus

Projections to the dorsal thalamus from systems other than the visual are relatively sparse in lower vertebrates. These other afferent fibers increase so greatly in mammals that the visual areas of the mammalian thalamus are relatively small in contrast to the expansion of nuclei concerned with other functions. The additional afferent systems of greatest importance are the auditory, cerebellar, tactile, and proprioceptive.

The medial geniculate body is a thalamic nucleus well differentiated only in mammals, although the primordium is found in lower vertebrates (Chapter 5). It receives auditory impulses from the inferior colliculus and discharges to a circumscribed neocortical region associated with audition. The projection of vestibular fibers in these pathways in mammals is uncertain.

A few fibers from the cerebellum terminate in the dorsal thalamus of all vertebrates, including such phylogenetically old species as the shark (Ebbesson et al., 1972). These fibers end diffusely in the poorly differentiated medial zone of the thalamus, but it is not certain if this area in elasmobranchs is homologous with the intralaminar nuclei or with the ventrolateral nucleus of the mammalian thalamus. Both receive cerebellar projections (from the dentate and other cerebellar nuclei) in mammals, although most terminate in the ventrolateral nucleus after decussating in the midbrain. The ventrolateral and ventro-anterior nuclei also receive the thalamic fasciculus from the globus pallidus in mammals, thus providing an anatomic region for the integration of cerebellar and striatal influence on muscle tone and posture. Efferent fibers ascend to the motor cortex. The red nucleus is another location where cerebellar and pallidal impulses are integrated, but in mammals, most rubral efferent fibers project rostrally to the ventrolateral thalamic nucleus, in contrast to the predominantly descending rubral pathway in lower vertebrates (Chapter 6). The red nucleus, at least the phylogenetically new parvocellular portion, thus becomes functionally incorporated into the ventrolateral thalamic nucleus, although the red nucleus retains its anatomic location in the midbrain. The connections of the basal ganglia are discussed in Chapter 12.

A few scattered fibers from the spinal cord overlap with the cerebellar projections in the thalamus of the shark (Ebbesson et al., 1972). Ascending fibers originating in the spinal cord of the frog were traced only as far rostrally as the tegmentum of the midbrain (Ebbesson, 1969), but projections from that region to the telencephalon were found by Vesselkin et al. (1971). This poorly differentiated area in anuran amphibians is probably the primordium of the ventroposterior nuclear complex of mammals, the large terminal for fibers of the medial lemniscus, spinothalamic, and secondary ascending trigeminal tracts. Because of its extreme caudal location in amphibians and reptiles, this somatic sensory nucleus may not originally have been part of the diencephalon, but was secondarily incorporated into the visual thalamus, similar to the incorporation of somatic sensory projections into the optic tectum, and perhaps even analogous to the functional incorporation of the red nucleus into the ventrolateral thalamic nucleus of mammals. This condition in amphibians is also accompanied by a more caudal extension of the visual thalamus into the midbrain than is found in mammals.

In frogs, a system of ascending fibers in the dorsal columns of the spinal cord, composed of processes of neurons of the dorsal root ganglia, project to the cerebellum (Chapter 6). Similar fibers ascend ipsilaterally in the dorsal columns of the spinal cord and terminate in clusters of neurons at the caudal end of the medulla in reptiles, birds, and mammals. These neurons comprise the somatotopically arranged gracile and cuneate nuclei. Neurons of these nuclei have processes that decussate and ascend in the brainstem as the medial lemniscus, a large fiber bundle in mammals. The ascending fascicles are accompanied by fibers of the spinothalamic and secondary ascending trigeminal tracts, but the fibers of these two tracts do not mix. The termination of the fibers in reptiles and birds is incompletely known, but in mammals, they end in the large ventroposterior nuclei of the thalamus. The dorsal columns of the spinal cord and medial lemniscus are reduced in size in snakes, compared with other reptiles, probably associated with lack of limbs. They are small also in birds, perhaps reflecting the decreased sensory function of the skin when feathers are present. Fibers from receptors in hair follicles form a particularly large proportion of the dorsal columns in mammals (Norton, 1969), although proprioception is also an important function carried in the dorsal columns (Calne and Pallis, 1966).

Several other thalamic nuclei are distinct in mammals, but have not been identified in other vertebrates. These include the anterior nucleus, having connections with the mammillary body, cingulate gyrus, habenula, and hippocampus; the dorsomedial nucleus, having connections with the basal ganglia and with other thalamic nuclei. The midline and intralaminar thalamic nuclei are associated with the reticular formation and are discussed in Chapter 11.

Some efferent thalamic fibers descend in all vertebrates. They project to many centers of the brainstem, but are even less completely understood than are the ascending connections. The known projections are discussed in association with the specific systems involved. Thalamic fibers ascend to telencephalic centers in even the lowest vertebrates, but in mammals, these efferent connections of the thalamus are massive, associated with the great proliferation of the cerebral cortex.

Evolution of mechanisms of vision

The visual system of lower vertebrates, such as the frog, is organized for recognition of a few stereotyped patterns. Discrimination of food is determined by size and movement. The frog will starve to death if surrounded by food that is not moving; conversely, it will attempt to eat any small, dangling, or moving object. Stationary details of the environment are ignored by the frog and perhaps are not even "seen" as we understand vision. This phenomenon may be related, in part, to the lack of a macula or fovea in the retina of the frog. Escape from enemies is accomplished by simply leaping toward the darkest part of the visual field. Most aspects of life are governed by other senses in the frog.

The brain of the frog may be activated by four patterns of visual images (Lettvin et al., 1959). These patterns are sharp edges with contrast, the curved edge of a dark object, the movement of edges, and focal or general dimmings produced by movement or rapid darkening within the total visual field. The frog responds best to intermittent movement of the convex edge of a small dark object. The object is remembered when it stops moving, but the memory is abolished if obscured momentarily by a shadow or if attention is distracted by another moving stimulus. The response is not affected by movement in the background or gradual changes in the background illumination. The arrangement is ideal for the detection of insects while the wind gently blows the surrounding grass and flowers.

A separate group of fibers in the optic nerve deals with each of the four patterns detected by the frog. These fibers are mixed within the optic nerve. The retinal field is projected as four separate layers of nerve endings in the optic tectum, and each layer corresponds to one of the four basic patterns (Lettvin et al., 1959). These layers of synapses are probably all within the intermediate gray and white layer of the optic tectum.

The severed optic nerve of the frog regenerates (Sperry, 1944, 1951), unlike the result of a similar lesion in higher vertebrates. This regeneration does not occur randomly. The fibers reconstitute the original retinographic projections, then terminate in the proper location in the optic tectum to re-establish the original organization of the visual system (Lettvin et al., 1959). The amphibian retina becomes irreversibly polarized early in ontogenetic development, however, so that experimental rotation of the eye does not change the original retinotopic projections upon the optic tectum (Stone 1960; Edds, 1967). The optic nerve of the goldfish has a similar capacity to re-establish retinotopic innervation in the rostral half of the optic tectum when the caudal half of the tectum is ablated (Yoon, 1972).

The arrangement of the neocortex serving vision in mammals differs somewhat from that of the optic tectum (superior colliculus) of either mammals or lower species. Mechanisms of visual perception in the dorsal nucleus of the lateral geniculate body and calcarine cortex, however, are reminiscent of the less complex condition in the optic tectum

of the frog. The visual mechanisms in the cat and monkey were elucidated by Hubel and Wiesel (1959, 1962, 1963, 1968). Both mammalian
species were similar, although the monkey had greater precision. The
mechanism of vision in man is probably similar.

Individual neurons of the calcarine cortex specifically respond to
stimulation by white light in restricted areas of the retina. The most
effective stimuli are edges or linear borders separating areas of different
brightness, slits or narrow rectangles of light, and dark bars against a
light background. Specific excitation by small convex edges as occurs in
the frog was not found. Single cortical neurons respond maximally
when an appropriate stimulus moves across the receptive field, but the
linear stimulus must be in a specific orientation. The shape and axis of
the stimulus are critical and constant for the activation of a particular
neuron of the cortex but differ for other cortical neurons. The axis may
be oriented in the vertical, horizontal, or oblique plane. Inhibitory as
well as excitatory fields are adjacent to each other and also are oriented
in the perpendicular axis, as with a polarizing effect. Summation occurs
within either excitatory or inhibitory fields, simultaneous illumination
of the antagonistic fields results in mutual cancellation of effects. Illumination of the entire receptive field with diffuse light causes little or
no response.

The calcarine cortex of mammals is subdivided into discrete regions
or columns extending from the surface of the brain to the subcortical
white matter. All neurons within each column respond to stimuli in the
same axis within the retinal receptive field. Some cortical columns are
round or oval in cross-section, but most are elongated and narrow. The
diameter is about 0.5 mm in the cat and is smaller in the monkey. In
some parts of the calcarine cortex, the columns are arranged in a regular manner, with a progressive gradual shift in the orientation of the
columns. In other regions of the cortex, however, adjacent columns are
randomly oriented with respect to one another. The smallest receptive
fields are near the fovea centralis; the fields tend to be larger in the
periphery of the retina.

Within each cortical column are the projections of several simple
receptive fields, as described, and also of more complex fields in which
the response to a stimulus cannot be predicted from the arrangement of
excitatory and inhibitory regions. Neurons of the more complex fields
tend to be in laminae II, III, V, VI and are binocularly activated in the
monkey; cells of the simple receptive fields are generally deep in layer

III and layers IV-A and IV-B (Hubel and Wiesel, 1968). About 80 per cent of all neurons of the calcarine cortex of the cat are influenced independently by the two eyes. In binocularly influenced neurons, the two receptive fields have the same orientation of axis and are situated in corresponding parts of both retinas are stimulated simultaneously (Hubel and Wiesel, 1962).

The superior colliculus of mammals has an organization similar in some respects to that of the calcarine cortex; vertical columns of neurons have specific axes of orientation (Michael, 1972 a,b). Different types of visual impairment result from lesions of the superior colliculus and of the cerebral cortex in the tree shrew, however (Jane et al., 1972).

Comparisons between the visual system as a biological pattern analyzer and similar man-made computer systems are discussed by Barlow et al. (1972).

Little is known about mechanisms of vision in birds. Many, particularly the birds of prey, have extremely sharp visual acuity. They probably perceive images as do mammals, rather than the limited number of specific patterns to which the frog responds.

Vision is particularly important to maintain proper orientation in flight. Between the world wars, the U.S. Army Air Corps became interested in the problem of spatial disorientation of pilots flying in clouds. Pilots were blindfolded and then required to walk, drive a car, or steer a boat in a straight line. In every case, the resulting path was a progressively tighter spiral. A similar series of experiments was then conducted with birds by releasing blindfolded pigeons from an airplane and observing the descent. The pigeons without exception demonstrated lack of control of flight, poor coordination, stalls, and spiral dives. Finally, holding the wings at a high dihedral angle, they descended to the ground in the same manner as a parachute (Ocker and Crane, quoted by Blodget, 1972). In birds, as in man, the visual system predominates over the vestibular as the primary mechanism of spatial orientation, although all animals are capable of adapting to blindness by greater reliance upon vestibular, auditory, and proprioceptive cues.

Stereoscopic vision

Almost all animals, including most mammals, have laterally directed eyes on the sides of the head. This arrangement allows panoramic vision but little or no overlap of the visual field of each eye. All primates, from the tarsier and lemur through man, have eyes directed forward, with overlap of all but the most lateral parts of the visual field. The overlap is associated with the partial decussation of the optic nerves in the chiasm, each side of the brain thus subserving one side of the composite visual field.

Even in lower vertebrates such as fishes, the small medial part of the visual field that overlaps anteriorly is associated with an analogous convergence of fibers in the midline of the optic tectum (Fig. 8-2). Cajal (1909-1911) indicated the need for crossed optic nerves in animals with panoramic vision, to maintain logical continuity of images from the two eyes (Fig. 8-3).

Stereoscopic vision is the fusion of images seen at a slightly different angle with each eye, to allow perception of depth. The overlap of the visual fields of primates and, to a lesser extent, of cats and some other mammals, allows stereoscopic vision. Depth perception in man is effective only for objects up to a few feet away, however, because at greater distances the difference in visual angle between the two eyes becomes insignificant. Depth beyond a few feet is therefore estimated by relative difference in size of objects and is based on visual experience.

It is uncertain if the second macula of birds, or even if the single macula of birds such as the owl, with eyes directed forward, results in stereoscopic vision. Overlap of visual fields and fusion certainly occur, but it is not yet proved that the optic tectum or visual hyperstriatum of birds can fuse the two images stereoscopically as the neocortex does in mammals. Many lizards move each eye independently of the other, or converge to focus both eyes simultaneously on the same object. Different neural pathways are needed, however, for panoramic and stereoscopic vision (Fig. 8-3).

Visual tracking and cerebral control of gaze

Mechanisms of tracking developed with the evolution of special receptors of distant information. Of these receptors, vision had distinct superiority over olfaction or chemical sensory systems. One advantage was that topographic projection of a receptive field allowed more precise localization than merely the general direction of a target, as ascertained by olfaction. This spatial localization allowed future movement of a target to be predicted from the pattern of past movement. Another advantage of vision over olfaction was that a greater number of targets could be recorded at the same time. Scanning was possible. Many objects could be seen that either were odorless or could not be detected by olfaction because of unfavorable water currents. Dispersion of light rays also was much less than the diffusion of chemical particles in water. Perhaps the greatest advantage of vision, however, was the negligible latent period for light to reach the eye even at great distances, contrasted with the long interval before an odor reached the olfactory epithelium. The rapid detection of targets was advantageous to both predator and the evading prey.

Mammals track objects by visual fixation and movement of the eyes to center images in the visual field. Because a macula does not differentiate in the retina of amphibians or of many other vertebrates, the periphery of the retina in these animals has the same visual acuity as the center (Polyak, 1957). Tracking in these creatures is therefore a form of scanning, accomplished by following the movement of an object across the entire visual field, without shifting the eyes. Compensatory movements of the eye occur in response to changes in position of the body of the animal, such as with a frog sitting on a rotating water lily. The eyes and retinal images are thus actively stabilized by both vestibular and visual reflexes.

The anatomic basis of ocular movements in man and other primates was reviewed by Carpenter (1971). Conjugate gaze is subserved by a frontal and occipital "eye field" in each hemisphere. The frontal eye field lies rostral to the primary motor strip, near the area for the face, but is not characterized histologically by a single cytoarchitectonic pattern. It is divided into upper and lower portions, each arranged as the reverse of the other (Crosby, 1953; Lemmen et al., 1959). The frontal eye field is a center of lateral gaze, mediating voluntary eye movements to the contralateral side. It is not dependent upon vision and actually inhibits visual fixation momentarily to allow the eyes to shift and refixate.

An occipital center for conjugate eye movements in the horizontal plane is not as localized as in the frontal lobe. The occipital eye field also differs anatomically from the frontal in having the two sides connected by fibers passing through the corpus callosum (Carpenter, 1971). Electric stimulation of a wide region of occipital lobe results in deviation of the eyes away from the stimulated side; the lowest threshold for this response in the monkey is found in the cortex bordering the calcarine fissure (Walker and Weaver, 1940), although the threshold for excitation is higher in the occipital than in the frontal lobe. One explanation of the ocular responses from the occipital lobe is that the animal tested is merely trying to look at a visual phenomenon produced by electric stimulation. The occipital eye field, however, may be concerned with visual fixation upon stationary or moving objects within the visual field, and with the tracking of these objects.

The presence of specific centers in the cerebral cortex for eye movements has also been denied and ocular motor function stated to be widely distributed over the cortex (Pasik and Pasik, 1964). Experimentally in monkeys, conjugate deviation of the eyes to the opposite side is elicited by electric stimulation of almost any part of the lateral hemisphere, and even of the corpus striatum (Wagman, 1964; Mettler, 1964). Clinically, focal epileptic phenomena limited to one hemisphere may be expressed, in part, by forced conjugate deviation of the eyes to the opposite side, even though the epileptic focus is not in the eye fields. Conversely, destructive lesions in monkeys or in man, as with infarcts in the distribution of the middle cerebral artery, often initially cause conjugate deviation of the eyes to the same side. Some compensation occurs later in most patients. The study of ocular movements in a patient 11 years after hemispherectomy, revealed deficiency of voluntary gaze to the side of the remaining hemisphere (Troost et al., 1972a) and deficiency of tracking to the opposite side (Troost et al., 1972b).

Our understanding of localization and somatotopic organization of other nonassociative functions in the cerebral cortex of man and other advanced mammals suggests that localization of voluntary ocular movements is likely. Associative fibers connect most areas of neocortex with each other, hence it is not surprising that artificial stimulation of almost any area of the hemisphere may be conducted to an "eye field" as well as to other areas. Ocular movements are more easily and consistently elicited from the region of the frontal eye field than elsewhere, however (Wagman, 1964). If diffuse, epileptic discharges may involve the eye field; foci of epileptic activity do not elicit ocular movements until the frontal eye field is involved by progressive spread of the epileptic focus.

Although oculomotor function may not be as limited to circumscribed cortical areas as once thought, the concept of a frontal eye field is probably more correct than the view that this function totally lacks focal organization in the neocortex. If this concept of eye fields is valid, the occipital eye field related to tracking is phylogenetically older and develops earlier embryologically than the frontal eye field subserving voluntary gaze. Perhaps this aspect explains why children learning to read often prefer to underline words with their finger; a child finds it easier to track the movement of the finger along the line of words than to move his eyes voluntarily along the line. Cerebral infarcts involving the frontal eye fields in man result in disorders of voluntary lateral gaze, and a similar mechanism has been postulated to explain the clinical features of congenital ocular motor apraxia (Altrocchi and Menkes, 1960). The absence of tracking in newborn infants is probably related to their inability to fixate visually.

The problem of vertical eye movements is more complex than that of horizontal eye movements because vertical eye movements require the balanced coordinated contraction of at least two ocular muscles. In addition, vertical movements have not been elicited as consistently from the frontal lobe in primates as have horizontal movements. Upward movement of the eyes occurs after stimulation of the inferior lip of the calcarine fissure, and downward movement with stimulation of the superior lip. This distribution corresponds to the somatotopic projection of the visual fields upon the calcarine cortex. It is difficult to be certain that the monkeys in this experiment were not simply looking toward visual stimuli produced in the primary visual areas.

The cortical eye fields initiate balanced contraction of the individual muscles of each eye. This phenomenon is similar to the coordinated contraction of several muscles in voluntary movements of the extremities. The participation of the cerebellum in ocular movements is uncertain. The eye fields differ from most motor areas of the cortex, however, in producing conjugate movements, simultaneously involving different muscles in the two eyes.

Submammalian vertebrates with well-developed foveas are also capable of visually tracking moving objects, but lack the neocortical centers of man. Whether this function emanates from the optic tectum, thalamus, or telencephalon of these animals is not fully known. The interstitial nucleus (of Cajal) and the nucleus of Darkschewitsch may also be important in the mediation of vertical eye movement (Carpenter, 1971).

Visual tracking may also be initiated and mediated by subcortical structures, even in mammals. Jane et al. (1972) demonstrated that in the tree shrew, one type of visual attention and possibly identification are tectal functions, the cortex acting in response to received visual information to inhibit inappropriate responses. Casagrande et al. (1972) found a difference in visual responses after lesions of the superficial and of the deep layers of the optic tectum in the tree shrew. Superficial lesions produced deficits in discrimination of form; deeper lesions produced an additional inability to track. In mammals, and especially man, the superior colliculus receives many projections from the area corresponding to the frontal eye fields (Kuypers and Lawrence, 1967), but most corticotectal fibers arise in the occipital lobe (Altman, 1962; Garey et al., 1968).

Parinaud's syndrome in man is paralysis of gaze above the horizontal plane. It usually occurs in patients with tumors of the pineal. Because the pineal lies anterior to and above the superior colliculus in man, the mechanism of palsy of upward gaze has been attributed to pressure on the superior colliculus, particularly involving the afferent corticotectal fibers concerned with tracking eye movements, and of tecto-oculomotor fibers (Crosby et al., 1962). Ablation of the superior colliculus in the monkey fails to alter eye movements, however (Pasik and Pasik, 1964). It is probable that occipitopretectal or occipitotegmental fibers not entering the superior colliculus mediate vertical eye movements, as with a similar path for lateral gaze. Lesions of the superior colliculus similarly failed to alter the blink reflex in response to sudden bright light, and did not induce spontaneous nystagmus or interfere with optokinetic nystagmus in the monkey (Pasik and Pasik, 1964). These experiments do not disprove the concept that the superior colliculus mediates reflexes related to eye movements in primates; they do, however, demonstrate that alternate pathways for these reflexes are present. Because of the connections of the superior colliculus in primates it is suggested that this structure in some way regulates eye movements, or is part of one pathway for visual tracking. The mechanism of Parinaud's syndrome remains speculative, although it is still a clinically useful sign.

9

Epithalamus and hypothalamus

The dorsal structures of the diencephalon comprise the epithalamus. They include the habenula, pineal body (epiphysis), paraphysis, and parietal eye. The latter two structures are discussed in Chapters 2 and 8, respectively.

Habenula

The habenulae are paired structures in all vertebrates. Each habenula is divided into two nuclei, the medial being more densely cellular in man.

The habenulae are well developed in the most primitive vertebrates and are relatively large in animals with little forebrain. The importance of the relation to the olfactory system is shown by the great development in species relying heavily on the sense of smell to find food, such as sharks and bloodhounds, and the underdevelopment in animals with poor olfactory sense, such as birds and aquatic mammals.

A striking feature of the habenula is the asymmetric development of the two sides, an unusual characteristic in the central nervous system. The habenulae of myxinoids are fused to form a large midline body in the dorsal diencephalon. Microscopically, right and left habenulae can be distinguished, but the right is much larger than the left, and the number of efferent fibers from the right is greater. Two nuclei within each habenula are present. In petromyzonts, the right habenula predominates but in elasmobranchs the left is larger; the two sides are macroscopically distinct in both. The habenulae in teleosts are smaller than in elasmobranchs, and mild asymmetry persists in most species, the right larger in some, the left in others. Among amphibians and reptiles, the two habenulae are variable in symmetry. In urodeles, they are nearly equal (Herrick, 1948), but in the frog (Kemali and Braitenberg, 1969) the left is considerably larger than the right. In birds and mammals, habenular symmetry is also variable. In man, the habenulae are small and equal in size.

The habenula receives fibers from the forebrain, particularly from olfactory centers, as well as fibers from the hypothalamus, preoptic area, thalamus, optic tectum, and parietal eye. It discharges over a principle pathway and several smaller pathways to the midbrain and thalamus. The fiber connections are constant in all vertebrates, although in fishes the course of habenular fibers differs from that of other vertebrates because of eversion of the piscine forebrain.

The afferent connections of the habenulae are (1) the septohabenular tract, composed of lightly myelinated fibers from the septal nuclei and paraolfactory area (Chapter 12) which partially decussate in the anterior commissure, travel in the medial forebrain bundle, and turn dorsally to the habenula in the stria medullaris. Further partial decussation occurs in the habenular commissure before the fibers are distributed to the habenular nuclei; (2) the amygdalohabenular (lateral corticohabenular) tract and the hippocampohabenular (medial corticohabenular) tract, ending mainly in the lateral habenular nucleus of the same side after coursing in the stria terminalis; (3) preopticohabenular and hypothalamohabenular tracts, accompanying the septohabenular fibers in the stria medullaris; (4) thalamohabenular fibers from the dorsal thalamus (Herrick, 1948; Schnitzlein, 1962); (5) tectohabenular fibers from both optic tecti, some fibers decussating in the habenular commissure; (6) interpedunculohabenular fibers travel in the fasciculus retroflexus to the lateral habenular nucleus in the rat and cat (Massopust and Thompson, 1962). Fibers from the neocortex of higher vertebrates to the habenula have not been found.

The largest efferent path from each habenula is the heavily myelinated habenulo-interpeduncular tract, also known as the fasciculus retroflexus (of Meynert). This large tract arises from the lateral and medial habenular nuclei and passes over the caudal pole of the dorsomedial nucleus of the thalamus, where some habenular fibers terminate. The tract then passes through the red nucleus without synapse, to end in the inter-peduncular nucleus of the midbrain. The fasciculus retroflexus also may include fibers from the dorsal and medial thalamic nuclei in mammals (Plante, 1972).

Other efferent habenular connections of smaller size are the reciprocal habenulotectal pathway and habenulotegmental fibers to the dorsal tegmental nucleus of the midbrain, a terminal also for many fibers from the interpeduncular nucleus. Habenular connections with the pineal have been suggested but not proved (Schnitzlein, 1962).

The habenular commissure lies posterior to the habenulae and contains many decussating fibers of tracts distributed to both habenulae. It also connects the amygdaloid nucleus of one side with the hippocampus of the other, these fibers not actually entering the habenulae (Crosby et al., 1962). It is uncertain whether the habenular nuclei of the two sides interconnect. In adult man, calcification sometimes occurs in the wall of the third ventricle adjacent to the habenular commissure. This focus of calcification is sometimes interpreted in radiographs of the skull as pineal calcification (Stauffer et al., 1953), but the distinction is not of clinical significance because both are in the midline in close proximity and can be used to determine if midline structures have shifted. The pineal itself may also calcify. The reasons for these calcifications are unknown.

The habenulopeduncular tract (fasciculus retroflexus) is the first forebrain tract to become myelinated in the human fetus, beginning early in the seventh fetal month and complete by term (Yakovlev and Lecours, 1967). The stria medullaris myelinates at term (Rorke and Riggs, 1969).

Interpenduncular nucleus

The name interpeduncular nucleus is descriptive of the location of this structure between the cerebral peduncles in the posterior part of the midbrain in man and other mammals. It is most prominent and is probably more important, however, in lower vertebrates lacking cerebral peduncles. In those species, it occupies a similar position in the midbrain and isthmus.

The interpeduncular nucleus is a single, elongated structure in the midline without demarcation of the two sides from each other. The principle afferent connection is the paired habenulo-interpeduncular tract or

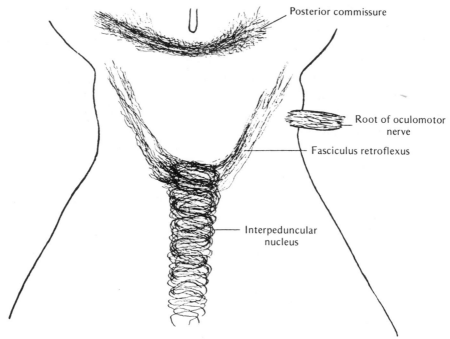

Figure 9-1 Horizontal section of the midbrain of a salamander. Spiral arrangement of habenulo-interpeduncular fibers of the fasciculus retroflexus within the interpeduncular nucleus as they descend to the caudal end of this structure; root of oculomotor nerve; posterior commissure. Drawing of Golgi impregnations (Herrick, 1948).

fasciculus retroflexus, possibly including thalamo-interpeduncular fibers. The asymmetry of the habenulae in most lower vertebrates is associated with disparity in the size of this tract on the two sides. After entering the interpeduncular nucleus, most fibers form a compact spiral, each fiber decussating many times and having numerous synapses along the course. This spiral extends the entire length of the interpeduncular nucleus (Fig. 9-1). Some fibers undergo only a few turns of the spiral or terminate without decussating. The spiral arrangement within the interpeduncular nucleus is unique in the central nervous system. It has been described in detailed studies of many species, including the salamander (Herrick, 1948), frog (Kamali and Braitenberg, 1969), and several mammals (Cajal, 1909-1911).

Other less numerous afferent connections of the interpeduncular nucleus include fibers from the mammillary bodies, olfactory structures of the forebrain, secondary visceral and gustatory centers of the medulla, basal optic tract, and tegmentum of the midbrain. The interpeduncular nucleus is small but still present in anosmatic animals, probably associated with the small size of the habenulae in these species. In mammals a magnocellular portion of the interpeduncular nucleus can be distinguished; it is connected to the nucleus of the dorsal raphé in the midbrain and to the dorsal and medial thalamic nuclei (Plante, 1972).

Efferent fibers of the interpeduncular nucleus enter the reticular formation of the midbrain and medulla, particularly the dorsal tegmental nucleus. Other fibers descend to motor nuclei of the medulla in the dorsal longitudinal fasciculus. An ascending interpedunculo-diencephalic pathway in mammals also has been described (Massopust and Thompson, 1972; Plante, 1972).

In salamanders and probably in most other lower vertebrates, highly branched processes of ependymal cells of the midbrain extend into the interpeduncular nucleus. These ependymal processes participate, together with tufted dendritic and axonal endings, in the formation of glomeruli (Herrick, 1948). These glomeruli are similar to those of the olfactory bulb (Chapter 12). The nature of ependymal participation in the metabolism of synapses in these structures is not known. Glomeruli are an efficient arrangement for the convergence, summation, and reenforcement of impulses. Axonal endings are not only of extrinsic connections but also of neurons within the interpeduncular nucleus. Because of the spiral course of the entering habenular fibers and the organization of the glomeruli, each fiber entering the spiral may synapse with most neurons of the interpeduncular nucleus (Herrick, 1948). Somatotopic organization or even lateralization is unlikely, therefore, and the interpeduncular nucleus probably functions as a single integrated structure serving both sides of the body, or for nonlateralized visceral activity.

Hypothetic function of habenulo-interpeduncular system

The habenula may be the highest correlative center in the central nervous system of many lower vertebrates. It receives converging fibers from centers under olfactory influence, from centers related to the viscera, from the hypothalamus and preoptic area, and also receives fibers relaying exteroceptive information from the thalamus and optic tectum.

In lower vertebrates, fibers of the tactile as well as of the visual system project to the optic tectum (Chapter 8).

Herrick (1948) proposed that the habenulae and interpeduncular nucleus were the principle components of a system that controlled feeding behavior in lower species. This system coordinates the activities of salivation, gastric secretion, and intestinal motility with somatic motor functions of the tongue, jaws, and facial muscles. He suggested that the habenulo-interpeduncular tract and mammillo-interpeduncular tract were mainly inhibitory components of an equilibrated dynamic system in which the basal forebrain bundles (Chapter 12) were the activating components. This concept implies that olfactomotor impulses descend in the basal forebrain bundles, and that the habenulae and mammillary bodies selectively inhibit either these impulses or conflicting activities, depending on the circumstances. Pathways converge on the interpeduncular nucleus for final relay along those reticulobulbar and reticulospinal tracts related to feeding and to other activities associated with olfaction and taste.

An analogy between the cerebellum and interpeduncular nucleus was also proposed by Herrick (1948). Neither the cerebellum nor the interpeduncular nucleus is capable of initiating motor activity or behavioral patterns. The relatively large size of the habenulae and interpeduncular nucleus in urodelan amphibians, such as the salamander, may be related to the shy and inhibited behavior of these animals, and the long latency period between the anticipation of eating and actual consumption. In lower species, the interpeduncular nucleus may also have inhibitory influences on other aspects of patterned behavior, such as mating.

Dominance of one cerebral hemisphere over the other is generally regarded as almost unique in the nervous system of man. This concept is correct in terms of speech, handedness, and some higher associative functions. The habenulae are asymmetrically developed in even the most primitive vertebrates, the cyclostomes. The principle of dominance of one side of the brain over the other therefore probably is an old phenomenon phylogenetically. The interpeduncular nucleus may be an integrating center for the two sides of the brain. Cerebral dominance in man, however, is not associated with unequal size of the cerebral hemisphere.

In mammals, the habenulae become supplanted in importance by the neocortex. The importance of the habenulae to man is further diminished by the relative insignificance of olfaction. The habenulae may be important in man only in the neonatal period and early infancy, when the hypothalamus and habenulae direct the feeding reactions that occupy the infant while awake. Neonates frequently show discrimination in taste by preferring milk and rejecting glucose in water. The lack of importance of the cerebral cortex in feeding activity of the human newborn is exemplified by the ability of infants with anencephaly, hydranencephaly, and extensive porencephaly to suck, swallow, and perform visceral functions necessary to digestion. Indeed, many of these infants are not identified as abnormal while they are in the newborn nursery or for several months.

Pineal body

The pineal body, also known as the "epiphysis," is an unpaired structure lying in the midline of the epithalamic region. It is attached by glial bridges to the habenular commissure rostrally and the posterior commissure caudally. The pineal develops embryologically as a vesicular evagination or, less commonly, as a compact bud from the dorsal ependymal wall of the diencephalon. The lumen, when present, communicates with the third ventricle and usually closes as the animal matures, although in some teleosts and anurans, this opening is maintained throughout life. Ascending the phylogenetic series of vertebrates, the lumen is progressively reduced by cellular proliferation during ontogenesis, culminating in the compact pineal body of mammals (Oksche, 1965). The pineal stalk in lower vertebrates is often long. The distal end of the pineal body forms the parietal eye in some species (Chapter 8).

Two types of cells differentiate from the primordial neuroepithelial cells, from which the embryonic human pineal develops (Kappers, 1955). One type matures into astrocytic cells with processes. The other type becomes the pinealocytes, arranged in nests and solid cords within the glial matrix. Processes of the pinealocytes surround blood vessels. Meninges envelop and invade the developing pineal, creating connective tissue septae. Degenerative changes in the human pineal, in the form of glial plaques, cysts, and calcium and magnesium concrements, begin in the second decade.

The comparative anatomy of the pineal in various vertebrates is considered in detail by Tilney and Warren (1919), Oksche (1965), van de Kamer (1965), Quay (1965a), and Anderson (1965). The pineal is present in most, but not all, vertebrates. It is lacking in myxinoids, torpedoes (an elasmobranch), crocodilians, and in many mammals. In the elephant and rhinoceros, it is small and vestigial.

Sensory neurons are found in the pineal of submammalian vertebrates, including petromyzonts, most fishes, amphibians, and lizards, but not in those species in which the pineal becomes glandular. The axons of these neurons form bundles entering the habenular commissure, the posterior commissure, or both, but the sites of termination are unknown (Kappers, 1965). Afferent nerve connections of the pineal in lower vertebrates often are best developed during embryonic stages, degenerating later (Oksche, 1965). Among mammals, particularly primates, the pineal contains a few neurons. Autonomic fibers enter the pineal. Although they may merely be aberrant fibers of little functional significance (Kappers, 1965), they probably are postganglionic sympathetic fibers from the superior cervical ganglion (Mollgaard and Moller, 1973). The dense network of autonomic nerve fibers enter the pineal body either by vascular plexuses or by two nervi conarii. In primates, the nervi conarii also may contain preganglionic parasympathetic fibers which synapse with pineal nerve cells, constituting an intramural ganglion. Separate small ganglia (of Marburg and Pastori) adjacent to the human fetal pineal also have been described and may be parasympathetic ganglia innervating the vessels of the pineal body (Mollgaard and Moller, 1973). Connections between the pineal and habenula have been suggested but not demonstrated. Evidence is also lacking of hypothalamopineal connections (Kappers, 1965). A nerve carrying impulses from the human pineal to a cluster of neurons near the subcommissural organ has been described (Mollgaard and Moller, 1973).

A transformation of the function of the pineal body from a sense organ to that of a gland is first encountered in turtles and snakes. Glandular characteristics are further developed in birds and mammals, in whom the pineal body is variable in shape, and hollow, follicular, or solid. A lobular structure is prominent in some species of mammals, including man.

Some lower vertebrates have another smaller but similar structure. It disappears in most teleostean fishes and in terrestrial vertebrates. This parapineal body (parietal body, accessory pineal body) usually lies just rostral to the pineal. It develops embryologically in the same way.

The pineal has fascinated philosophers and students of anatomy since ancient times (Kappers, 1965). Descartes, the seventeenth-century philosopher and mathematician, thought that the pineal was the "seat of the soul," but he based his theory on the conclusions of ancient Greek philosophers. Many anatomists of the eighteenth and nineteenth centuries thought the pineal functioned as a regulator of the flow of cerebrospinal fluid through the aqueduct. In the early twentieth century, it was suggested that the pineal regulated the outflow of venous blood from the choroid plexuses of the lateral and third ventricles, thereby controlling the production of cerebrospinal fluid. Pineal extracts have been used in the therapy of mental disease, particularly schizophrenia.

An endocrine function of the pineal has been suggested for many years. The pineal now is known to produce melatonin, a hormone that acts antagonistically to melanin-stimulating hormone on melanophores of amphibians (Bagnara, 1965, Novales and Novales, 1965) and on melanocytes of mammals (Wurtman and Axelrod, 1965). In addition, a substance elaborated by the pineal takes part in the metabolism of water and electrolytes, in the secretion of adrenocortical hormones (Clementi et al., 1965; Palkovitz, 1965), and in the inhibition of gonadotropin secretion by the pituitary (Thieblot, 1965; Moszkowska, 1965; Thieblot and Blaise, 1965). Some of the gonadotropin-inhibiting effect may be related to serotonin produced by the pineal (Jouan and Samperez, 1965). Sexual precocity has been observed in some children with pineal tumors. It has been suggested this change may be related to the effects of obstructive hydrocephalus or transmitted pressure on the hypothalamus from the enlarging pineal (Russell and Rubinstein, 1971), but this explanation does not account for the overwhelming male preponderance.

A rare pineal tumor resembling a chemodectoma was found in a 17-year-old girl (Hughes and Smith, 1955). They thought that the normal human pineal and carotid bodies were similar and suggested that the pineal may be a chemoreceptor organ.

Continuous light inhibits the pineal of the rat, particularly at puberty (Roth, 1965; Quay, 1965b). The influence of light on the pineal may be mediated through the parietal eye of lower vertebrates (Chapter 8), or through autonomic fibers of the pineal of mammals. These autonomic fibers are derived largely from the superior cervical sympathetic ganglion (Kappers, 1965), the same source of sympathetic fibers for the pupillary light reflex of the paired lateral eyes. The functional relation of the pineal body to the parietal eye in lower vertebrates has been a topic of speculation for many years, but it remains poorly understood.

The degenerative changes occurring in the human pineal after puberty suggest that its function is more important during early life, analogous to that of the thymus.

Hypothalamus

The comparative anatomy of the hypothalamus and the relations with other centers in various vertebrates were extensively reviewed by Crosby and Woodburne (1940) and Crosby and Showers (1969). The human hypothalamus was discussed by Nauta and Haymaker (1969). The following account is based on the observations of these various authors.

The striking feature of the evolution of the hypothalamus is the similarity of its nuclear differentiation and fiber connections throughout the phylogenetic series.

The hypothalamus is little differentiated in cyclostomes and urodelan amphibians, except that the gray matter separates into a poorly laminated medial and a nonlaminated lateral region. Teleosts and mammals have the largest hypothalamus. Most of the hypothalamic nuclei can be recognized, although the degree of development differs among species of fishes and terrestrial animals. These nuclei include the ventromedial, suprachiasmatic, diffuse supraoptic hypothalamic nuclei, and the anterior hypothalamic area. The dorsomedial hypothalamic nucleus and the dorsal hypothalamic area are poorly differentiated in reptiles and birds, and cannot be distinguished in lower vertebrates.

The posterior hypothalamic nucleus and the mammillary body with its subdivisions can be identified in reptiles, birds, and mammals, and is probably primordial in most lower vertebrates, particularly anuran amphibians and teleosts. The mammillary body in man is large compared to that of other primates (Crosby et al., 1962). In the rat, it is a band of gray matter continuous in the midline, rather than the conspicuous bulges on the surface of the brain as in man (Zeman and Innes, 1963). The supramammillary commissure (posterior hypothalamic decussation) and its associated nucleus are developed in amphibians and other terrestrial vertebrates.

The tuber cinereum is a protuberance on the surface of the brain between the optic chiasm and the mammillary bodies. The infundibular stalk arises from it. In lower vertebrates, such as fishes and amphibians, the tuber cinereum includes most of the hypothalamus. In man, it contains certain hypothalamic nuclei of both medial and lateral zones.

The division of the hypothalamic nuclei of man into zones and sub-groups was considered by Christ (1969), and Nauta and Haymaker (1969).

Preoptic area

A preoptic area rostral to the optic chiasm is recognized in all verte-brates (Crosby and Woodburne, 1940). This area can be divided into a periventricular region, and the medial preoptic nuclei. Although not part of the hypothalamus proper, and possibly even of telencephalic origin, the preoptic area is intimately related to the hypothalamus, both anatomically and physiologically.

The periventricular region is laminated and divided into nuclei, one containing small neurons and the other large ones. The small neurons are oriented parallel to the wall of the third ventricle. The nucleus be-comes progressively larger as the phylogenetic series is ascended. The large neurons of the periventricular region contain colloidal neurosecre-tions in the cytoplasm. These cells are scattered in the posterior periven-tricular region in lower vertebrates, but in reptiles and higher verte-brates, they progressively differentiate into the supraoptic and paraven-tricular nuclei (Crosby and Showers, 1969). Even in some teleosts, they cluster into two distinct groups.

Neurosecretory cells exist even in cyclostomes (Bentley and Follett, 1962) and have been found in amphibians (Gershenfeld et al., 1960). The chemical composition of the collodial neurosecretory material in the large periventricular cells is similar in all vertebrates (Scharrer and Scharrer, 1954; Sawyer, 1961). These data suggest an early evolution of neural control of endocrine function, common to all vertebrates. Neuro-secretory cells also are found in the brains of some insects (Larsen and Broadbent, 1968), indicating that cerebral control of some endocrino-logic functions is almost universal in the animal kingdom.

The medial preoptic area is distinguished from the periventricular nuclei throughout phylogeny by a lack of lamellae. In lower vertebrates, it consists merely of a few scattered cells.

Neurosecretory cells similar to those of the preoptic area are also found in the spinal cord of some fishes. The original discovery of neuro-secretion was made by Speidel (1917) in studying the spinal cord of the skate.

Infundibulum and saccus vasculosus

An infundibulum composed of fibers connecting the supraoptic and paraventricular nuclei to the neurohypophysis (pituitary) extends from the ventral surface of the diencephalon, although it does not protrude in cyclostomes as it does in higher vertebrates. The infundibulum is simply a fiber tract surrounding a recess of the third ventricle in terrestrial vertebrates, but fishes have associated neural tissue.

A prominent ventral mass of the hypothalamus surrounds the infundibulum even in cyclostomes. This hypothalamic tissue forms paired structures extending caudally, ventral to the midbrain, in elasmobranchs, teleosts, and other classes of fishes. These structures are called the inferior lobes of the hypothalamus. The ependymal-lined infundibular recess extends through the center of each inferior lobe and communicates rostrally with the third ventricle. The inferior lobes of fishes have unique connections with the cerebellum in addition to diencephalic projections.

The neurohypophysis lacks neurons, but has special astrocytes, called pituicytes, upon which the descending fibers of the infundibulum terminate (Polak and Azcoaga, 1969).

The adenohypophysis develops embryologically as a diverticulum of the roof of the mouth (Rathke's pouch) in all vertebrates. Adult cyclostomes and a few primitive holostean fishes still retain this primordial communication with the mouth. The adenohypophysis of fishes is simple, and it is separated from the neurohypophysis by a vascular septum. The glandular epithelium of the adenohypophysis differentiates into distinct parts, specialized in specific hormonal production in terrestrial vertebrates. A simple hypophyseal portal system is first found in amphibians and controls the adenohypophysis by means of hematogenous neurosecretory substances from the hypothalamus. In amphibians, the glandular part of the hypophysis envelops the neurohypophysis and extends caudally, rather than rostrally, as in man.

Fishes have a specialized midline structure in the posterior part of the infundibulum, associated with the inferior lobes. This structure is the saccus vasculosus or infundibular organ (Dammerman, 1910; Dorn, 1955; Altner and Zimmerman, 1972). It is highly vascularized. Convoluted walls of ciliated, cuboidal epithelium and neurosensory cells with hair-like processes project into a lumen that is continuous with the infundibular recess of the third ventricle. Axons of the neurosensory cells form a fiber layer in the wall of the saccus vasculosus and inferior lobes.

This tract of the saccus vasculosus decussates in the posterior wall of the infundibulum. Some fibers terminate in a nucleus of the saccus vasculosus to distribute impulses to hypothalamic nuclei and the tegmentum of the midbrain. Other fibers from the saccus vasculosus pass to the dorsal thalamus without synapse.

The saccus vasculosus is undeveloped in cyclostomes. It is best differentiated and largest in fishes of the deep sea, but smaller in those living in shallow, fresh water. The saccus is absent in amphibians and other terrestrial vertebrates. Herrick's (1948) designation of the highly vascular neurohypophysis of the salamander as the saccus vasculosus does not correspond to the homologous structure of fishes.

The saccus vasculosus probably perceives intraventricular fluid pressure as a function of depth in water. It influences the size of the swim bladder through autonomic nerves (Chapter 10) and hydrostatic mechanisms. The static function of the hypothalamus is evident not only by the fiber relations to the saccus vasculosus, but also by the reciprocal connections between the inferior lobes and the cerebellum (Kappers et al., 1936).

The infundibulum of lungfishes is transitional between that of fishes and of amphibians (Romer, 1970), corresponding well to their place in the scheme of evolution. The inferior lobes of the hypothalamus are reduced to thin sheets of tissue, and a saccus vasculosus is absent. The adenohypophysis is differentiated into the primordial pars intermedia and pars distalis of terrestrial vertebrates.

Connections of hypothalamus and preoptic area

The hypothalamus and preoptic area receive fibers from most parts of the forebrain and diencephalon in lower vertebrates, but fibers from olfactory centers and from the gustatory nuclei of the medulla predominate. These connections persist in man. Efferent fibers to various motor centers and reticular formation in the brainstem, as well as to the thalamus and to forebrain olfactory and limbic centers, are a constant feature throughout phylogeny. The hypothalamus does not receive fibers from the major somatic sensory pathways.

The medial forebrain bundle (Chapter 12) is present in all vertebrates. It is an ascending and descending system of thinly myelinated fibers connecting the olfactory and limbic centers of the forebrain (hippocampus, anterior olfactory nucleus, and septal area) with the preoptic and hypothalamic regions, and the tegmentum of the midbrain. Some fibers cross in the anterior commissure. Fibers arising in the hypothalamus also ascend in the medial forebrain bundle to the septal nuclei to further correlate gustatory and visceral impulses with olfactory information. Hypothalamic fibers pass caudally in the medial forebrain bundle to terminate in the subrubral and deep tegmental gray matter of the midbrain. Some of these hypothalamotegmental fibers in mammals are thought to regulate body temperature (Crosby and Woodburne, 1951; Kahn et al., 1969), although many probably mediate hypothalamic influence on autonomic centers of the brainstem and spinal cord (Zeman and Innes, 1963).

In cyclostomes and fishes, the preoptic area and rostral hypothalamus are related to the primordial hippocampi also by scattered, partially decussated fascicles composing one element of the fornix (Chapter 12). As the fornix enlarges in amphibians and reptiles, fibers to the preoptic area and hypothalamus increase in number.

The amygdaloid nucleus is present in primordial form in cyclostomes. It differentiates into basolateral and corticomedial portions in fishes and in all higher vertebrates (Droogleever-Fortuyn, 1961; Schnitzlein, 1962; Chapter 12). Fibers mainly from the corticomedial portion pass medially to enter the preoptic area and anterior hypothalamus in all vertebrates. In mammals, the amygdalopreoptic and amygdalohypothalamic tracts compose the stria terminalis, passing as an arc along the tail, body, and head of the caudate nucleus to the anterior commissure, where many of the fibers decussate; others pass above or below the commissure to enter the preoptic and hypothalamic nuclei of both sides. A few reciprocal connections also likely occur in mammals (Nauta and Haymaker, 1969).

Efferent fiber projections of the hypothalamus remain constant throughout phylogeny. Some have already been mentioned. The diencephalic periventricular fiber system consists of fibers originating in the various nuclei of the hypothalamus. They spread along the wall of the third ventricle to enter the thalamus or course caudally as the dorsal longitudinal fasciculus (of Schuetz) to synapse in various brainstem centers. These centers include the Ediger-Westphal nucleus, optic tectum, periaqueductal gray matter, reticular formation, and motor nuclei, particularly those concerned with visceral function, such as the salivatory nuclei, dorsal motor nucleus of the vagus, and cardiovascular and respiratory centers of the reticular formation in the medulla. The dorsal longitudinal fasciculus supplements other slower hypothalamic pathways that reach the visceral motor nuclei of the brainstem through the polysynaptic reticular formation. Ascending gustatory components of the dorsal longitudinal fasciculus terminate in the hypothalamus (Fox, 1941; Thompson, 1942).

Fibers arising in the visceral sensory and gustatory centers of the medulla and ascending to the mammillary bodies and hypothalamic nuclei are known in mammals as the mammillary peduncle. They are present in all vertebrates including cyclostomes. This peduncle is prominent in fishes with a highly developed gustatory system. A diffuse, uncrossed, ascending gustatory system, in addition to the mammillary peduncle, occurs in fishes except cyclostomes. Secondary and tertiary gustatory pathways from the nucleus solitarius to comparable nuclei of the midbrain are relayed to the hypothalamus. These projections are found in teleosts and urodeles and, in less developed form, in frogs and some lizards, but not in birds. The tegmentomammillary tract in mammals may be homologous to the secondary and tertiary gustatory-hypothalamic pathways of fishes.

The mammillary bodies have two principle pathways of discharge: the mammillotegmental tract, consisting of lightly myelinated fibers to the deep tegmental nuclei of the midbrain and to the interpeduncular nucleus (Herrick, 1948), and the mammillothalamic tract (bundle of Vicq d'Azyr), composed of heavily myelinated fibers terminating in the anterior nuclei of the thalamus. Reciprocal connections from each of these areas to the mammillary bodies are also present. The tracts are uncrossed. They are largest in mammals, and less well developed in birds, reptiles, amphibians, and fishes.

Fibers arising in the hypothalamus and preoptic area reach the habenula by way of the stria medullaris in all vertebrates.

In submammalian vertebrates, fibers of the optic tract terminate directly in the preoptic area and hypothalamus. This connection is prominent in some fishes (Ebbesson, 1968). Information on vision and color is presumably used by the hypothalamus to mediate color changes in skin for camouflage in animals with cutaneous chromatophores, such as the chameleon and some fishes. This projection from the retina could not be demonstrated in the cat (Lin and Ingram, 1972) and probably is also absent in man and other mammals.

The ventral peduncle of the lateral forebrain bundle contains a few pallidohypothalamic fibers in all vertebrates.

The supraoptico- and paraventriculo-hypophysial tract extends through the infundibulum to the posterior lobe of the pituitary in all vertebrates. The neurons of origin and axons of the tract contain neurosecretory granules. Some fibers from other hypothalamic nuclei accompany the tract. The unique infundibular portal system and other infundibular mechanisms of transport are discussed by Haymaker (1969). Hypothalamic control of the pituitary and the secretion of various hormones in birds is reviewed by Nalbandov and Graber (1969), and in mammals by Harris and George (1969) and Sawyer (1969).

Some neocortical fibers project directly from the frontal lobes in mammals (Nauta and Haymaker, 1969), but the neocortex is related to the hypothalamus mainly through connections of thalamus and structures of the limbic system.

Small fibers interconnect adjoining hypothalamic and supraoptic nuclei. Many course in the medial forebrain bundle. Some fibers of the supraoptic decussation may be hypothalamic commissural fibers or interrelate thalamus and hypothalamus of opposite sides in the pathways of emotional expression (Papez, 1937).

Functions of hypothalamus

Highly developed species with more discriminatory ability have a greater number of hypothalamic responses than do less well developed animals. The common functions in all vertebrates are (1) the correlation of gustatory, visceral, and olfactory impulses. The magnitude of this relation differs with the relative importance of taste or smell in the individual species; (2) control of the autonomic nervous system, both sympathetic and parasympathetic. Hypothalamic control over autonomic centers of the brainstem and spinal cord is mediated by two pathways: the periventricular diencephalic fiber system descends the brainstem in the dorsal longitudinal fasciculus; and the hypothalamotegmental pathway in the medial forebrain bundle. These tracts synapse in the gray matter of the descending reticular formation of the midbrain. Influence is thus exercised over centers of vasomotor and respiratory control, pupillary tonus, piloerection, genital function, urinary bladder control, gastric secretion, intestinal motility, bronchial constriction, and other functions. In general, sympathetic autonomic reactions are elicited by stimulation of the posterior nuclei of the hypothalamus; stimulation of the anterior nuclei results in parasympathetic responses in mammals; (3) the regulation of appetite (Stevenson, 1969); (4) the regulation of somatic growth in childhood by controlling secretion of growth hormone (Harris and George, 1969); (5) the regulation of water and electrolyte metabolism by production of antidiuretic hormone (ADH), control of salt craving and thirst, and regulation of secretion of adrenocorticotropic hormone (ACTH); (6) the regulation of endocrine activity through control of the pituitary. At least nine polypeptides have been isolated from hypothalamic tissue; each selectively stimulates or inhibits the release of anterior pituitary hormones (Schally et al., 1973); (7) an incompletely understood function related to the limbic system (Chapter 12) in the synthesis and expression of affect, mood, and emotion (MacLean, 1969); (8) part of reticular activation (Chapter 11); and (9) the regulation of body temperature in homeothermic animals, such as birds and mammals (Myers, 1969).

The separation of animals into cold-blooded (poikilothermic) and warm-blooded (homeothermic) groups is arbitrary. All vertebrates have a limited range of temperatures in which they can maintain a metabolic rate consistent with their usual activity and without excessive stress. When the ambient temperature falls below the minimum of that range, the animal must either move to a warmer environment or hibernate. Cold-blooded frogs thus bury themselves in the mud for the winter; bears also undergo an extended sleep for the winter months, although they are "warm-blooded" mammals. Birds and mammals maintain a more constant body temperature than do lower vertebrates, but young mammals, including human newborns, also have poor control of body temperature relative to the environment. Adult monotremes and marsupials still regulate their body temperatures at low levels (27° to 33°C) and have poor mechanisms for coping with either endogenous or environmentally induced heat stress (Bakker, 1971). Early mammal-like reptiles may have been similar in this respect. Evidence is accumulating that some modern reptiles also have mechanisms of maintaining relatively constant body and cerebral temperatures (Zitko et al., 1972).

It is speculated that dinosaurs became extinct because they were warm-blooded creatures at the onset of the ice age (Bakker, 1972). Dinosaurs were too large to escape the change in climate by hibernating in burrows or other warm habitats available to small, homeothermic creatures; dinosaurs also were unable to withstand prolonged drops in body temperature, unlike turtles, lizards, and other poikilothermic animals. Large tropical mammals with naked skin, such as the rhinoceros, hippopotomus, and elephant, in existence today would probably die from exposure to prolonged severe cold in the same way that the large, naked dinosaurs of the tropical Mesozoic era became extinct.

Some pituitary hormones may have different effects among vertebrates. Prolactin is a substance causing lactation in pregnant and postpartum female mammals. A similar or identical hormone also is found in submammalian vertebrates lacking mammary glands (Nicoll and Bern, 1968; Licht and Nicoll, 1969). A prolactin-like substance is even produced by fishes, although it differs from that of lungfishes and all terrestrial vertebrates (Nicoll and Bern, 1968). Prolactin in amphibians may be a type of growth hormone; mammalian prolactin inhibits thyroxine-induced resorption of the tail in bullfrog tadpoles, although mammalian growth hormone lacks a similar effect (Bern et al., 1967). Prolactin may also influence the metabolism of water and electrolytes in amphibians. The condition in lower vertebrates suggests that human prolactin may have other effects in addition to the influence on the mammary glands.

Many hypothalamic functions became modified by the development of telencephalic structures, but the hypothalamus is the central correlating and controlling organ for the internal environment in both the most primitive and the most advanced vertebrates.

Associative activity of diencephalon

The diencephalon is one of the primary correlative regions of the brain throughout phylogeny of vertebrates. The optic tectum and thalamus correlate somatic sensory (exteroceptive) information regarding the external environment (Chapter 8). The hypothalamus correlates visceral (interoceptive) information of the internal environment with gustatory and olfactory information to directly influence visceral function and synthesize appropriate visceral motor and secretory responses.

The conventional concept of diencephalic structures as "way-stations" to the correlative cerebral cortex is probably not justified. The theory is appealing if only the human brain is examined, but the study of comparative neuroanatomy reveals that many vertebrates function well with little development of the telencephalon. They can achieve conditioned learning, possess memory, and make simple but appropriate judgments when decisions are needed. The participation of the telencephalon of fishes and amphibians in correlative function is poorly understood.

The development of telencephalic structures allows refinement and amplification of the correlative processes that are accomplished almost entirely in the diencephalon of lower vertebrates but the telencephalon does not replace the diencephalon as the *primary* corrlative area. It is probably correct to consider the integrated function of diencephalic and telencephalic structures, rather than to attempt to separate them. The hypothalamus enlarges and differentiates as the phylogenetic series is ascended, to more critically analyze visceral information and to provide more autonomic responses.

Higher integration and synthesis of complex feeding patterns, even in mammals and to some extent in man, occur in the diencephalon. The "social smile" of the young infant is probably a visual-hypothalamic reflex which can be blocked by certain other factors mediated by the hypothalamus, such as hunger or mood. Much of what had formerly been attributed to "instinct," especially in birds, is now known to be learned behavior. Instinct as a neurologic concept is discussed in Chapter 12.

Man has exalted his highly developed neocortex but tends to derogate cerebral activity originating in subcortical centers as "reflexive." Reflex may be defined as an involuntary, reproducible reaction to a given stimulus. Association, as defined in neurologic terms, is the gathering of all relevant data available, discriminating the relative importance of each, comparing them with each other and with past experience, and then determining appropriate responses. A prediction of the consequences of each course of action is a higher associative function; the extent to which this occurs in lower vertebrates is difficult to determine.

By this definition, discriminatory diencephalic function is not reflexive, but associative. No two situations with many variables, however, are identical. A fish, sensing another unfamiliar fish, must decide whether to eat it, ignore it, or swim away lest he be eaten. The decision probably is made in the diencephalon. To call it reflexive is misleading. Evidence is lacking, however, that the diencephalon is capable of performing those higher associative functions termed "intellect" or "the mind," which, in their phylogenetic development, distinguish mammals from other vertebrates, primates from other mammals, and man from other primates. These functions include the ability to plan a sequence of indirect actions to achieve a goal, symbolism, abstraction, imagination, conscience, and social concerns.

10
Autonomic nervous system

Evolution of autonomic structure and function

All living things must preserve their internal environment to sustain life. Neural control of visceral function is almost universally found in the animal kingdom. This control of visceral activity is autonomic. Autonomic nerves associated with spinal nerves are sympathetic and those derived from branchial nerves are parasympathetic. In higher vertebrates, the sacral part of the spinal cord also gives origin to parasympathetic nerves. Sympathetic and parasympathetic components are anatomically mixed. Their separation is of little physiologic significance in lower vertebrates but becomes increasingly important as the distribution of the two components overlaps in terrestrial vertebrates. Antagonistic functions develop with this anatomic change. Neural modification of visceral activity evolved early. Even amphioxus has some autonomic control.

Smooth muscle of the gastrointestinal tract, urinary bladder, and blood vessels as well as secretory glands and the heart have an intrinsic functional capability not dependent upon neural stimulation. Neural excitation or inhibition of visceral muscles and glands, however, is an efficient way to coordinate visceral activity with external information and internal requirements. Primitively, the viscera are innervated by only one autonomic source, either sympathetic or parasympathetic, except the stomach. This structure is innervated by the two sources in most lower vertebrates, but the effects of both sympathetic and parasympathetic (vagal) stimulation are excitatory and additive, rather than antagonistic. In its most complete form, the autonomic nervous system consists of a balanced antagonism between sympathetic and parasympathetic innervation of the same organs. The impulses of each have opposite effects upon the activity of the end organs; either may dominate at one time, depending on the activity of cerebral centers. This antagonism between excitation and inhibition is first found in advanced amphibians and becomes progressively more developed, involving many organs in higher vertebrates.

The peripheral portion of the autonomic nervous system, both sympathetic and parasympathetic, is organized throughout phylogeny as a series of two neurons. The cell body of the first neuron lies within the spinal cord or brainstem. The cell body of the second neuron lies in the wall of the visceral end-organ, usually isolated from other neurons. This primitive arrangement is retained in the parasympathetic system of all vertebrates, including man. Some regional specialization occurs, however, exemplified by the submucosal and myenteric plexuses (of Meissner and Auerbach) in the gut. These intestinal plexuses are primordial in elasmobranchs, and well developed in anurans (Gunn, 1951). The sympathetic system, in contrast, becomes organized as segmental ganglia, containing the relocated and concentrated cell bodies of the terminal neurons in the series. The ganglia are secondarily joined with each other by longitudinal fibers to form trunks. Adjacent ganglia of the cervical region tend to fuse.

In the lowest vertebrates, the sympathetic system has a limited distribution to the viscera, including gastrointestinal tract, urogenital system, and splanchnic blood vessels. As the phylogenetic series is ascended, however, the sympathetic system extends into the head and peripherally to cutaneous vessels and glands. Parasympathetic distribution remains confined to the viscera and eyes and does not include the body wall or skin. Cutaneous glands and vessels thus continue to have only sympathetic innervation in man.

Sympathetic ganglia in the sacral and caudal regions of lower vertebrates are connected with corresponding segmental nerve roots. A sacral parasympathetic system is present only in amphibians and higher vertebrates. In amphibians, sacral sympathetic and parasympathetic systems are both present. The sacral and caudal extension of the sympathetic system disappears in higher vertebrates.

All vertebrates have parasympathetic components of the vagus and other branchial nerves. The extent of visceral distribution of the vagus increases in phylogeny.

Autonomic function and physiologic responses in lower vertebrates were reviewed by Nicol (1952). Responses by visceral organs to drugs are strikingly similar in lower and higher vertebrates. Acetylcholine, pilocarpine, and eserine (physostigmine) thus cause increased tone and peristalsis in the smooth muscle of the gastrointestinal tract and contraction of the muscle of the urinary bladder in fishes and amphibians, as well as in mammals. Atropine blocks these effects. Epinephrine, in contrast, causes relaxation of smooth muscle. These data suggest a similarity in neurotransmission throughout phylogeny, but the results of electric stimulation of autonomic nerves and ganglia are conflicting and often differ among investigators. In general, electric stimulation of splanchnic (sympathetic) nerves in lower vertebrates increases peristalsis and tone in the gastrointestinal tract and causes contraction of the gall bladder. Vagal stimulation also produces contractions of the gastric musculature, but it has no effect on intestinal tone or motility. In mammals, the vagus usually facilitates and the sympathetic nerves inhibit movement of the gastrointestinal tract. One explanation is that the function of the autonomic component changes in evolution, but this concept is unlikely in view of the similarity of pharmacologic reactions. An alternative possibility is that electric stimulation of autonomic nerves does not reproduce physiologic effects.

Autonomic effects on secretion by mucosal glands in the gastrointestinal tract are not known in lower vertebrates. Gastric secretion in elasmobranchs is a continuous process, and stimulation of the vagus fails to elicit a response.

The heart is innervated only by the vagus in lower vertebrates. Stimulation of this nerve results in bradycardia, as in higher vertebrates. Sympathetic fibers are present in anuran amphibians and higher vertebrates. Stimulation of these nerves accelerates the heart rate and also increases the force of contraction.

Cyclostomes lack intraocular muscles. In elasmobranchs and lower teleosts, such as the eel, the constrictor muscle of the iris contracts in direct response to light and is not under neural control, a phenomenon perhaps related to the retinal origin of the iris (Chapter 8). The radial or dilator muscle of the iris is innervated by parasympathetic ciliairy nerves. Electric stimulation of the oculomotor nerve causes dilatation of the pupil. In higher teleosts, the cranial extension of sympathetic fibers reciprocally controls the iris. Parasympathetic fibers cause pupillary dilatation and sympathetic fibers cause constriction of the pupils (Young,

1931b). Amphibians, or their crossopterygian ancestors, also developed reciprocal neural control of the muscle in the iris, but with reversed innervation compared to that developed by teleosts. In modern amphibians and in all higher terrestrial vertebrates, the parasympathetic oculomotor nerve thus innervates the pupillary constrictor, and the sympathetic nerves innervate the pupillary dilator (Pick, 1970). The opposite pupillary innervation of fishes and terrestrial vertebrates exemplifies divergent evolution with similar functional results.

Both epinephrine and acetylcholine act on the peripheral and splanchnic vessels in lower vertebrates to cause vasoconstriction and increased blood pressure.

In spite of the anatomic similarities between the autonomic nervous systems of amphibians and higher vertebrates inculding man, there are important functional differences. Frogs do not respond to changes in environmental temperature by a generalized sympathetic discharge, as do mammals. Blood is not shifted from one part of the body to another by selective vasoconstriction and vasodilatation, and frogs do not shiver with skeletal muscles; instead they bury themselves in mud at the bottom of a pond to hibernate (Pick, 1970). The profuse sympathetic discharge with which higher vertebrates prepare themselves for fight or flight is also not characteristic of amphibians (Pick, 1970).

Comparative anatomy of peripheral autonomic system

The comparative anatomy of the autonomic nervous system of protochordates and lower vertebrates was reviewed by Young (1931a, 1933), Nicol (1952), and Pick (1970).

The origin of the autonomic nervous system may be found not only in amphioxus, but also in other protochordates even less differentiated or more aberrant than amphioxus. In the acorn worm (balanoglossid), a diffuse network of nerve fibers extends throughout the alimentary tract and other viscera, but the central nervous system is so poorly developed that conclusions are speculative about the central origin of these fibers and their relations to other neural centers (Silén, 1950).

The sympathetic ganglia and nerves of all vertebrates, as well as the dorsal root ganglia are derived from the neural crest. Ontogenesis is reminiscent of phylogenesis; it is therefore understandable that the visceral motor nerves of amphioxus originate from the dorsal spinal nerves of both the branchial and post-branchial regions. The fibers ram-

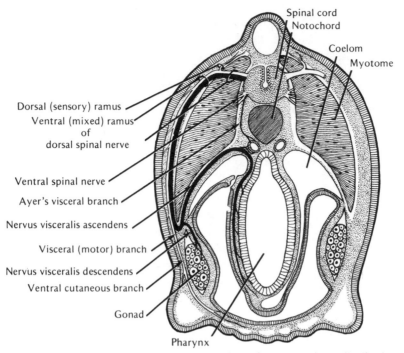

Figure 10-1 Diagrammatic cross-section of amphioxus to show distribution of visceral efferent (autonomic) nerves, emerging from the spinal cord in the dorsal root (Pick, 1970, after Boveri and Hatscheck, 1904).

ify in the walls of the gill arches, serosa, gonadal pouches, intestine, and hepatic cecum (Fig. 10-1). They also innervate visceral blood vessels, a pair of small muscles enveloping the gut just behind the pharynx, and the anal spincter. Plexuses in the intestinal wall are composed of stellate neurons and anastomosing, layered networks of nerve fibers. Although Nicol (1952) thought that the entire visceral motor system of amphioxus was homologous with the sympathetic nervous system of vertebrates, the rostral autonomic nerves are probably parasympathetic, because they are associated with the large series of branchial nerves of this animal, the forerunners of the vagus (Chapter 4). Segmental sympathetic ganglia do not differentiate in amphioxus.

In petromyzonts, as with amphioxus, the separate dorsal and ventral spinal roots do not unite after emerging from the spinal cord. Preganglionic sympathetic fibers arise from the dorsal roots and some neurons with which they synapse form scattered, poorly organized ganglia in the dorsal wall of the body. Longitudinal connections between ganglia are lacking. Terminal sympathetic ganglion cells are also found in the enteric plexus, the buccal and branchial mucosa, connective tissue about the kidneys and excretory ducts, and in the walls of venous sinusoids, dorsal cardinal veins, segmental veins, and smaller vessels. The later phylogenetic relocation of terminal sympathetic neurons in specialized ganglia suggests that the original condition of neurons scattered within the walls of end-organs is the more primitive; it is retained by the parasympathetic system in higher vertebrates. Chromaffin tissue is widely distributed along large veins and the dorsal body wall in cyclostomes and is innervated by sympathetic nerves.

The facial nerve of cyclostomes contains parasympathetic fibers related to the control of branchial, or gill arch, circulation (Lindström, 1949). Parasympathetic components of the vagus are distributed to the heart, jugular vein, and pharyngeal wall, where they synapse with scattered neurons in the walls to form terminal plexuses. Unconfirmed evidence suggests that one or more branches of the vagus may supply the intestine distal to the pharynx and esophagus. If this innervation occurs, some of the terminal neurons embedded in the intestinal wall are parasympathetic.

The arrangement of visceral nerves in *Ammocoetes,* a larval petromyzont, is between amphioxus and adult lampreys in complexity (Pick, 1970). The vagal nerve is formed by the fusion of several segments.

Elasmobranchs have better developed and more extensive sympathetic and parasympathetic systems than do cyclostomes. Sympathetic nerves no longer emerge from the dorsal roots, but rather from the ventral roots, as in all higher vertebrates. White communicating rami are sympathetic preganglionic fibers that separate from the ventral roots and terminate in sympathetic ganglia. The ganglia are segmentally arranged on both sides, each ganglion corresponding to one ventral root. The absence of gray communicating rami, however, is associated with the absence of autonomic innervation of dermal structures in elasmobranchs (Young, 1933). Occasional isolated neurons or small ganglia occur along the proximal course of the sympathetic nerves, a transitional condition between the primitive location of autonomic neurons in the walls of end-organs and their final location in the segmental ganglia in advanced vertebrates. Large, paired gastric ganglia in the wall of the posterior cardinal sinus near the subclavian artery on each side are connected by white communicating rami with several anterior spinal nerves of the corresponding side. The gastric ganglia are formed embryologically by the fusion of several anterior ganglia, a feature that recurs in phylogeny and increases in advanced vertebrates. Posterior to the gastric ganglia, small bilateral segmental ganglia receive preganglionic fibers from the corresponding ventral root of the spinal cord. Longitudinal fibers connecting the chain of sympathetic ganglia on each side are few and inconstant. Postganglionic fibers are not as well myelinated, but they are more numerous than preganglionic fibers, indicating that each preganglionic axon synapses with several postganglionic neurons. This relation persists throughout phylogeny. The sympathetic system is absent in the tail of elasmobranchs. This lack is probably a secondary modification because transient caudal sympathetic ganglia occur in the embryos of these species. Postganglionic sympathetic fibers comprise the anterior, middle, and posterior splanchnic nerves. They generally accompany blood vessels to the viscera, genital organs, and vascular walls. The head and heart in elasmobranchs lack sympathetic innervation.

Each sympathetic ganglion is accompanied by an aggregate of chromaffin tissue, but the largest masses of this tissue occur in the suprarenal area and in association with the gastric ganglia, forming the "axillary body" on each side. This structure may be the homolog of the carotid body in man. Sympathetic neurons are present among the chromaffin cells. Postganglionic fibers synapse with chromaffin cells in elasmobranchs and other lower vertebrates, in contrast with mammals in whom preganglionic fibers synapse directly on chromaffin cells in the adrenal medulla (Young, 1933; Hollinshead, 1936). A few sympathetic neurons, however, are still found within the adrenal medulla of man.

Elasmobranchs are the lowest vertebrates having a parasympathetic system arising in the midbrain. Preganglionic fibers of the visceral motor component of the oculomotor nerve synapse in the ciliary ganglion in the orbit. Postganglionic ciliary nerves are distributed to orbital blood vessels and to intraocular muscles. Only the ciliary ganglion is organized in the entire parasympathetic system of lower vertebrates, but reptiles and mammals acquire additional ganglia (otic and submaxillary) to innervate salivary glands. In some reptiles, the oral salivary glands become highly specialized as poisonous glands but retain the same innervation.

The autonomic nervous system of holostean fishes, such as the sturgeon, resembles that of elasmobranchs. Many new features, as well as better organization of the sympathetic ganglionic trunks, appear in teleosts. Sympathetic ganglia are connected to spinal nerves by both white rami of myelinated preganglionic fibers and gray rami of unmyelinated postganglionic fibers (Young, 1931a). The teleostean autonomic system therefore approaches that of terrestrial vertebrates in organization and complexity.

In teleosts, the sympathetic system has a well-differentiated, bilaterally symmetric pair of trunks: segmental ganglia are joined by longitudinal fibers. The trunks extend from the first spinal nerve to the end of the tail, although the two trunks fuse between the kidneys to form a single chain for a few segments. In addition, postganglionic fibers of the cervical sympathetic ganglia and some preganglionic fibers extend into the head. Sympathetic ganglia also are associated with the ganglia of the vagal, glossopharyngeal, facial, and trigeminal nerves and with the ciliary ganglion. Fibers pass between the cranial sympathetic ganglia and the parasympathetic cranial nerves, so that the sympathetic and parasympathetic systems become anatomically indistinct and inseparable in the cranial region. The cranial extension of the sympathetic system is lacking in lower vertebrates but is a constant feature in all higher animals. Sympathetic ganglia no longer occur in the head in mammals, however; postganglionic fibers to cranial structures in mammals are derived entirely from cervical sympathetic ganglia.

Postganglionic fibers of more posteriorly located sympathetic ganglia in teleosts are distributed directly to the viscera in splanchnic nerves. Gray communicating rami are absent in elasmobranchs but are present in teleosts in addition to the white communicating rami. The fibers of the gray rami emerge as a bundle from each sympathetic ganglion and reenter the ventral spinal root to be distributed with general somatic sensory fibers to dermal vessels and chromatophores in the skin. In teleosts, the sympathetic distribution is thus extended farther both cranially and peripherally than in cyclostomes, elasmobranchs, and urodeles. Preganglionic fibers no longer all terminate in the ganglion of the corresponding segment but may travel to higher or lower levels in the sympathetic trunk. The communicating rami of the first two cervical sympathetic ganglia contain mostly postganglionic fibers; most of the preganglionic fibers to these ganglia arise in more caudal segments. In mammals, the communicating rami of the cervical sympathetic ganglia are completely lost.

The swim bladder is an air-filled diverticulum of the gut in some teleosts. It functions as a hydrostatic organ for control of depth in water, and also as a resonating membrane for the perception of sound (Chapter 5). The volume of gas in the swim bladder is controlled by sympathetic and vagal fibers as with the stomach (Young, 1931a; von Ledebur, 1937). These autonomic impulses are influenced by pressure perceived in the saccus vasculosus (Chapter 9).

The submucosal and myenteric plexuses of teleosts are better developed than in elasmobranchs and indicate regional specialization in the parasympathetic system.

All major elements of the sympathetic system of reptiles, birds, and mammals are already present in the highly organized sympathetic nervous system of amphibians, particularly that of anurans. Differences among higher vertebrates are more quantitative than qualitative.

Paravertebral sympathetic trunks, composed of segmental ganglia and longitudinal fibers, extend the entire length of the spine. Postganglionic fibers are distributed to visceral, urogenital, vascular, and dermal structures, as well as passing into the head from cervical sympathetic ganglia. White and gray communicating rami are present. Occasional duplication of the sympathetic trunks occurs in some locations in urodeles, but is inconstant.

Parasympathetic fibers emerge from the sacral cord in anuran amphibians, unlike the condition in fishes. The fibers do not form communicating rami or distinct ganglia and do not enter the sympathetic trunk. They are distributed to the rectum, urinary bladder, and genital organs, where they synapse with ganglion cells embedded in the walls of these organs. The structures receiving sacral parasympathetic fibers also receive postganglionic fibers of the sympathetic system, establishing an anatomic basis for balanced antagonism. Sacral sympathetic ganglia disappear in mammals, but the urogenital organs, rectum, and distal colon retain sympathetic innervation from lumbar ganglia.

The heart receives sympathetic fibers, in addition to the phylogenetically old parasympathetic innervation, in anurans and all higher vertebrates. The peripheral distribution of nerves to the heart in representative vertebrates was systematically investigated by Hirsch (1970), although he did not study the central origin of the preganglionic fibers. A system of ganglion cells with both coarse and thin myelinated fibers is distributed along the aortas, epicardium, and endocardium in the hagfish. The myocardium of this myxinoid contains a plexus of terminal nerve fibers similar to, and almost as extensive as, that occurring in the hearts of more advanced fishes and amphibians. Among teleosts, amphibians, reptiles, birds, and mammals, including man, a common pattern prevails in the structure and distribution of the nerves innervating the myocardium. Many large nerves mostly originating in vagal ganglia have small branches forming an extensive subendocardial plexus. The myoneural connections of the terminal fibers are perimysial, not intracellular, an arrangement similar to the myoneural junction of skeletal muscle. Subtle structural differences are common in the pattern of innervation of the heart among different orders and species of mammals.

The hearts of all vertebrates have an intrinsic conduction system composed of specialized myocardial fibers. In advanced vertebrates, this system includes the sinoatrial and atrioventricular nodes, bundle of His, left and right bundle branches, and fibers of Purkinje. Lower vertebrates have less complete systems because the interventricular septum is absent. The specialized myocardial cells of the conduction system are richly supplied with autonomic nerves, as are the papillary muscles, although muscle fibers of the general myocardium also receive direct innervation (Hirsch, 1970).

The peripheral autonomic innervation of the lung in different vertebrates was studied by Hirsch and Kaiser (1969). The relatively large amount of smooth muscle in the lungs of amphibians, reptiles, and birds comprise an intrinsic muscular apparatus for expansion and compression during breathing. Mammals, in contrast, have a pleural space, a large amount of supplementary muscle in the thoracic wall and neck, and a muscular diaphragm. These structures expand and compress the lung even more efficiently. Smooth muscle in the lungs of mammals is therefore largely limited to the walls of bronchioles, and the autonomic innervation of the lungs is correspondingly less extensive. Both vagal and sympathetic fibers innervate the lungs in all terrestrial vertebrates.

Coelacanths and lungfishes (Dipnoi), the closest living descendants of the crossopterygians, have a loosely organized autonomic system similar to that of elasmobranchs, without cranial or peripheral extensions of the sympathetic system (Holmes, 1950; Nicol, 1952). It is remarkable that, although teleostean fishes and terrestrial vertebrates evolved along different and independent lines, the autonomic systems developed similarly. This phenomenon is unlikely to have occurred by chance. It is more probable that a placoderm or another early common ancestor had already begun to develop the advanced modifications of the autonomic nervous system.

Chromaffin tissue is widely distributed, particularly near and within sympathetic ganglia of most vertebrates. In mammals, particularly man, it becomes almost exclusively limited to the adrenal medulla, carotid bodies, glomus jugulare, and organ of Zuckerkandl (chromaffin tissue found in late fetal and early postnatal life at the origin of the inferior mesenteric artery). Even in man, collections of chromaffin cells are encountered occasionally within or near sympathetic ganglia, remnants of a distribution that was at one time extensive.

Central autonomic regulatory centers

Visceral regulatory centers are widespread within the central nervous system. The dominant correlative and associative regions for visceral function are the hypothalamus and the limbic system of the forebrain, although the insular region of the cerebral cortex may also influence visceral activity. The reticular formation of the brainstem regulates some visceral activities as well, particularly cardiac and respiratory function.

Preganglionic efferent fibers of the cranial parasympathetic system originate in the Edinger-Westphal nucleus of the oculomotor complex, and visceral motor nuclei associated with branchial nerves, such as the salivatory nuclei and the dorsal motor nucleus of the vagus. Preganglionic sympathetic fibers originate in the intermediolateral columns of the spinal cord. Sacral parasympathetic fibers also arise in that location. These centers are discussed in other chapters.

Possible relation of phylogeny to peripheral autonomic syndromes

Several syndromes of autonomic dysfunction are known. Among these are familial dysautonomia of Riley-Day, in which a decreased number of neurons is present in the sympathetic ganglia and dorsal spinal root ganglia (Pearson et al., 1971, 1973). Deficiencies of dopamine-beta-hydroxylase (Smith et al., 1964; Weinshilboum and Axelrod, 1971) and of choline acetyltransferase (Mittag et al., 1973) in many patients with this disease are probably related, at least in part, to lack of development of autonomic neurons. In another disorder, orthostatic hypotension has been correlated at necropsy with degeneration of preganglionic autonomic neurons of brain and spinal cord (Shy and Drager, 1960; Schwarz, 1967). Adie's syndrome of the myotonic pupil may also be accompanied by postural hypotension and absent muscle stretch reflexes. Neuronal degeneration in the ciliary ganglion has been shown in Adie's syndrome

(Harriman and Garland, 1968), and the accompanying clinical features suggest a lesion also in the sympathetic and dorsal root ganglia.

The dorsal root ganglia and sympathetic ganglia are embryologic derivatives of the neural crest and also have a common phylogenetic origin. The origin of the ciliary ganglion is obscure, however. It is absent in cyclostomes who lack intraocular muscles and is developed in elasmobranchs and in all higher vertebrates. It is one of the few parts of the parasympathetic system that morphologically resembles sympathetic ganglia; some sympathetic fibers to the eye actually pass through it.

These autonomic syndromes do not correspond to the normal condition in any known living creature. The derivatives of neural crest are among the first neural components to differentiate both ontogenetically and phylogenetically, and they are well-developed primordia even in amphioxus. The diseases of autonomic degeneration suggest that some metabolic features of the neural crest are unique and are selectively impaired in these cases. This condition contrasts with the more common pattern of many degenerative diseases of the nervous system, in which phylogenetically recent structures are selectively affected (Chapter 1). It would be interesting to examine the neural plexuses in the walls of end-organs of such patients to determine if a phylogenetically primitive or normal human pattern prevails.

11
Reticular formation

Reticular formation of brainstem

The reticular formation of the human brain is an irregular column of neurons extending from the medulla through the tegmentum of the pons and midbrain. It is continuous with the intralaminar nuclei of the dorsal thalamus. This column is sometimes regarded as poorly differentiated gray matter because the boundaries are uncertain and anatomically distinct clusters of neurons are rare. Physiologically, however, the reticular formation is as highly specialized as any part of the central nervous system.

The organization of the reticular formation is well suited to the function of sleep cycles, generalized arousal, and the maintenance of consciousness. Dendrites of individual neurons extend over large areas, creating many synapses with collateral fibers of ascending and descending tracts, and adjacent nuclei. Short and long axons provide both slow and rapid conduction and numerous interconnections.

The anatomy of the reticular formation was studied in the cat by Nauta and Kuypers (1958). They found the following major connections: (A) A widespread pathway extending the length of the brainstem, containing numerous axons originating in the medial regions of the medulla and pons, mixed with other diffuse fiber systems, including ascending spinal and trigeminal pathways. The axons are distributed to extensive regions of the tegmental reticular formation, periaqueductal gray matter, optic tectum and pretectal area, intralaminar thalamic nuclei, and subthalamic region. Most of the fibers ascending to the diencephalon originate in areas rostral to the inferior olives; (B) The smaller neurons of the lateral part of the medullary reticular formation give origin to a lateral fasciculus that serves as an intrinsic association system, although some fibers ascend to the diencephalon; (C) An extensive region of the mesencephalon projects to the hypothalamus, preoptic area, and medial septal nucleus by the dorsal longitudinal fasciculus. The origin of these fibers includes the ventral part of the periaqueductal gray matter and the more distinct reticular nuclei known as the dorsal tegmental nucleus, deep tegmental nucleus, and ventral tegmental area of Tsai. It is reciprocally connected with the limbic system. The mesencephalic reticular formation is part of a neural mechanism of homeostatic control over some endocrine and autonomic functions; (D) Direct projections to the caudate nucleus and putamen arise in the mesencephalic tegmentum near the red nucleus.

The extent of these connections of the reticular formation in submammalian vertebrates is almost unknown. The gray matter surrounding the cerebral aqueduct is part of the mesencephalic reticular formation in mammals. It is less distinct in reptiles and birds, and not clearly demarcated in amphibians and fishes.

The descending reticulospinal pathways are discussed in Chapter 7. The direct reticulospinal tract is a phylogenetically new pathway found in mammals. Lower vertebrates have polysynaptic pathways, but similar functions may be served by vestibulospinal, tectospinal, and other direct motor pathways from the brainstem.

The reticular formation is the substrate of a polysynaptic pathway of ascending and descending impulses throughout phylogeny. Lower vertebrates probably depend on these pathways more than do advanced species because the direct motor pathways from the brain to the spinal cord are fewer and smaller, and motor nuclei differentiate from reticular neurons in phylogeny (Chapter 7). The reticular formation remains useful in generalized responses even in man, because of the extensive connections. For example, collateral fibers of ascending sensory pathways synapse with reticular neurons, and account for the generalized arousal response to tactile stimuli in sleeping or obtunded patients.

In addition to functioning as a pacemaker of sleep and wakefulness, the reticular formation also is active in regulation of the autonomic nervous system. The medullary portions of the reticular formation near the nuclei of the facial, glossopharyngeal, and vagal nerves are particularly important in the vital functions of the cardiovascular and respiratory systems.

The reticular formation thus provides a mechanism of divergence whereby specific impulses may be disseminated throughout the central nervous system and evoke generalized responses. It also provides a pathway from almost any part of the brainstem, such as the vestibular nuclei, to almost any other, even in the absence of direct fiber tracts. Many other functions of the reticular formation are not known to be related to phylogenetic considerations.

Phylogeny of sleep

All vertebrates experience cycles of activity and inactivity. In lower species, "sleep" is difficult to define as the term applies to man, but even amphioxus buries itself in the sand and is inactive during the day, emerging to filter-feed only at night. Little is known about sleep in fishes.

Sleep may be divided into two basic stages in marsupial and placental mammals (Jouvet, 1967). These two alternating patterns of deep (slow-wave) sleep and paradoxical or active sleep recur several times each night. Each stage is characterized by specific electroencephalographic features: deep sleep has slow, synchronous, cortical electric activity; paradoxical sleep is associated with fast, low voltage, asynchronous cortical activity similar to that of wakefulness. Rapid eye movements and dreaming occur during paradoxical sleep.

Paradoxical sleep comprises 20 per cent of total sleep in adult man and in carnivores, 15 per cent in rodents, and only 6.6 per cent in ruminants; newborns of each species of mammals have two to three times more paradoxical sleep than do the adults (Rechtshaffen et al., 1963). Only 0.5 per cent of the total sleep of birds is paradoxical, however, and reptiles have no paradoxical sleep observed electroencephalographically (Rechtshaffen et al., 1963). In hens, chicks, and pigeons, the electroencephalogram in sleep resembles that of mammals, although spindles (sigma waves) are lacking; avian paradoxical sleep is extremely short, lasting about ten seconds, and is accompanied by acceleration of the electric activity of the hyperstriatum, reduction in tone of cervical muscles, bursts of phasic ocular movements, and bradycardia (Jouvet, 1967).

Jouvet (1967) suggested that the phylogenesis of sleep mechanisms is related to the evolution of reticular dopaminergic neurons in the pontine tegmentum and median raphé. The process governing deep sleep, in contrast, is mediated by serotonergic neurons.

The parts of the mammalian reticular formation effecting arousal are located in the midbrain (Moruzzi and Magoun, 1949). Reticular activity in the pons results in paradoxical or active sleep; pontine inhibition by the medullary reticular formation results in deep sleep (Moruzzi, 1964). The reticular formation of the brainstem is thus the central pacemaker of cycles of sleep and wakefulness and also influences states of consciousness in illness.

Reticular formation of diencephalon

The mammalian intralaminar nuclei are diffuse groups of neurons in the internal medullary lamina of the thalamus. They are characterized by extensive and diffuse connections with the reticular formation of the brainstem, spinal cord, cerebellum, and optic tectum (Ebbesson et al., 1972). The influence on intralaminar thalamic nuclei by the reticular formation of the brainstem is shown by the frequency with which seizures occur in epileptic patients during the induction of sleep or arousal. The clinical manifestations are associated with the production of bisynchronous spike-and-wave discharges (Pollen, 1968).

The intralaminar nuclei may be regarded as a diencephalic extension of the reticular formation. They are not recognized with certainty in submammalian vertebrates, although some groups of thalamic neurons even in sharks have similar afferent connections and may be homologous (Ebbesson et al., 1972). The midline nuclei of the thalamus are similarly not differentiated morphologically, or are identified on the basis of connections in submammalian species (Ebbesson et al., 1972).

The massa intermedia is a structure within the third ventricle, bridging the thalami of the two sides. Although it has been termed the "thalamic adhesion," this designation is inappropriate because it infers that the massa intermedia is something other than gray matter composing part of the midline thalamic nuclei. The massa intermedia is large in some mammals, such as the horse (Fig. 11-1), and in some primates it almost fills the third ventricle. In man, it is relatively small, but variable in size in different individuals, and may even normally be lacking in some (Rosales et al., 1968). When it is absent, the nuclei are incorpo-

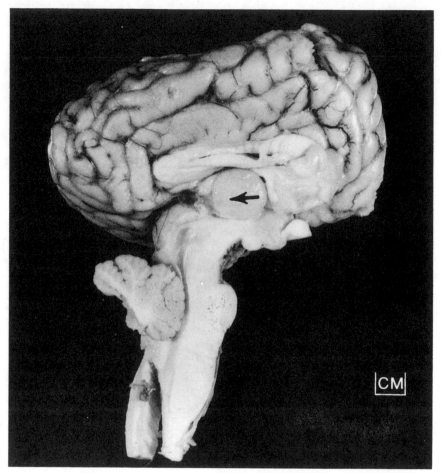

Figure 11-1   Mid-sagittal section of the brain of a horse, demonstrating large size of massa intermedia (arrow) relative to that of man. The structure almost fills the third ventricle, resembling a tumor. The posterior part of the cerebellum was torn away.

rated into the medial walls of the thalami and do not meet in the midline. In the monkey, a few commissural fibers connecting the lateral posteroventral thalamic nuclei of the two sides by passing through the massa intermedia were described (Glees and Wall, 1948), but none have been demonstrated in man (Toncray and Krieg, 1946). There is therefore little evidence to conclude that the presence of a massa intermedia in man may reduce the paralytic effects of a lesion in the motor cortex by providing a link between the ascending pathways of the two sides of the body to permit bilateral motor cortical influence (Lumpey, 1972). Electric stimulation of the anterior part of the massa intermedia in cats produces bilaterally synchronous spike-and-wave discharges in the cerebral cortex, similar to those associated with petit mal epilepsy in man (Hunter and Jasper, 1949).

The centromedian nucleus becomes progressively developed within the internal medullarly lamina of higher mammals (Walker, 1966). Its connections with the corpus striatum suggest a correlative function of this nucleus between the reticular formation and the neostriatum.

The intralaminar thalamic nuclei project to extensive areas of cerebral cortex in mammals, but data are not available for other vertebrates. Even in mammals, the details of these projections have not yet been ascertained and the evidence is largely electrophysiologic (Morrison and Dempsey, 1942). Because of the wide extent of these projections they are often regarded as nonspecific. The concept of "nonspecific" thalamic projections originate in Herrick's descriptions of the diffuse ascending projections of the poorly differentiated thalamus of unspecialized vertebrates, such as the salamander. The concept is also applied to man in describing the generalized activating properties of the reticular formation, the impulses being relayed to the cortex by the intralaminar thalamic nuclei. The concept also persisted in clinical neurology as the idea of "centrencephalic" epilepsy. This term has been used to describe bilaterally synchronous polyspike-and-wave discharges in the electroencephalogram. The epileptogenic focus in such cases is assumed to be in a midline pacemaker in the brainstem and diffusely projected to the cortex of both hemispheres by nonspecific thalamic relay (Jasper and Kershman, 1941). The actual extent of interconnections between the two sides of the brain in the reticular formation is probably great, but it needs further experimental documentation.

The zona incerta (peripeduncular nucleus) is a band of gray matter lying dorsomedial to the subthalamic nucleus in man. It is primordial in reptiles and birds, larger in lower mammals, and best developed in man and other advanced mammals. The poorly understood zona incerta and the nucleus of the field of Forel are regarded as another part of the reticular formation (Truex and Carpenter, 1970).

Locus coeruleus

The locus coeruleus (laterodorsal tegmental nucleus) is in the pons of all mammals, and in birds (Russell, 1955). Its presence in lower vertebrates is uncertain, but it probably is derived from the superior reticular nucleus of fishes, amphibians, and reptiles (Kappers et al., 1936; Russell, 1955). The nucleus is distinct in most mammals because of the accumulation of melanin within the neurons, particularly in higher primates. The significance of this neuromelanin and that in neurons of the substantia nigra is discussed in Chapter 12.

Afferent connections of the locus coeruleus include fibers from: (A) The trigeminal nucleus, including the chief sensory and mesencephalic nuclei; (B) A diffuse interstitial plexus that lies in the tegmental reticular formation, extending the length of the pons and medulla, and probably includes visceral sensory projections; (C) Collaterals of the dorsal longitudinal fasciculus; (D) Collaterals of the lateral lemniscus; (E) Possibly the amygdala. Efferent connections of the locus coeruleus are limited to a descending uncrossed tract terminating in the reticular formation around the inferior olivary complex (Russell, 1955).

Russell (1955) concluded that the locus coeruleus is the "pneumotaxic center." He proposed that it serves a relay function in the cortical and subcortical facilitation of control over autonomic functions. Trigemino-coeruleal fibers thus may be part of the mechanism of respiration involving facial and masticatory muscles. Connections from the lateral lemniscus of the auditory system may explain the sudden reflexive inspiration observed in the startle reaction after a sudden loud noise. The concept that the locus coeruleus is an important reticular center in the regulation of sleep cycles is unproved.

12

Forebrain and some related structures

Origin of forebrain

The evolution of the forebrain or telencephalon is unlike that of most other parts of the central nervous system. Instead of progressive differentiation of structure in successively higher classes of vertebrates, each class has evolved specialization of different structures of the forebrain. The resultant form of the cerebral hemispheres in the most advanced species of each class only remotely resembles the forebrain in advanced species of others. Primitive species of each class, however, resemble each other more closely.

The forebrain probably is not an intrinsic portion of the primitive neural tube, as are the medulla, midbrain, and diencephalon. In mammalian embryos it is derived from paired lateral outgrowths at the rostral end of the neural tube (Fig. 12-1). Even in adult man, the most rostral extension of the embryonic neural tube is still demarcated at the anterior limit of the diencephalon by the lamina terminalis and the velum interpositum. A telencephalon is totally lacking in amphioxus, further suggesting that the forebrain is a secondarily developed structure, and not part of the original neural tube.

Recent discoveries in the thalamotelencephalic connections in submammalian vertebrates pose questions not previously considered about the phylogenetic origin of the forebrain. Ascending thalamocortical projections in man and other mammals are entirely ipsilateral. In the shark, corresponding pathways decussate completely, however (Ebbesson and Schroeder, 1971). One interpretation of this contrast is that the ascend-

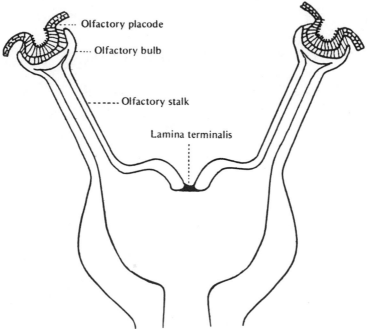

Figure 12-1 Drawing of outgrowths of the rostrolateral walls of the forebrain in the direction of the developing placodes of olfactory epithelium. This simple, traditional explanation is challenged by the recent finding that ascending thalamotelencephalic projections completely decussate in the shark (see text) (Kappers, Huber and Crosby, 1936).

ing fibers from the diencephalon originally formed a bilateral projection in an ancestral vertebrate; the ipsilateral connections were lost in the evolution of modern sharks, and the contralateral pathways disappeared in evolving mammals (Ebbesson, personal communication). More data regarding thalamic connections in other vertebrates are needed for further refinement of this theory.

The traditional concept of the inseparability of thalamus and cerebral cortex may be further challenged by considering the "diffuse versus discrete" fiber connections among various mammals (Jane and Schroeder, 1971). Auditory and somatosensory pathways overlap greatly in the dorsal thalamus of the hedgehog, but project discretely to the medial geniculate body and ventroposterior nucleus, respectively, in more advanced species. The visual pathways, in contrast, are quite discrete even in the hedgehog, and the projections of the lateral geniculate body to cerebral cortex are equally specific and not diffuse. The parcellation of sensory projections to specific and exclusive neurons of the dorsal thalamus precedes the specialization of cortical regions in the evolution of mammals, and the thalamus thus is the highest center for analyzing specific sensory information in many mammals. The cortex in these animals probably serves to inhibit inappropriate responses selectively, as demonstrated in the visual system of the tree shrew (Jane et al., 1972).

Throughout phylogeny, the thalamus has few descending fibers; its efferent discharge is almost entirely projected into the forebrain; neither structure functions completely independently of the other, particularly in higher mammals. In man the interdependence of diencephalon and telencephalon extends even to speech. This unique human capability is usually regarded as one of the most complex functions of the cerebral cortex, but the importance of the ventrolateral nucleus of the thalamus in speech has also been demonstrated (Ojemann and Ward, 1971).

The evolution of the forebrain as a secondary neural structure occurred when filter-feeding protochordates became active seekers of food. The earliest true vertebrates, therefore, probably had already developed a forebrain.

Figures 12-2 and 12-3 are simplified diagrams illustrating the relative development of structures of the forebrain in each major class of vertebrates. The general configuration of the cerebral hemisphere, namely, that portion of the forebrain posterior to the olfactory bulbs and tracts, and the position and shape of the lateral ventricles are a result of the differential growth of the various structures. Differentiation of selective structures of the forebrain characterizes each class of vertebrates.

In the primitive condition, the lateral outgrowths of the anterior end of the neural tube have dorsal and ventral walls of approximately equal size. In cyclostomes, elasmobranchs, and in all terrestrial vertebrates, both dorsal and ventral walls grow medially to form a pair of tubular, inverted cerebral hemispheres. The walls of each hemisphere thus surround an extension of the third ventricle to form the lateral ventricle on each side. In higher vertebrates, differential growth of the original walls greatly modifies the shape of the hemispheres. The two hemispheres may be separated from each other as in most reptiles, may be fused by a thin layer of ependyma as in some amphibians, or the neural tissue of the medial walls of the two hemispheres may be continuous. Commissural fibers join the hemispheres at the junction of the diencephalon in all vertebrates.

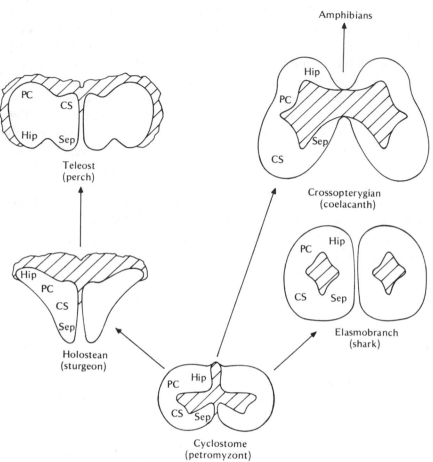

Figures 12-2 and 12-3   Relative position of homologous structures in a coronal section of the forebrain of representative species of each class of vertebrate. In holostean and teleostean fishes, the everted forebrain results from the lateral growth of
structures. This condition creates an external ventricle covered dorsally by an ependy-

In bony fishes, the growth of the primitive telencephalon is lateral
rather than medial, resulting in an everted forebrain (Niewenhuys,
1969). A lateral ventricle thus is not formed, and the third ventricle
is continuous with the space over the everted forebrain. The cerebrospinal fluid is contained by an expanded ependymal membrane over the
dorsal surface of the brain (Fig. 12-2). The everted condition of the

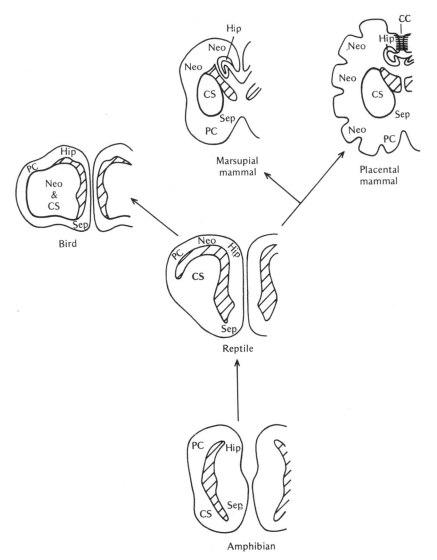

mal sheet. Most other vertebrates have inverted forebrains resulting from medial growth, forming a lateral ventricle within each hemisphere. The arrows indicate the progression in evolution. Precise boundaries of each structure are poorly understood in most submammalian vertebrates. Corpus callosum (CC); hippocampus (Hip); neocortex (Neo); piriform cortex (PC); septum (Sep); corpus striatum (CS).

forebrain makes fishes good experimental animals for the intraventicular instillation of various substances, because the needle does not have to pass through cerebral tissue.

The generalized inverted cerebral hemisphere of amphibians has four major portions surrounding the lateral ventricle (Fig. 12-3): (A) the medial wall is composed of the septum, and archicortex (hippocampus and amygdala); (B) the lateral wall is composed of the corpus striatum, and paleocortex (olfactory tubercle and piriform cortex). The neocortex is first recognized in reptiles in the region between the hippocampus and piriform cortex, but the primordium of this important structure may be contained within the telencephalon of lower vertebrates as well. All other structures of the forebrain are derived from these basic components.

Cephalization and cerebral plasticity

"Cephalization" is a term denoting an evolutionary trend toward progressive phylogenetic development of centers in more rostral parts of the brain, to allow expanded functions in systems already primarily organized for reflexive activity. The forebrain evolved to permit refinement and flexibility of function through greater associative capacity; it evolved to satisfy a need for a functionally plastic structure. The older centers were so highly organized for reflexes that further development and enlargement of these older structures could not offer plasticity without sacrificing reflexes that were still needed.

In cephalization, phylogenetically old centers are supplemented rather than replaced. Both simple and conditioned reflexive responses are kept. Additional pathways incorporating old structures may develop in higher species, paralleling other new pathways that bypass these old structures.

Cephalization leads to progressive dependence upon the function of the forebrain. Ability to regress and exclusively use phylogenetically old centers is lost. An opossum with a lesion of the visual area of the cortex may still retain useful vision if the optic tectum remains intact; a similar lesion in man causes blindness. Unilateral ablation of the motor cortex or corticospinal tract in the rat results in transient impairment of walking; a similar lesion in man leads to permanent spastic hemiplegia. For these reasons, the relation between old and new centers within a functional system is perhaps studied better in lower mammals than in man.

The same plasticity or adaptability of the forebrain even makes it possible for different classes of vertebrates to accomplish similar function in different structures, such as association in the corpus striatum of birds and in the neocortex of mammals. The highly developed corpus striatum of birds is not entirely homologous with just the striatum of mammals because the structure in birds may incorporate some of the primordial neocortex of reptiles. This same feature of plasticity makes generalizations about function based on the study of one species highly speculative when applied to another, and less reliable than in more constant parts of the nervous system.

Association, instinct, and limbic system

Association was defined in Chapter 9 as the sequence of gathering relevant data, discriminating the relative importance of each, comparing them with each other and with past experience, and determining appropriate responses. Higher associative functions include a prediction of the consequences of each course of action, deductive problem-solving, and abstract and creative thinking. Association fibers are intrinsic fibers remaining within a structure or connecting areas of cortex to form an integrated whole.

Instinct, in contrast, is here defined as a genetically determined pattern of behavior. This definition specifically excludes conditioned reflexes and learned behavior, sometimes attributed to instinct. Instinctive behavioral characteristics are generally well suited to the specialized features of the body in the evolution of each species; individuals or species with inappropriate behavior in relation to their physical capabilities do not survive unless these behavioral patterns are soon modified by experience and learning.

The anatomic substrate of instinct is as difficult to localize in the brain as is memory. The genetic basis of instinct suggests that this phenomenon may be associated with specific neural organization. The coordinated behavioral patterns determined by instinct probably originate in centers similar to those where memory is stored. Because instinct governs most behavior in lower vertebrates, its anatomic substrate must be a phylogenetically old structure and present in even the lowest species. It is probable, however, that secondary centers of instinct may also have developed in recently evolved structures of the forebrain, as a type of cephalization.

It is likely that most instinct originates in the hippocampus. This structure is well developed throughout phylogeny. It is not primarily concerned with a particular special sense or with primary motor activity. The habenula may direct feeding activities in lower vertebrates (Chapter 9). The importance of instinct in relation to the reticular formation remains to be defined. Both the habenula and the reticular formation have direct and indirect connections with the hippocampus and related structures. The hippocampus is related to the neocortex in mammals, both by direct connections and also through the mammillary bodies and thalamus.

Little evidence exists that the limbic lobe of Broca, including the hippocampal complex, cingulate gyrus, amygdala, and septum, is an important component of the olfactory system of lower vertebrates as suggested by Herrick, or that these structures in man assume a unique function related to emotion, mood, and libido. Connections of these structures with the olfactory bulbs are lacking and projections from secondary olfactory centers are few throughout phylogeny. Although lower vertebrates do not display the large variety of subtle moods of human beings, or perhaps man is not sufficiently sensitive to the recognition of emotion in fishes and reptiles, states of contentment, excitement, anger, and fear may be observed in almost all animals.

It is reasonable to postulate that if emotion indeed resides in the limbic system of man, then it probably also has an anatomic substrate in homologous structures of other vertebrates. Papez (1937) suggested an anatomic basis for emotion by considering the hippocampus to be the center of feelings of emotion, and the fornix the major pathway over which these feelings could be expressed by the production of autonomic phenomena in the hypothalamus and mammillary bodies. According to Papez's scheme, the cingulate gyrus disseminated impulses to neocortical areas. The projection of impulses from the mammillary body to the anterior thalamic nuclei (mammillothalamic fasciculus), then to the cingulate gyrus, and finally back to the hippocampus provided a feedback loop of the limbic system.

The limbic structures are related to olfaction in species other than man only with respect to the relative importance of olfaction as one of several special senses in those animals. Olfactory impulses enter the limbic system through the amygdala. That the hippocampus is the site of origin of emotion and mood is in accord with the previously stated hypothesis that the hippocampus is the primary center of instinct. Emotion and instinct are closely related and influence each other to a great extent, particularly with regard to characteristics of temperament peculiar to individual species of animals. Differences in personality among individuals of a single species probably are also in part genetically determined.

Other functions of the limbic structures may include regulation of some visceral activities and control of reticular activating influences upon the neocortex (Green, 1964). In addition, the hippocampus and mammillary bodies are implicated in the storage of recent memory. The evidence for this hypothesis was reviewed by Kahn and Crosby (1972), who proposed that the impairment of memory in patients with Korsakoff's syndrome is associated with involvement of these structures. Probably all vertebrates are capable of limited memory, even if only to serve as a basis for simple conditioned reflexes in the most primitive species.

The original function of the telencephalic outgrowths of the neural tube may have been related to the special sense of olfaction. Most of the forebrain of even the lowest presently living species is however, non-olfactory. Early concepts of the extent and importance of olfactory structures in the evolution of the telencephalon have been greatly modified (Allison, 1953; Heimer, 1969). Our understanding of function of most of the forebrain in lower vertebrates is less than our knowledge of the human brain.

Olfaction and mechanism of tracking

The lowest living vertebrates, the cyclostomes, have an olfactory system. It is similar to other special sensory systems in being bilateral and symmetric. Olfaction was a significant addition to the tactile receptive ability of protochordates, not only informing the earliest vertebrates about the environment but allowing this information to be perceived without physical contact. The olfactory epithelium was probably the first receptor of distant information; it is simple and well developed in living lower vertebrates. Although early investigators described an olfactory placode and a single median olfactory nerve in amphioxus, that interpretation is probably incorrect (Chapter 2). It cannot as yet be determined if all special senses evolved together or sequentially.

The neural organization that accompanied the development of olfactory receptors allowed animals to find food by the mechanism of tracking. Tracking is so successful a process that it evolved similarly in the other systems of reception of distant information, vision and hearing. Tracking is dependent upon the ability to discriminate changes in intensity of a continuous stimulus, relative to movement of the target. It allows information regarding distance to be correlated with time; direction of movement and a prediction of future movement of a tracked object can then be computed. Olfaction is the simplest special sense in the neural organization of tracking. It does not involve comparison to two sides as does auditory localization, nor does it depend on precise somatotopic projection as does visual tracking. Also, the number of competitive odors in the background is generally less than distracting stimuli in audition or vision. Complex aspects of olfactory tracking, however, are also demonstrated by inability of fishes to correctly localize a source of odor without a differential rate of flow of water (Kleerekoper, 1967).

The rhinencephalon includes the primary and secondary olfactory structures of the forebrain. The term has been used to include structures of the limbic system because of the earlier belief that these were also primarily olfactory in function. The constancy of neural olfactory structures and their connections throughout vertebrates is particularly remarkable because of the early phylogenetic appearance of these structures in the telencephalon, the part of the brain with the greatest variations among species. Because man is among those vertebrates that do not generally rely upon olfaction for tracking food, recognizing enemies, or mating, the importance of this special sense in the evolution of cerebral structure and behavior is difficult to appreciate.

Olfactory structures are phylogenetically retrogressive or even secondarily lacking in some vertebrates, including most birds, whales, and primates.

Olfactory receptors

A pair of nasal cavities and a specialized sensory epithelium, the olfactory placode, are differentiated in all vertebrates except a few in whom the primary olfactory structures have been lost in evolution. The nasal cavities open to the outside through a median orifice above the mouth in petromyzonts, or within the pharynx in myxinoids. Teleosts and other bony fishes have a pair of olfactory pits lying on the dorsal surface of the head, removed from the currents of water entering the mouth for respiration.

In elasmobranchs, a pair of olfactory pits open into large sacs formed by specialized epithelium on the ventral side of the snout. The current of water entering the mouth passes over these olfactory sacs. The olfactory epithelium in elasmobranchs, such as sharks, is in the current of water intended for respiration. This condition is unlike that of teleosts but similar to that of lungfishes and of terrestrial vertebrates, in whom air instead of water passes over the olfactory epithelium before entering the respiratory structures. The arrangement of neural structures of the inverted forebrain of elasmobranchs is also more similar to that of lungfishes and primitive terrestrial vertebrates than to that of bony fishes. This evidence corroborates other indications that elasmobranchs and teleosts evolved independently.

Internal nares opening into the roof of the mouth in lungfishes and primitive amphibians correspond to the choanae of more advanced animals. External nares open on the snout of all vertebrates that breathe air. In the phylogenetic series of air-breathing animals, nasal cavities are subdivided into compartments by increasingly complex bony structures and folding of the mucous membranes. Turbinate bones are large and complex in most mammals, but they are reduced in primates to simple, scroll-like structures, the conchae. Paranasal air sinuses, particularly ethmoturbinates, develop in marsupial and placental mammals. They support much of the olfactory mucosa. The nasal structure in lower tetrapods has been reviewed by Parsons (1967), that of birds by Stager (1967), and that of mammals by Moulton (1967).

The olfactory epithelium consists of columnar, basal, and sensory receptor cells. The latter bipolar neurons have peripheral "rods" or processes with sensory hairs. Slender axons of these receptors cells form fascicles of the olfactory nerve in the submucosa. The ultrastructure of the olfactory epithelium was described by de Lorenzo (1970).

The olfactory epithelium of the nose is moistened by watery products of mucosal glands in air-breathing vertebrates. Lacrimal secretions from the conjunctival sac also enter the nasal cavity in adult amphibians and most advanced animals. Bowman's glands are thought to participate in olfaction by coating the processes of receptor cells; they occur in most terrestrial animals.

The complex structure of the olfactory organ in many mammals probably is not necessary for olfactory discrimination; man can probably recognize as wide a range of odors as other mammals, although the threshold of sensitivity to odors is considerably higher than in macrosmatic mammals, such as the bloodhound. The molecular and physiologic basis of the detection and discrimination of odors has been discussed in several symposia (Pfaffman, 1969; Wolstenholme and Knight, 1970; Ohloff and Thomas, 1971).

Vomeronasal organ

The olfactory sac of elasmobranchs, some teleosts, and lungfishes is divided into two compartments, each with a separate nerve supply. The medial sensory area is the vomeronasal organ (accessory olfactory organ; organ of Jacobson). In sedentary fishes such as the flounder, the accessory nasal chamber may function as a contractile sac for the replacement of sea water in the olfactory cavity, to prevent the accumulation of debris and also to bring odors in contact with the olfactory epithelium (Kapoor and Ojha, 1972, 1973).

The vomeronasal organ is a highly developed diverticulum in anurans. In snakes and lizards, the vomeronasal organ on each side is a blind sac, opening through the hard palate into the mouth, completely separated from the nasal cavity. The two prongs of the forked tongue insert into this pair of palatal openings, allowing odorous particles adherent to the tips of the tongue to thus be sensed. Most mammals have a vomeronasal organ opening into the nasal cavity or into the nasopalatine canal (Moulton, 1967), but it is atrophic or absent in the adult stage of birds and higher primates. It is present in the human embryo.

The submucosa of the vomeronasal organ is highly vascular. The mucous membrane is similar to olfactory epithelium. The central connections of the vomeronasal organ are similar to those of the primary olfactory system.

Olfactory bulbs

The olfactory bulbs are paired structures with a similar laminated architecture in all vertebrates. They develop phylogenetically and embryologically as rostral extensions of the pair of telencephalic masses. In cyclostomes, they constitute the entire rostral half of the forebrain. The olfactory bulbs are consistently near the olfactory epithelium. In many fishes and in animals with long snouts, the bulbs lie far rostral to the rest of the forebrain, connected by long peduncles of myelinated fibers, and scattered neurons and glia. The formation of the olfactory bulb is similar in vertebrates with either everted or inverted hemispheres of the forebrain.

The lateral ventricles extend into the olfactory bulbs in most vertebrates, but in man and other higher primates this narrow ventricular extension is obliterated in the adult and is usually patent only in fetal life.

Even in adult man, however, vestigial ependymal cells or even ventricular spaces may be seen as vestiges of the olfactory ventricles within the olfactory bulb.

The projection of the olfactory epithelium onto the bulb has spatial localization (LeGros Clark, 1951), but it is not as precise as that of the retina onto the lateral geniculate body. Olfactory discrimination is effected more by the synaptic organization of the olfactory bulb than by responses of peripheral olfactory receptors (Shepherd, 1972).

Axons of the receptor cells of olfactory epithelium make synapses with small granular neurons in the olfactory bulb of petromyzonts. In more advanced fishes, many of these primitive granular cells are differentiated into large triangular mitral cells. In amphibians and higher vertebrates, the primary olfactory synapses are made exclusively with mitral and tufted cells. The latter are modified mitral cells. These primary synapses occur in glomeruli, specialized spherical synaptic zones composed of the convergence of axons from many olfactory receptor cells upon dendrites of fewer mitral cells. It is estimated that in each glomerulus of the rabbit, 26,000 olfactory nerve fibers converge upon 24 mitral cells and 68 tufted cells (Allison and Warwick, 1949). The glomerulus is thus well adapted for spatial summation and contributes to the acuity of the sense of smell. Each mitral cell is associated with two or more glomeruli in reptiles and with larger numbers of glomeruli in lower vertebrates, but in mammals each mitral or tufted cell has a single dendrite, ending in one glomerulus. Diffuse connections are thus replaced by closed, more specific pathways. As greater specificity of these connections evolves, increasing integration within the olfactory bulb is effected by the development of periglomerular neurons in amphibians and higher species. These neurons connect adjacent glomeruli. Granular and small stellate neurons progressively increase to integrate olfactory impulses with afferent impulses from other structures of the basal forebrain. These connections are few in fishes, and are numerous in reptiles and mammals. Associative fibers confined to the olfactory bulb, particularly recurrent collaterals of mitral cells, also increase progressively in phylogeny. The conclusion of early investigators that commissural fibers connect the two olfactory bulbs through the anterior commissure has not been confirmed (Heimer, 1969).

The ultrastructural organization of synapses, and specificity of types of connections within the olfactory bulb is almost identical in all classes of vertebrates (Andres, 1970). Dendrodendritic synapses in the glomeruli of mammals mediate inhibitory feedback onto the principal relay neurons, the mitral and tufted cells; this feedback also involves the periglomerular cells (Shepherd, 1972).

The various layers of cells and fibers in the olfactory bulb are similarly arranged in all vertebrates. The relatively poor lamination in man is consistent with the regression of the olfactory system in primates. Lamination of the olfactory bulb as well as of the piriform cortex is poorly developed in petromyzonts, but remarkably well differentiated in myxinoids, indicating that some other features of the brains of myxinoids are retrogressive and not simply related to an early stage of evolution.

Neurons of the vomeronasal organ project axons to the olfactory bulb in fishes, and to a small but distinct accessory olfactory bulb on each side, in most terrestrial vertebrates. The architecture of the accessory olfactory bulb is similar to that of the main bulb in amphibians and most reptiles (Allison, 1953; Hoffman, 1963; Andres, 1970). The simple structure of the accessory bulb in mammals is comparable to that of the main olfactory bulb of amphibians, in which each mitral cell has many dendrites ending in several glomeruli. The size and differentiation of the accessory bulb is proportionate to that of the vomeronasal organ. It, too, is well developed in the human embryo, but disappears in adult man.

Secondary olfactory centers

The cerebral hemispheres in the lowest vertebrates with inverted forebrains contain basal, lateral, and medial "olfactory" areas. These regions persist in all classes of vertebrates, and similar connections are maintained. Only a portion of these areas is concerned with olfaction, however.

The distribution of fibers from the olfactory bulb in the shark is ipsilateral and is confined to a region on the lateral and ventrolateral surface of the forebrain (Ebbesson and Heimer, 1970). The major part of the telencephalon in this cartilaginous fish is devoid of olfactory connections, although it was once thought to represent a model "olfactory brain" of lower vertebrates.

The massive basal olfactory area of lower vertebrates is the olfactory tubercle of mammals, or anterior perforated substance of man. This structure is derived from paleocortex. Only the anterior part has olfac-

tory connection; the posterior part is related to the preoptic and hypothalamic nuclei.

The lateral olfactory area corresponds to the piriform cortex. The homologous region in man and other mammals is given the deceptive designation of prepiriform cortex; the region just posterior to the prepiriform cortex is then called the entorhinal cortex, although it lacks
olfactory connections and is relatively large in man and other micros-
matic primates. In spite of the constant pattern of the rhinencephalon
throughout phylogeny, the confusing terminology makes the understanding of homologous relations a difficult task. The piriform (prepiriform) cortex is probably the only cortical center that has specific
olfactory function. It is the most important secondary olfactory center.

The medial olfactory area of lower vertebrates is homologous with the
septum, hippocampus, and the primordium of the neocortex, none of
which has significant olfactory connections.

A thin layer of neurons underlies the piriform cortex along the lateral
ventricle. This deep cerebral layer of neurons is designated by many
names in different vertebrates, including the lateral olfactory nucleus,
epistriatum, olfactostriatum, paleostriatum, intercalated nucleus, nucleus
accumbens, and nucleus of the stria terminalis. This nucleus arches over
the lateral forebrain bundle in submammalian species, and over the internal capsule in mammals. It is continuous at one end with the nucleus
of the anterior commissure and the medial preoptic area, and at the
other with the central amygdaloid nucleus.

The anterior olfactory nucleus, largely a nonolfactory structure, is in-
appropriately named, as is true of the naming of many other structures
of the rhinencephalon. This nucleus has poorly defined borders and consists of scattered neurons along the course of the olfactory tract, but few
of these fibers synapse with the neurons. It comprises the rostral part of
the prepiriform cortex of mammals, and the anterior part of the olfactory tubercle.

The olfactory tract conveys impulses from the bulb to other structures
of the forebrain. The tract may be divided in most animals into lateral
and medial (including intermediate) bundles of fibers. Of greater importance, however, is the separation of fibers of the olfactory tract into
superficial cortical and deep subcortical projection systems in all classes
of vertebrates. Most fibers travel in the lateral olfactory tract to the piriform (prepiriform) cortex, to part of the anterior olfactory nucleus, to
part of the olfactory tubercle, and to the medial amygdaloid nucleus.

These thick fibers are the axons of mitral cells of the ipsilateral olfactory bulb, and are among the most heavily myelinated in the brain. Fibers of the deep projection system are thin and lightly myelinated axons of tufted cells. They may partially decussate in the anterior commissure and enter the stria terminalis to be distributed to the lateral olfactory nucleus and to the central amygdaloid nucleus; other thin fibers pass to the medial preoptic area.

Fibers from the accessory olfactory bulb terminate in the anterior olfactory nucleus and in the central amygdaloid nucleus. Details of the distribution of olfactory fibers in various vertebrates are discussed by Allison (1953), Scalia (1968), Scalia et al. (1968), Heimer (1969), and Ebbesson and Heimer (1970).

Experimental data suggest that the subcortical projection system is concerned primarily with the simple recognition of odors; the superficial cortical system involves the use of olfaction in conditioned reflexes and in responses requiring judgment.

Tertiary olfactory centers

Two major pathways relay olfactory impulses from the secondary olfactory areas of the cerebral hemispheres to the diencephalon where visceral activity is initiated. These two pathways are the olfactohypothalamic and the olfactohabenular tracts. In fishes and other animals in whom the optic tectum is an important integrative region, olfactotectal fibers are also conveyed in the olfactohabenular tract. Some secondary olfactory fibers cross in the habenular commissure of amphibians (Scalia et al., 1968) and of reptiles (Heimer, 1969), but this decussation has not been demonstrated in mammals (Scalia, 1968; Heimer, 1969).

The piriform cortex projects bilaterally to the insular cortex or island of Reil (Allison, 1950). Olfaction in mammals is therefore related to a region of the neocortex, as it true of other senses. Taste also has neocortical localization in the para-insular region, adjacent to that of olfaction and near that of somatic sensation from the tongue (Patton, 1950). Taste and olfaction thus are correlated in the neocortex as well as in the hypothalamus.

Other fibers travel from the piriform cortex and also from the amygdala through the stria terminalis to the medial preoptic region (Allison, 1950). The tertiary connections of the olfactory system are incompletely known.

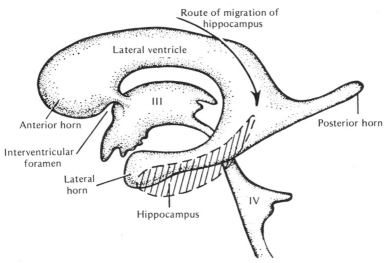

Figure 12-4   Cerebral ventricles of man. The hippocampus develops as a dorsal structure forming the medial part of the cerebral hemisphere in lower terrestrial vertebrates. In advanced mammals, however, the hippocampus is rotated back and down
into a ventral position by the great expansion of the neocortex (Romer, 1970).

Archicortex: hippocampus and amygdala

The archicortex in all vertebrates consists of hippocampus and amygdala. The hippocampus comprises the dorsomedial part of the inverted,
unspecialized forebrain of amphibians. In reptiles, the hippocampus differentiates into a loosely laminated structure. In many species, a dorsal
portion homologous with Ammon's horn (cornu Ammonis) may be recognized, and a dorsomedial portion is homologous with the dentate gyrus of mammals. In birds, the dentate gyrus is smaller and Ammon's
horn is relatively larger than in reptiles.

   In lower mammals, the hippocampus still occupies a primitive dorsal position in the medial wall of the hemisphere. As the neocortex and
corpus callosum develop, the lateral wall of the hippocampus is rolled
medially from above. The subsequent shift causes the formation of the
hippocampal sulcus. Continued growth of the neocortex displaces the
hippocampus back and down in the medial side of the temporal lobe
in man (Fig. 12-4). Transitional positions persist in many other mammals. The hippocampal migration may be disturbed in human cases of
agenesis of the corpus callosum (Kirschbaum, 1947). The great growth

of the neocortex in the normal human embryo, as well as in phylogeny, also causes the hippocampus to roll on itself so that the cortical layer of Ammon's horn is pushed between the separated limbs of the V-shaped dentate gyrus.

As the hippocampus is displaced in phylogenesis from the dorsal position, the efferent fiber projections are maintained by lengthening these fibers, creating a compact bundle, the fornix (inferior or ventral fornix), on either side. The columns of the fornix arch under the corpus callosum, along the migratory path of the hippocampus. The fibers of the fornix are axons of the large pyramidal cells of the hippocampus. These fibers spread over the ventricular surface of the hippocampus, forming the alveus and then converge to become the fimbria. They then proceed caudally under the splenium of the corpus callosum. The fibers of the fornix pass forward and bifurcate, some arching in front of and others behind the anterior commissure. The fornix distributes hippocampal fibers to the mammillary bodies, rostral part of the hypothalamus, lateral preoptic area, septum, and anterior and intralaminar thalamic nuclei. A few fibers reach the tegmentum of the midbrain. Hippocampal commissural fibers also cross between the columns of the fornix on the ventral surface of the corpus callosum. They are known as the superior or dorsal fornix, or psalterium in man. Although the importance of the fornix in man is poorly understood, each human fornix contains more fibers than either the optic nerve or the pyramidal tract.

The principal afferent connections of the hippocampus are from the septum as a relay of visceral and hypothalamic impulses, and from the cingulate gyrus. Some cingulate fibers synapse in the entorhinal area before the impulses are conveyed to the hippocampus.

The amygdala are archicortical structures with only rudimentary lamination in some parts. Several nuclei differentiate within the amygdala, some early and others late in phylogeny. The amygdala gather olfactory impulses and other visceral information essential to the function of the limbic system. Direct fibers from the olfactory bulb terminate in the corticomedial amygdaloid nuclei, and olfactory fibers originating in the piriform cortex end in the basolateral amygdaloid nuclei; fibers from the rostral hypothalamic nuclei project to all amygdaloid nuclei except the central nucleus (Cowan et al., 1965).

The central amygdaloid nucleus is found in all vertebrates. It is a continuation of the lateral olfactory nucleus (nucleus of the stria terminalis). The medial amygdaloid nucleus is primordial in lower vertebrates, and is well developed in reptiles, birds, and mammals. A cortical portion is found only in mammals. The basolateral amygdaloid nuclei are developed only in mammals and are the best differentiated part of the amygdala in man. This portion is continuous with the overlying hippocampus. Although it probably functions as an associative area of the limbic system, it lacks the lamination characteristic of cerebral cortex.

In addition to intimate relations with the hippocampus, fibers also pass from the basolateral amygdaloid nuclei into the fornix to terminate in the mammillary bodies and surrounding hypothalamic nuclei. The most prominent efferent pathway from the amygdala, however, is the stria terminalis. It projects to the preoptic and anterior hypothalamic nuclei, habenula, and to the contralateral amygdala. A ventral amygdaloid projection in man also passes to the preoptic and hypothalamic regions, septum, olfactory tubercle, substantia innominata, dorsomedial thalamic nucleus, and to the ventral insula, claustrum, and rostral neocortical gyri of the temporal lobe (Truex and Carpenter, 1970).

Mesocortex

The cerebral tissue surrounding the hippocampus in adult man and other mammals is transitional in architecture between archi- and neocortex. Six laminae can be distinguished. The main structures of mesocortex include the hippocampal gyrus. This structure is adjacent to the hippocampus. The hippocampus proper consists of Ammon's horn, the dentate gyrus and related fibers. Other mesocortical derivatives are the parahippocampal gyrus including the uncus in man, the cingulate gyrus (fornicate gyrus), entorhinal area (anterior part of parahippocampal gyrus), and para-olfactory area or paraterminal gyrus next to the lamina terminalis. These structures are present in all mammals, but cannot be distinguished from primordial neocortex in reptiles.

The organization of mesocortex is similar to that of neocortex in that white matter is internal to the more superficial gray matter. The primitive condition of archicortex resembles the arrangement in the spinal cord and brain stem; the layer of fibers (alveus) lies outside the gray matter.

The indusium griseum (supracallosal gyrus) is a thin layer of neurons dorsal to the corpus callosum along its entire length in man, between the corpus callosum and cingulate gyrus. Smith (1897, 1910) thought that the indusium griseum was a remnant of hippocampus produced

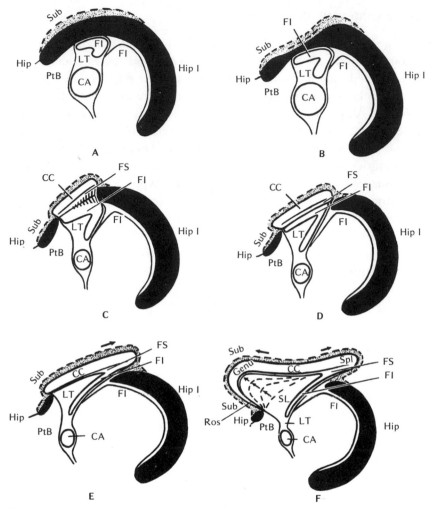

Figure 12-5 Diagram of medial aspect of cerebral hemisphere to show the evolution of the corpus callosum and septum pellucidum. (A) condition in monotremes and marsupials: hippocampus (black) and subiculum (stippled) lie dorsal to lamina terminalis; (B) hypothetic intermediate stage: hippocampal infolding brings subiculum closer to lamina terminalis; broken line in subiculum indicates position of incipient fibers of corpus callosum; (C) condition in hedgehog and bat: corpus callosum develops by penetrating subiculum; most of hippocampus beneath corpus callosum is obliterated; (D) except for small precommissural remnant, hippocampus lies entirely behind corpus callosum; (E) condition in rodents: splenium of corpus callosum expands as more fibers are needed; (F) condition of primates and other advanced mammals: rostral portion of corpus callosum expands and forms an arc, drawing the frontal part of lamina terminalis into the concavity to become part of the septum pellucidum; neural component is derived from paraterminal body. Subiculum above corpus callosum is induseum griseum in man. See text for further details. Arrows indicate direction of expansion; broken lines in the septum pellucidum are successive positions of the genu of the corpus callosum. Anterior commissure (CA); corpus callosum (CC); inferior fornix (FI); superior fornix (FS); lamina terminalis (LT); paraterminal body (PtB); rostrum (Ros); splenium (Spl); septum pellucidum (SL); subiculum (Sub) (Abbie, 1939).

during its caudal migration. This view was further expounded by Kappers et al. (1936). Abbie (1939), however, demonstrated that the corpus callosum consistently develops dorsal to the hippocampus in all mammals and that the indusium griseum is actually a lip of subiculum everted by the penetrating callosal fibers in following the most direct course between the two neocortical hemispheres (Fig. 12-5). The subiculum is a mesocortical structure just dorsal to the hippocampus. The part of the subiculum ventral to the callosal fibers migrates with the hippocampus to become the hippocampal gyrus.

The mesocortical structures are intimately related to the hippocampus by extensive reciprocal connections, and are part of the limbic system. The cingulate gyrus also receives many fibers from the anterior nuclear group of the thalamus, conveying visceral and gustatory impulses from the hypothalamus and mammillary bodies. The entorhinal area relates the hippocampal to the cingulate gyrus. This area is small in lower mammals, better developed in carnivores and primates, and largest in man (Rose, 1927). Neither the entorhinal area nor the cingulate gyrus receives primary or even secondary projections from olfactory structures (Allison, 1953). The cingulate gyrus has both afferent and efferent connections with almost all parts of neocortex in man (Schneider et al., 1963). It is therefore the principal intermediary between hippocampus and neocortex.

Septum

The septum, in the ventromedial portion of the hemispheres of the forebrain, is differentiated in all vertebrates. It is large and subdivided in most fishes. Medial and lateral septal nuclei are large in amphibians, but are even better developed in reptiles and in lower mammals. In some species, other, smaller septal nuclei also differentiate.

The connections of the medial and lateral septal nuclei are similar, and they are summarized together. Reciprocal fibers connect the septum with the hippocampus, and with the preoptic and hypothalamic nuclei (Raisman, 1966). Fibers to and from these diencephalic centers travel in the medial forebrain bundle. A few septal fibers also descend to the tegmentum of the midbrain and the interpeduncular nucleus. The medial septal nucleus is continuous posteriorly with the nucleus of the diagonal band of Broca. The latter receives hypothalamic fibers and a few afferents from the olfactory tubercle and piriform (prepiriform) cortex.

The septal nuclei give rise to fibers of the stria terminalis which terminate in the amygdala and habenulae.

On the basis of its connections, therefore, the septum may be regarded functionally as an intermediate structure between the originally overlying hippocampus, and the preoptic and hypothalamic nuclei. It is also a correlative center relaying visceral information to the hippocampus, amygdala, habenula, and interpeduncular nucleus. The frequent statement that the septum is an olfactory structure cannot be substantiated, although a few olfactory impulses may reach the septum from the olfactory tubercle. A few fibers from the olfactory bulb pass through the septum to the preoptic area, but they do not terminate in the septum.

The primitive corpus callosum lay flat on the lamina terminalis. Abbie (1939) proposed that with the upward and forward expansion of the corpus callosum in mammalian phylogenesis, the lamina terminalis was drawn up into the concavity of the corpus callosum and formed the septum pellucidum (Fig. 12-5). Other authors (Kappers et al., 1936) suggested that the septum itself was drawn forward and thinned. They denied that the interseptal space was lined by ependyma. The caudal part of the medial septal nucleus of the frog may be homologous with the neural component of the human septum pellucidum (Hoffman, 1963).

The septum pellucidum of man is composed of two thin leaves of gliotic neural tissue with occasional scattered neurons. The leaves may be fused, but an interseptal space, the cavum septi pellucidi persists in 85 per cent of normal adults as a small slit or large space (Hughes et al., 1955). This interseptal space is lined by ependyma (Liss and Mervis, 1964), and it is often connected with the ventricular system, as shown by the frequency of filling with air during pneumoencephalography even in neonates (Larroche and Baudey, 1961). A combination of the theories would explain the histologic nature of the septal leaves as neural tissue lined by ependyma and derived from the lamina terminalis. The cavum septi pellucidi may be continuous with the third ventricle, or the lamina terminalis may completely separate the cavum from the anterior end of the ventricle. The open cavum septi pellucidi described by Thompson (1932) as occurring in ungulates, carnivores, and primates, was really the recess beneath the frontal end of the corpus callosum (Abbie, 1939). The human septum pellucidum is absent in association with agenesis of the corpus callosum (Kirschbaum, 1947) and is intimately related to and dependent upon the preceding and concomitant growth of the corpus callosum during embryogenesis (Rakic and Yakovlev, 1968). Cysts and other developmental anomalies of the septum pellucidum in man were discussed by Dooling et al. (1972).

The precommissural portion of the septum of reptiles is homologous with the para-olfactory area (paraterminal body or gyrus; subcallosal gyrus) of mammals, rather than with part of the septum pellucidum. The para-olfactory area of man is not atrophic as is the septum pellucidum but is large and has the same connections as the septum of lower vertebrates.

Neocortex

The neocortex is usually defined in terms of a six-layered structure of the mammalian telencephalon. A homologous primordium of neocortex may comprise part of the forebrain of all vertebrates, however. This primordium was not recognized by most comparative neuroanatomists until recently because of the difficulty in tracing fine, lightly myelinated fibers by older techniques and because of the rigid definition of neocortex as a laminated structure. The familiar association of neocortex with man and other mammals has perhaps also had a retarding effect on the development of new phylogenetic concepts regarding the origin of this important cerebral structure.

The primordial neocortex, a formation between the hippocampus (archicortex) and piriform cortex (paleocortex) is first recognized in reptiles. It is poorly demarcated from the surrounding older cortical structures, and the area is therefore designated in reptiles as the general cortex. The differentiation of the neocortex in birds is difficult to determine because part is probably incorporated into the corpus striatum; the superficial avian cortex is sparse. Neocortex characterizes the mammalian brain, and comprises a large part of the cerebral hemispheres of even the lowest mammals. The developing neocortex pushes ventrally on the piriform cortex to form the rhinal sulcus, the line of demarcation between the two cortical areas.

Although the hippocampal and rhinal sulci are present in all mammals, the neocortex itself is smooth (lissencephalic) in most lower species. Further expansion of the surface area of the cortex results in the development of convolutions, the gyri, characteristic of the neocortex of most mammals. The pattern of gyri and sulci is relatively constant in individual species and is most complex in higher primates, especially man.

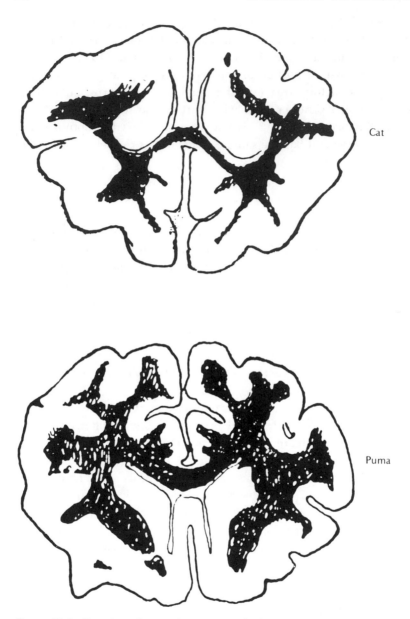

Figure 12-6   Drawing of coronal section of the brain of a puma (mountain lion) reduced until it is the same size as the coronal section of the brain of a domestic cat. The comparison shows the relatively increased amount of white matter in larger animals of the same order. The relation is similar between quantities of cortical gray matter and subcortical white matter in comparing the brain of a child with that of an adult (Kappers et al., 1936).

The complexity of the convolutional pattern of the cortex, however, is not an infallible measure of the place of each species on the phylogenetic scale. The Australian spiny anteater, *Echidna*, has a well-convoluted cortex (Lende, 1969), although this animal is a monotreme. The cytoarchitecture of this cortex is not as complex as in advanced placental mammals, however.

Increase in the surface of the cortex is not directly proportional to the size of the brain. Small animals may have a greater cortical surface than larger species within the same order. In general, however, the smallest mammals have a lissencephalic and relatively thick cortex with few myelinated fibers; larger animals generally have gyrencephalic brains with a relatively thin cortex and much subcortical white matter (Fig. 12-6). The increase in surface area provided by the development of convolutions satisfies a need not met by a simple increase in thickness of the cortical gray matter.

Lissencephaly is also a term applied to the extreme form of pachygyria, a developmental disorder of the human brain resulting from arrest of normal migration of neurons into the cortex. This abnormal brain is smooth. It has few, if any, gyri and grossly resembles the normally lissencephalic brain of the 22-week human fetus (Larroche, 1967) or of some adult lower mammals, such as the rat or rabbit. Microscopic examination of the cortex, however, reveals that the orderly lamination of the cortex is lacking or interrupted in human lissencephaly. Children with such brains are almost always mentally retarded, may have anomalies elsewhere in the body, and often die in infancy. Hanaway et al. (1968) indicated that in pachygyria the pathologic process characteristically involves only the neocortex and not the phylogenetically older cortical structures. The phenomenon is not simply related to an insult occurring at a specific time after development of the archicortex and before development of the neocortex. Radioautographic studies of the developing mouse brain indicate that neuronal migration from the neuroepithelium to the neocortex, hippocampus, and corpus striatum is almost simultaneous (Angevine, 1963; Angevine and Sidman, 1961, 1962; Sidman and Angevine, 1962).

The comparative patterns of convolutions in the mammalian cerebral cortex were the object of detailed studies during the early part of the twentieth century. The cortex of all mammals is laminated. Archi- and paleo-cortex (collectively called "allocortex") have three layers with an organization similar to that found elsewhere in the central nervous system. Afferent fibers synapse with receptive and correlative granular cells; impulses are then conveyed to large effector neurons. Three transitional layers of neocortex are similar in the human fetus. Six layers are eventually formed. These layers have a similar organization throughout the neocortex of the late human fetus, but shortly before birth the architectural pattern of the adult brain emerges. Lower mammals, too, have few histologic differences between various areas of cortex; regional specialization also occurs in phylogenesis.

Differences of predominance of layers and of neuronal composition in different gyri are the foundation of meticulous mapping of the cortex, termed "cytoarchitectonics." Attempts have been made to correlate these histologic findings with physiologic studies to delineate the histologic counterpart of function. The results of that approach are described in most standard textbooks of human neuroanatomy. Success has been limited, particularly in "associative areas" of cortex.

Cytoarchitectonic evidence suggests that the generalized six-layered neocortex of primitive mammals evolved simultaneously from both hippocampal and piriform cortices (Sanides, 1969). As the first stage in the development of laminated neocortex, the archicortex forming the medial side, and the paleocortex of the lateral side of the cerebral hemisphere probably gave origin to cortex with an architecture intermediate in complexity between three and six layers. This intermediate cortex surrounded the primitive cortex of origin. A second zone of further differentiated neocortex formed as an additional concentric ring. This latter zone became the parahippocampal structures on the medial side such as the cingulate gyrus, and the insular cortex laterally. A third ring of further differentiated neocortex then appeared; these paralimbic and parainsular cortices became sites of specialized sensory and motor functions. Part of the parainsular region also became an auditory center, and a cortical visual center developed in the paralimbic zone. Lower placental mammals, such as the hedgehog and the bat, have poorly differentiated neocortical laminae, lacking thick granular layers and large pyramidal cells; these animals have progressed only as far as the paralimbic and parainsular stage of neocortical evolution (Sanides, 1969).

Some neocortical areas are unique in man, being undeveloped in even the highest anthropoid apes. Most notable among these is the pars opercularis and triangularis of the inferior frontal gyrus, corresponding to Broca's speech area. The phenomenon of cerebral dominance in man is not normally associated with asymmetry of the two hemispheres.

The central or Rolandic fissure separates the frontal and parietal lobes of the human cortex. The precentral gyrus is predominantly motor, and the postcentral gyrus is mainly a somatic sensory area, but the separation of function is incomplete. A few sensory projections from the thalamus terminate in the motor cortex, and some motor fibers of the corticospinal tract arise in the sensory cortex. Lende (1969) studied the somatotopic pattern of the neocortex of lower mammals and found that lower placental mammals have an extensive overlap of somatic sensory and motor areas. Only the most frontal part of the cortex is almost purely motor, and the most caudal portion is almost exclusively sensory. In marsupials, a single large primary cortical area is organized in overlapping sensory and motor fields; a spatial counterpart of the precentral motor area of man is lacking. Lende (1969) also found that primary cortical areas of vision and hearing overlapped in marsupials and insectivores, but to a lesser extent than the somatic sensory and motor areas. The visual cortex of these lower mammals is at the dorsal posterior pole of the cortex; the auditory area lies ventral to the visual cortex (Fig. 12-7).

The cortical areas of vision, audition, somatic sensation, and motor function in lower mammals are homologous only with the corresponding primary areas of advanced vertebrates. Secondary or associative neocortex develops as the cortical mantle progressively expands in higher mammals. In Pick's disease, selective degeneration involves the secondary associative areas of neocortex, and spares the phylogenetically older regions of primary sensory and motor neocortex, paleocortex, and archicortex.

Although the somatotopic organization of the neocortex is similar in most placental mammals, each species has a different proportion of cortex associated with specialized parts of the body. Welker and Seidenstein (1959) showed that the racoon has an individual sensory gyrus for each finger and volar area of the paw (Fig. 12-8); this animal relies heavily on tactile sensations in the paws, and the sensitivity is greatest when the paws are wet. It is probably for this reason that the racoon moistens its food in water before eating it.

Monotremes have evolved a cortical organization unlike that of marsupial and placental animals. The visual, auditory, somatic sensory and motor fields are grouped closely over the posterior pole of the hemisphere, with unique spatial relations. Although associative cortex is not found between these primary areas, the "frontal" cortex, rostral to these primary areas, is relatively more extensive than in any other mammal, including man (Fig. 12-7; Lende, 1969).

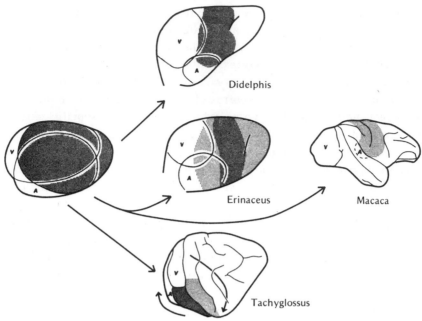

Figure 12-7   Evolution of specificity of function in cortical regions. Vertical hatch: somatic sensory. Horizontal hatch: somatic motor. Cross hatch: somatic sensory-motor. Visual and auditory borders indicated by arcs which extend through other areas to show amount of overlap. Symbols V and A positioned on nonoverlapping portions. Left, primordial cortex with largely superimposed visual, auditory and somatic sensory-motor areas. *Didelphis* is an opossum, a marsupial; *Erinaceus* is a hedgehog, a primitive placental mammal; *Macaca* is a monkey; *Tachyglossus* is a monotreme. Arrows around cortex of *Tachyglossus* indicate direction of rotational displacement (Lende, 1969).

The insular region is completely covered by the margins of the Sylvian fissure only in man, although it is partially enveloped in some other primates. In most mammals, the homologous insular region is superficial on the lateral side of the hemisphere. The anterior portion of the temporal lobes and the part of the frontal lobes rostral to the motor areas are well developed only in primates, and are greatly enlarged in man. The occipital poles of the hemispheres are also largest in man, a result mainly of an increase of the visual associative areas.

The primary visual area bordering the calcarine fissure differs architecturally from other areas of neocortex: a band of fibers divides lamina IV into superficial and deep layers. This line of Gennari is seen grossly

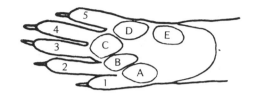

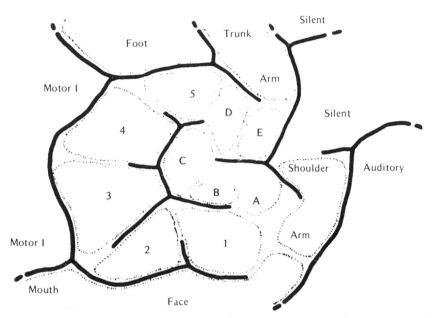

Figure 12-8   The racoon has an individual sensory gyrus for each finger and volar area of the paw. This pattern is associated with acute tactile sensitivity in the paws (Welker and Seidenstein, 1959).

on the cut surface of the cortex. The primary visual cortex therefore is called the "striate cortex."

The optic radiations are distributed retinotopically in space. The inferior retinal quadrants projects to the inferior lip of the calcarine fissure, and the superior quadrants to the superior lip. The macula projects to the occipital pole. Commissural fibers of the visual cortex pass in the splenium of the corpus callosum. Cortical regions surrounding the primary visual cortex are designated secondary or associative visual areas. They lack a line of Gennari.

The calcar avis is a longitudinal prominence in the medial wall of the occipital horn of the lateral ventricle in man. It is produced by the deep penetration of the calcarine fissure. The calcar avis is best developed in primates, but a primordial swelling also is found in the calcarine cortex of carnivores, even though the lateral ventricles in these animals usually lack occipital horns.

Motor pathways of neocortex

The phylogenetic development of the motor areas of the neocortex in mammals is associated with the simultaneous evolution of three major pathways influencing somatic motor function. The first is the cortico-neostriatal (corticocaudate and corticoputamental) pathway. Direct cortical projections to the pallidum are lacking, but both neostriatal structures discharge into the pallidum. The cortical projection to the substantia nigra may also be included in the category of corticoneostriatal pathways. The efferent pathway from the corpus striatum is the ansa lenticularis, descending to the red nucleus and tegmentum of the midbrain in lower vertebrates. In the phylogeny of mammals, progressively more pallidal efferent fibers enter the thalamus to recircuit through the motor cortex. These fibers constitute most of the pallidal efferent fibers in man.

The second motor pathway from the neocortex is the cortico-ponto-cerebellar tract discussed in Chapter 6.

The third important motor pathway of the neocortex is the heavily myelinated corticospinal tract. Corticobulbar fibers to the brainstem are included in this pathway. The corticospinal tract arises predominantly from pyramidal cells of the motor areas of neocortex, but some fibers also originate in the parietal lobe. The tract is small in monotremes, marsupials, and lower placental mammals. It enlarges progressively as the phylogenetic scale is ascended and is largest in primates, especially man. Most fibers decussate at the caudal end of the medulla and descend in the lateral funiculus of the spinal cord (Chapter 3). A smaller uncrossed component of the corticospinal tract in the anterior funiculus of the spinal cord decussates at the spinal segment of termination.

Fibers of the corticospinal tract do not synapse directly on motor neurons of the ventral horn, but rather on interneurons, which then synapse with the alpha motor neurons. It is not certain whether descending fibers synapsing with gamma motor neurons of the spinal cord also travel in the corticospinal tract.

Some direct corticobulbar fibers end in motor nuclei of the brainstem in man and other primates (Kuypers, 1958b), although this tract is absent in the cat (Kuypers, 1958a). In most mammals except primates, therefore, the corticobulbar pathway is still interrupted by one or more synapses in the reticular formation of the brainstem. The direct tract in primates supplements rather than replaces this phylogenetically older synaptic pathway.

The corticopontine, corticospinal, and corticobulbar tracts comprise much of the internal capsule and cerebral peduncles. They form the basal area of the pons, a structure distinguished only in mammals. The corticospinal tract is separated into numerous fascicles by the crossing corticopontine fibers and pontine nuclei, but the fascicles recombine on the ventral surface of the medulla to form the pyramids. This arrangement of fibers is constant in all mammals and can be recognized even in the lowest forms. A few fibers of a primordial corticospinal tract may be found in some reptiles.

Corpus striatum

A primordial pallidum (globus pallidus, paleostriatum) with large motor neurons gives rise to descending fibers in even the most primitive vertebrates. Only a portion of the cerebral hemisphere in lower vertebrates, traditionally regarded as corpus striatum, may actually be homologous with the pallidum of advanced species, however (Ebbesson and Schroeder, 1971).

The development of the caudate nucleus and putamen (collectively the neostriatum) parallels the development of the thalamus and neocortex. These neostriatal structures first appear in reptiles as the anterior part of the hypopallium (dorsal ventricular ridge), the portion of cortex of the lateral wall of the hemisphere between pallidum and piriform cortex. The hypopallium invaginates into the ventricle (Fig. 12-9) because of greater growth of the hippocampus and neocortex than of the ventrally situated pallidum (Smith, 1919). The hypopallium remains rostrally continuous with the general cortex of reptiles. The posterior part of the hypopallium contributes to the amygdala. The derivation of

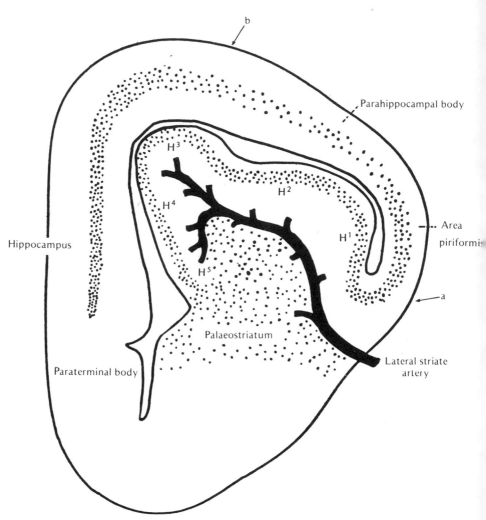

Figure 12-9   Development of hypopallium (primordial neostriatum) as invagination of lateral wall of hemisphere into lateral ventricle in lower reptile. Infolded column of cells of hypopallium (H^1-H^5); areas of change in arrangement of cells (a,b) (Smith, 1919).

the mammalian claustrum either from the posterior hypopallium of reptiles (putamen of mammals) or from the insular neocortex is controversial. The claustrum probably is part of one of these two structures, separated by sheets of myelinated fibers, the external and extreme capsules. Embryologically, the claustrum cannot "arise" from either the insular cortex or putamen because telencephalic structures lack proliferative capacity; they develop as cellular migrations from periventricular neuro-epithelium.

The pallidum in man is divided into inner and outer segments by a lamina of fibers that is largely intrinsic to the pallidum and connects the two segments. This distinct segmentation of the pallidum occurs only in advanced mammals, especially primates.

The neostriatum is large and well developed in birds. Other structures of the dorsal ventricular ridge, the hyperstriatum and ectostriatum, also appear to differentiate from the cephalic end of the hypopallium in birds. These unique avian structures may incorporate the primordial neocortex of reptiles and often thicken (Fig. 12-10). They become sec-ondarily divided, and parts are laminated in some birds. Embryologic studies of birds also suggest that derivatives of the dorsal ventricular ridge are homologous with the neocortex of mammals (Källén, 1962).

The forebrain of birds evolved in two directions; the most divergent modern species are owls and parrots (Fig. 12-11; Stringelin and Senn, 1969). Other birds exemplify intermediate stages in these two lines of evolution, the pigeon having a more generalized avian brain. The fore-brains of primitive birds (paleognaths) such as the ostrich represent an intermediate stage between reptiles and advanced birds. The best developed neostriatum among reptiles is in crocodiles. It resembles the primordial avian brain more than any other reptile. This feature is remi-niscent of the evolution of crocodilians and birds from a common sau-ropsid ancestor; the brains of dinosaurs also may have resembled those of modern birds for the same reason (Chapter 1).

The divergent pattern of the two lines of evolution of birds involves the relative predominance of the various striatal structures (Fig. 12-10). The pattern of lamination of the avian hyperstriatum is unlike that found in the mammalian cerebral cortex. Evidence of more primitive lamination resembling the hyperstriatum occurs in the corresponding neocortical regions of some reptiles. Much of the avian cerebral hemi-sphere is formed almost entirely by striatal structures. It is covered by a thin layer of poorly developed cortex. The amygdaloid complex forms the ventroposterior part of the lateral hemisphere of birds.

The corpus striatum becomes a deep structure within the hemispheres of mammals because of the great development of the neocortex and corpus callosum. Striatal structures are often termed "basal ganglia" by clinicians. The amygdala is sometimes regarded as the archistriatum, al-

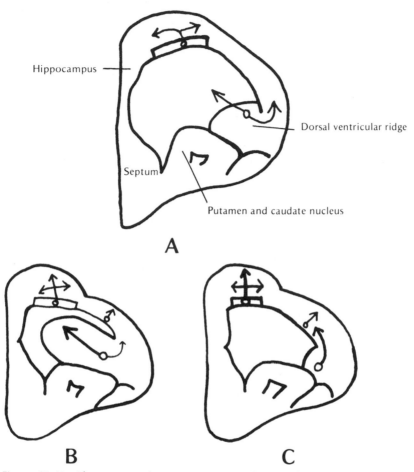

Figure 12-10 Theory to explain incorporation of primordial neocortex into corpus striatum of birds because of migration of neurons from (A) primitive hypopallial position into either (B) avian corpus striatum, or into (C) cerebral cortex of mammals (Karten, 1969).

though it is more properly considered part of the limbic rather than of the striatal system. The caudate nucleus and putamen are similar in structure and connections. They progressively enlarge and become separated in the phylogenetic series of mammals, although some continuity between the two structures is retained. In man, the connection is in the rostral portion.

The caudate, putamen, subthalamic nucleus, and substantia nigra

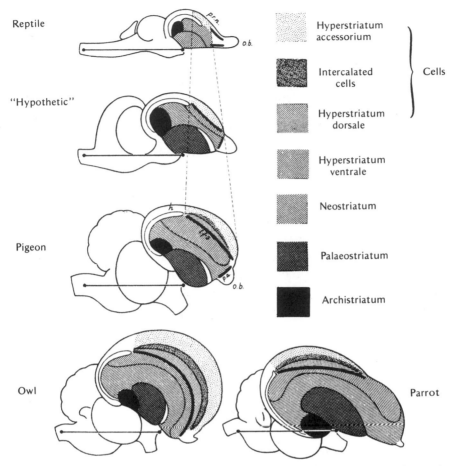

Figure 12-11 Divergent lines of evolution of the avian forebrain (Stringelin and Senn, 1969).

project to the pallidum, the source of efferent discharge of the entire striatal complex in all classes of vertebrates. Descending pallidotegmental fibers are reduced in number and replaced in importance by pallidothalamic fibers of the ansa lenticularis and the lenticular fasciculus in mammals. Impulses are projected from the thalamus to the neocortex. Impulses from the corpus striatum and cerebellum are correlated in the red nucleus, and, in mammals, in the ventrolateral nucleus of the thalamus.

The striatal complex coordinates motor activities and postural muscle

tone in all vertebrates, but the mechanism of action is poorly understood. Disease of parts of the corpus striatum in man results in various
abnormal involuntary movements, thought to be release phenomena
from interruption of inhibitory pathways. Attempts to reproduce such
syndromes in animals, however, have had little success. Our knowledge
of the functions of the corpus striatum in other mammals and in the
submammalian species is also deficient, although further investigation
of simple vertebrates may yield clues at least to the original function
of that area of the forebrain. Comparison of the corpus striatum of
snakes and turtles, for example, may reveal which parts subserve axial
and appendicular muscles, respectively, and have implications for the
understanding of the "extrapyramidal" disorders of man.

The highly developed corpus striatum of birds performs many functions similar to those of the neocortex in mammals, perhaps in part because of incorporation of the primordial neocortical tissue. In addition
to being a controlling motor center, visual and auditory fibers project
to the ectostriatum and hyperstriatum of birds in a precise pattern
(Karten, 1969); these are probably the most important associative area
of the avian brain.

Ventral thalamus

The ventral thalamus (pars ventralis thalami) is composed of scattered,
small collections of neurons dorsal to the hypothalamus as well as inter-
spersed among the descending fibers in the ventral peduncle of the
lateral forebrain bundle (ansa lenticularis in mammals). These neurons
in the latter location are also known as the entopeduncular nuclei.

It is uncertain if the origin of the ventral thalamus is diencephalic,
telencephalic, or a mixture of the two. It is closely related, both functionally and anatomically, to the corpus striatum. Neurons belonging to
the ventral thalamus are found in all vertebrates, but in no species do
the nuclei achieve the size or importance of the dorsal thalamus or
corpus striatum. The entopeduncular nuclei are better developed in
terrestrial vertebrates than in fishes; in mammals they contribute to the
formation of the substantia nigra and subthalamic nucleus. A small
nucleus also persists in mammals, retaining the name entopeduncular
nucleus.

The subthalamic nucleus (corpus Luysii) is recognized only in mammals. It is rudimentary in marsupials, rodents, and carnivores, and it is
largest in man (von Bonin and Shariff, 1951). The nucleus is closely re-

lated to the globus pallidus by reciprocal fiber connections. Lesions of the subthalamic nucleus in man result in hemiballism, violent choreic movements on the opposite side of the body.

The substantia innominata (of Reichert) is a poorly understood band of gray matter in man and some other mammals. It extends dorsal to the anterior commissure. Afferent connections are mainly from the putamen.

It was reported by early neuroanatomists that the nuclei of the ventral thalamus projected axons caudally to the midbrain, medulla, and spinal cord, but these connections await further verification. It is probable that the entopeduncular nuclei have both afferent and efferent fibers in the lateral forebrain bundle.

Substantia nigra

The substantia nigra (of Soemmering) differentiates as a nucleus in the midbrain of most reptiles (Huber and Crosby, 1933). It probably derives from the most caudal neurons of the entopeduncular nuclei, associated with the lateral forebrain bundle in lower vertebrates. The principal connections of the reptilian substantia nigra are with the optic tectum, probably serving to integrate optic reflexes into the increasingly complex motor system. The nucleus in birds is similar to that in reptiles.

The substantia nigra of marsupial (Woodburne, 1943) and placental mammals (Crosby and Woodburne, 1943a, b, c; Gillilan, 1943a, b) is divided into three parts. Pars lateralis is homologous with the entire substantia nigra of reptiles and birds. In man and other advanced primates, connections with the superior colliculus persist, and pars lateralis is smaller. The lesser size is proportionate to the decreased importance of the superior colliculus to vision. When vision is of secondary importance as in moles, bats, and other burrowing or nocturnal mammals, pars lateralis also is small.

Pars compacta is the largest part of the substantia nigra of most mammals. The phylogenetic development of this structure parallels the evolution of the neocortex.

Pars reticularis contains neurons scattered among the dorsal fibers of the cerebral peduncle. Embryologically, the nigral neurons arise from the neuroepithelium of the basal plate of the midbrain and migrate ventrally toward the cerebral peduncle (Shaner, 1936; Cooper, 1946; Hanaway et al., 1971).

Knowledge of the connections of the substantia nigra has been enhanced by intensive study associated with pharmacologic discoveries in the treatment of Parkinson's disease. This human disorder involves the substantia nigra more severely and consistently than other parts of the brain, although lesions may be widespread. Reciprocal nigral connections with the caudate and putamen, as well as nigropallidal projections, integrate the substantia nigra into the motor system of the corpus striatum. The function of the substantia nigra is uncertain. Disease of this nucleus is usually associated clinically with rigidity, tremor, bradykinesia, and impairment of postural reflexes.

The substantia nigra is poorly formed or atophic in developmental disorders of the forebrain of man, associated with absence or atrophy of the cerebral cortex, corpus striatum, and pallidum (Gamper, 1926), or in similar cases with only the pallidum intact (Edinger and Fischer, 1913; Jakob, 1923).

Neuromelanin

A constant feature of the human substantia nigra, shared by a few other nuclei of the human brain, is the accumulation of melanin within the cytoplasm of the neurons. Melanin is present in the substantia nigra of adult human albinos (Foley and Baxter, 1958; Kennedy and Zelickson, 1963; Marsden, 1965). Neuromelanin, therefore, may be formed in a different manner from melanin in the skin, eyes, and meninges, or albinism may result from local inhibition of melanin synthesis, not involving the brain (Marsden, 1965).

Melanin is found in man in nuclei other than the substantia nigra. These sites include the locus coeruleus, pontine nuclei, dorsal motor nucleus of the vagus, autonomic neurons of the intermediolateral column of the spinal cord, and scattered neurons throughout the tegmentum of the brainstem (Jacobsohn, 1909). The melanin-pigmented nuclei in adult man form a column in each side of the brainstem. This distribution corresponds, in general, to the visceral efferent column, the neurons of which also contain catecholamines (Bazelon et al., 1967). In some locations, such as the dentate nucleus of the cerebellum, melanosis occurs only rarely (Singer et al., 1974).

Melanin in the central nervous system is as ancient as amphioxus. The function of the pigmented cells within the spinal cord of amphioxus (Fig. 2-10), and even whether these cells are neurons, are not known. The suggestion that they are photoreceptors (Kapper et al., 1936) is not confirmed.

Neuromelanin occurs within neurons of the central nervous system of some urodelan amphibians and larval stages of anurans, but it disappears after metamorphosis (Adler, 1939). Similar granules in the somatic muscles of these amphibians also disappear with metamorphosis. Melanin is also present in the nervous system of some amphibian species lacking pigmentation elsewhere (Adler, 1939). Among mammals, most species lack neuronal melanin, but those that have it do not follow a precise phylogenetic sequence. It is present in the marsupial tree shrew, gray squirrel, armadillo, horse, deer, sheep, dog, cat, and in most primates (Scherer, 1939; Adler, 1942; Marsden, 1961). Comparisons of degree of pigmentation among various animals is not possible without knowing the age relative to the life span, but in general the lower mammals have the least neuromelanin. It is most constantly found in primates; man has the greatest amount of this pigment.

Marsden (1965) proposed that the deposition of neuromelanin in various motor centers of the brainstem of mammals is associated with decreased synthesis of catecholamines, as the activity of these nuclei shifts to more rostral centers in phylogenetic cephalization. Melanin is not present at birth or in young animals, and tyrosinase activity is greatest early in life. Tyrosinase is an essential enzyme in the production of both catecholamines and melanin. Neuromelanin deposition around particles of this enzyme within neurons may result in diminished enzymatic activity and consequently diminished synthesis of catecholamines. Gfeller (1965) suggested an alternative possibility that the pathway of synthesis of catecholamines is diverted to that of neuromelanin postnatally.

Melanin pigment in the central nervous system may be oxidized lipofuscin (Barden, 1969), although such speculation cannot be confirmed because the chemical structure of lipofuscin is not yet fully known. Neuromelanin is not seen in human nigral cells until approximately 18 months of age, after which time the granules in each neuron gradually increase in number and coalesce with advancing age (Foley and Baxter, 1956). Lipofuscin also steadily accumulates in neuronal cytoplasm with aging (Sarnat, 1968), although lipofuscin is more widely distributed throughout the nervous system, muscles, and other organs of the body. Neurons of a few nuclei of the human brain, such as the lateral geniculate body and inferior olivary nucleus, accumulate lipofuscin earlier and in greater quantity than do most other nuclei.

Basal forebrain bundles

In all vertebrates, the forebrain is reciprocally connected with caudal centers by contiguous longitudinal fascicles. The exact composition differs among species, in conformity with diverse behavioral patterns associated with these connections.

The medial forebrain bundle has thin, lightly myelinated fibers that descend from the olfactory bulb and from structures of the medial and ventral walls of the primitive hemipshere (septum and hippocampus) to the preoptic and hypothalamic nuclei and to the interpeduncular nucleus and tegmentum of the midbrain. Some fibers of the medial forebrain bundle decussate in the anterior commissure. Ascending connections intermingle among the descending fascicles. The dorsal fibers of the medial forebrain bundle include the precommissural portion of the fornix and the stria terminalis. The medial forebrain bundle is a visceral pathway in man and in all other vertebrates.

The lateral forebrain bundle is composed of heavily myelinated fibers related to structures of the lateral and dorsal walls of the primitive hemisphere. Descending fascicles from the pallidum are confined to the large ventral peduncle of the lateral forebrain bundle, and terminate in the thalamus, entopeduncular nuclei, and tectal and tegmental centers of the midbrain; some fibers may descend as far as the medulla in urodeles (Herrick, 1948). The descending fibers of the lateral forebrain bundle of amphibians, reptiles, and birds are the homologous predecessors of the ansa lenticularis, lenticular fasciculus, subthalamic fasciculus, pallidotegmental, and pallidorubral tracts of mammals. They therefore are the "extrapyramidal" motor system of man.

Lightly myelinated thalamocortical connections occur in amphibians and progressively increase in phylogeny, paralleling the evolution of the neocortex. These ascending fibers in lower vertebrates form the dorsal

Figure 12-12 Coronal sections of forebrain of (A) opossum and (B) mouse. The hippocampus is still a dorsal structure in both species. The marsupial opossum lacks a corpus callosum, a structure connecting corresponding associative regions of neocortex in the two cerebral hemisphere in all placental mammals. All vertebrates have an anterior commissure, however (not shown in these sections). In the mouse, as in other placental mammals, the commissural fibers just ventral to those of the corpus callosum are the hippocampal commissure; this connection is also present in the opossum, but is not seen at this level of section. The large nucleus in the dorsomedial position in these sections of both mammals is the habenula. Luxol fast blue and cresyl violet, (A) X 12; (B) X 20.

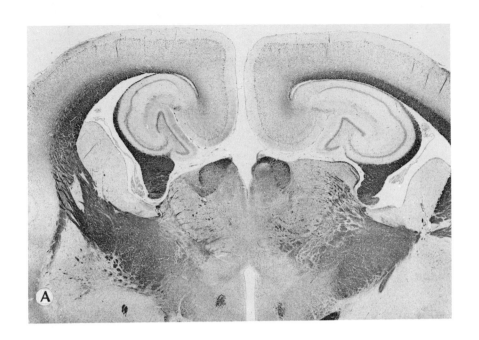

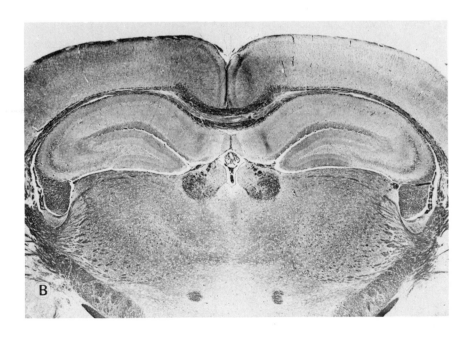

peduncle of the lateral forebrain bundle, or the thalamic radiations of mammals.

The stria medullaris arises in all parts of the medial side of the hemisphere and passes dorsally to the habenula and to structures of the opposite hemisphere in all vertebrates.

Commissural systems of forebrain

Two principal commissural systems are found in the forebrain of all vertebrates. Two bundles of fibers, the dorsal from the hippocampus, and the ventral from all other parts of the cerebral hemisphere, decussate in the closed anterior end of the primitive neural tube, the lamina terminalis. The hippocampal commissure (psalterium of man) and the anterior commissure persist throughout phylogeny, although fascicles may separate to form small and inconstant commissures in particular species, especially in fishes. In a few marsupials, some fibers of the anterior commissure pass through the internal capsule as the fasciculus aberrans. Fibers connecting similar areas of the basolateral amygdaloid nuclei, hippocampus, and neocortical temporal lobe comprise the largest components of the anterior commissure in primates, including man. The stria terminalis is the part of the anterior commissure that follows an unusual course along the medial side of the caudate nucleus from the corticomedial amygdaloid nuclei to the contralateral amygdala.

The corpus callosum is a large commissure connecting corresponding associative areas in the neocortex of the two hemispheres in all placental mammals (Fig. 12-12). Impulses from primary sensory and motor regions of the cortex are not transferred to the other hemisphere by the corpus callosum, however (Welker and Seidenstein, 1959). The corpus callosum does not develop in monotremes or marsupials, although the anterior commissure is large (Heath and Jones, 1965). The development of the corpus callosum in only placental mammals is probably related to the expansion of the associative areas of neocortex in these animals.

The hippocampus is still a dorsal structure in lower placental mam-

Figure 12-13   (A) Coronal section of human brain through head of caudate nucleus. This 5-year-old child had partial agenesis of the corpus callosum resembling the normal condition in marsupials and lower vertebrates. In addition, well demarcated fatty tumors (lipomas) lie near the midline just ventral to the cingulate gyri, replacing the corpus callosum and reducing the lateral ventricles to narrow slits. The child also had agenesis of the cerebellar vermis (Zettner and Netsky, 1960); (B) coronal section of normal human brain at similar level as (A) to show corpus callosum. Compare with Figure 12-12.

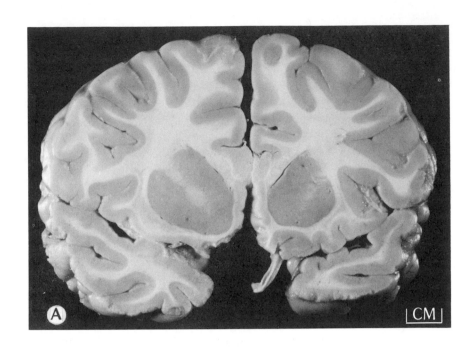

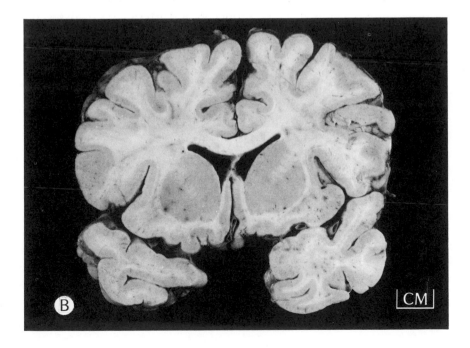

mals. The corpus callosum then develops as a commissure dorsal to the hippocampus (Fig. 12-5). The callosal fibers take the most direct route between the two hemispheres, passing through the subiculum. The most dorsal fimbria of the hippocampus and subiculum form the hippocampal commissure on the ventral surface of the corpus callosum (psalterium; dorsal or superior fornix). The hippocampal tissue between the small dorsal and large ventral fornices disappears in phylogeny as the hippocampus is displaced backward, leaving a small hippocampal remnant that does not migrate.

The phylogenetic development of the corpus callosum involves first a linear caudal extension in lower placental mammals. This development is followed by enlargement and arcuate expansion of the rostrum and genu of the corpus callosum in carnivores and primates, in association with the phylogenetic development of the neocortex.

The corpus callosum may fail to develop in some individuals (Fig. 12-13); patients with congenital absence of this structure may be seemingly normal although defective transfer of information between the hemispheres, and other subtle neurologic deficits may be detected by special examinations (Jeeves, 1965; Gazzaniga and Freedman, 1973). Other patients with callosal agenesis are mentally retarded. Because the vascular supply to the rostrum and splenium of the corpus callosum in man is from the anterior cerebral and posterior cerebral arteries, respectively, the careful evaluation of patients who have suffered occlusions of these vessels may yield more information about the functions of the corpus callosum. These functions relating the two neocortical hemispheres are discussed by Ettlinger (1965), Gazzaniga (1970), and Cuenod (1972).

The supraoptic commissure in man is an additional small bundle of thin fibers decussating above the optic chiasm. The dorsal fibers connect the subthalamic nucleus of one side to the contralateral globus pallidus (Carpenter and Strominger, 1967); the ventral fibers probably interconnect the medial geniculate bodies and possibly also some hypothalamic nuclei. The supraoptic commissure is present in fishes as well as in terrestrial vertebrates, but in some animals it is behind rather than above the optic chiasm. It is not known to include optic fibers in any species.

References

Abbie, A. A.: The origin of the corpus callosum and the fate of structures related to it, *J. Comp. Neurol.* 70:12-44, 1939

Abbie, A. A., and W. R. Adey: Motor mechanisms in the anuran brain, *J. Comp. Neurol.* 92:241-291, 1950

Achucarro, N.: On the evolution of the neuroglia and specially their relation to the vascular apparatus, *J. Nerv. Ment. Dis.* 48:333-342, 1918

Adelman, L. S., and S. M. Aronson: Intramedullary nerve fiber and Schwann cell proliferation within the spinal cord (schwannosis), *Neurology* 22:726-731, 1972

Adler, A.: Melanin pigment in the central nervous system of vertebrates, *J. Comp. Neurol.* 70:315-329, 1939

Adler, A.: Melanin pigment in the brain of the gorilla, *J. Comp. Neurol.* 76:501-507, 1942

Allison, A. C.: An investigation of the morphology of the mammalian olfactory system, thesis, Oxford University, 1950

Allison, A. C.: The morphology of the olfactory system in the vertebrates, *Biol. Rev.* 28:195-244, 1953

Allison, A. C., and R. T. Warwick: Quantitative observations on the olfactory system of the rabbit, *Brain* 72:186-197, 1949

Altman, J.: Some fiber projections to the superior colliculus in the cat, *J. Comp. Neurol.* 119:77-95, 1962

Altman, J., and M. B. Carpenter: Fiber projections of the superior colliculus in the cat, *J. Comp. Neurol.* 116:157-178, 1961

Altner, H., and H. Zimmermann: The saccus vasculosus, in *The Structure and Function of Nervous Tissue*, vol. 5, Academic Press, New York, 1972

Altrocchi, P. H., and J. H. Menkes: Congenital ocular motor apraxia, *Brain* 83:579-588, 1960

Amin, A. H., T. B. B. Crawford, and J. H. Gaddum: The distribution of substance P and 5-hydroxytryptamine in the central nervous system of the dog, *J. Physiol.* 126:596-618, 1954

Andersen, P., J. K. S. Jansen, and Y. Llyning: Slow and fast muscle fibers in the Atlantic hagfish (Myxine glutinosa), *Acta Physiol. Scand.* 57:167-179, 1963

Anderson, E.: The anatomy of bovine and ovine pineals, *J. Ultrastruct. Res.* suppl. 8, 1965

Andres, K. H.: Anatomy and ultrastructure of the olfactory bulb in fish, amphibia, reptiles, birds and mammals, in *Taste and Smell in Vertebrates* (Ciba Foundation Symposium), G. E. W. Wolstenholme and J. Knight, eds., Churchill, London, 1970

Angevine, J. B.: Autoradiographic study of the histogenesis in the hippocampal formation of the mouse, *Anat. Rec.* 145:201, 1963

Angevine, J. B., and R. L. Sidman: Autoradiographic study of cell migration during histogenesis of cerebral cortex in the mouse, *Nature 192*:766, 1961

Angevine, J. B., and R. L. Sidman: Autoradiographic study of histogenesis in the cerebral cortex of the mouse, *Anat. Rec. 142*:210, 1962

Arao, T., and E. Perkins: The nictitating membrane of primates, *Anat. Rec. 162*:53-70, 1968

Armstrong, J. A.: An experimental study of the visual pathways in a snake (Natrix natrix), *J. Anat. 85*:275-288, 1951

Bagnara, J. T.: Pineal regulation of body blanching in amphibian larvae, *Prog. Brain Res. 10*:489-506, 1965

Bairati, A., and F. Maccagnani: Richerche sulla glioarchitettonica dei vertebrati. I. Anfibi II. Ucelli. *Monit. Zool. Ital.* suppl. 58, 1950

Bakker, R. T.: Dinasaur physiology and the origin of mammals, *Evolution 25*:636-658, 1971

Bakker, R. T.: Anatomical and ecological evidence of endothermy in dinosaurs, *Nature 238*:81-85, 1972

Barden, H.: The histochemical relationship of neuromelanin and lipofuscin, *J. Neuropath. Exp. Neurol. 28*:419-441, 1969

Barlow, H. B., R. Narasimhan, and A. Rosenfeld: Visual pattern analysis in machines and animals, *Science 177*:567-575, 1972

Bazelon, M., G. M. Fenichel, and J. Randall: Studies on neuromelanin. I. A melanin system in the human adult brainstem, *Neurology 17*:512-519, 1967

Behrman, S., and B. D. Wyke: Vestibulogenic seizures. A consideration of vertiginous seizures with particular reference to convulsions produced by stimulation of labyrinthine receptors, *Brain 81*:529-541, 1959

Bender, M. B., and S. Shanzer: Oculomotor pathways defined by electric stimulation and lesions in the brainstem of monkeys, in *The Oculomotor System*, M. B. Bender, ed., Hoeber, New York, 1964

Bennett, M. V. L.: A comparative study of neuronal synchronization, in *The Thalamus*, D. P. Purpura and M. D. Yahr, eds., Columbia University Press, New York, 1966

Bentley, P. J., and B. K. Follett: The action of the neurohypophysial and adrenocortical hormones on sodium balance in the cyclostome, Lampetra fluviatilis, *Gen. Comp. Endocrin. 2*:329-335, 1962

Bern, H. A., C. S. Nicoll, and C. Strohman: Prolactin and tadpole growth, *Proc. Soc. Exp. Biol. Med. 126*:518-520, 1967

Birks, R., H. E. Huxley, and B. Katz: The fine structure of the neuromuscular junction of the frog, *J. Physiol. 150*:134-144, 1960

Bleier, R.: The relations of ependyma to neurons and capillaries in the hypothalamus: A. Golgi-Cox study, *J. Comp. Neurol. 142*:439-464, 1971

Bodenheimer, T. S., and M. W. Brightman: A blood-brain barrier to peroxidase in capillaries surrounded by perivascular spaces, *Amer. J. Anat. 122*:249-267, 1968

Boeke, J.: Infundibularorgan im Gehirne des Amphioxus, *Anat. Anz. 32*:473-488, 1908

Bok, S. T.: Die Entwicklung der Hirnnerven und ihrer zentralen Bahnen. Die stimulogene Fibrillation, *Folia Neuro-biol. 9*:475-565, 1915

Bolk, L.: *Das Cerebellum der Säugetiere,* Haarlem, De Erven F. Bohn, G. Fischer, Jena, 1906

Bone, Q.: The central nervous system in Amphioxus, *J. Comp. Neurol. 115*:27-51, 1960

Bons, N.: Nise en évidence du croisement incomplet des nerfs optiques au niveau du chiasma chez le canard, *C. R. Acad. Sci.* (Paris), *268*:2186-2188, 1969

Boord, R. L.: The anatomy of the avian auditory system, *Ann. N.Y. Acad. Sci. 167*: 186-198, 1969

Boyd, I. A.: The motor innervation of mammalian muscle spindles, *J. Physiol. 159*: 7-9, 1961

Boykin, F. C., D. Cowen, C. A. J. Iannucci, and A. Wolk: Subependymal glomerate astrocytomas, *J. Neuropath. Exp. Neurol. 13*:30-49, 1954

Brawer, J. R.: The fine structure of the ependymal tanycytes at the level of the arcuate nucleus, *J. Comp. Neurol. 145*:25-42, 1972

Brightman, M. W.: The intracerebral movement of proteins injected into blood and cerebrospinal fluid of mice, *Prog. Brain Res. 29*:19-40, 1967

Brightman, M. W., and T. S. Reese: Junctions between intimately apposed cell membranes in the vertebrate brain, *J. Cell. Biol. 40*:648-677, 1969

Brightman, M. W., T. S. Reese, Y. Olsson, and I. Klatzo: Morphologic aspects of the blood-brain barrier to peroxidase in elasmobranchs, *Prog. Neuropathol. 1*:146-161, 1971

Brodal, A.: Reticulo-cerebellar connections in the cat: An experimental study, *J. Comp. Neurol. 98*:113-154, 1953

Brodal, A., and E. Hauglie-Hanssen: Congenital hydrocephalus with defective development of the cerebellar vermis (Dandy-Walker syndrome), *J. Neurol. Neurosurg. Psychiat. 22*:99-108, 1959

Brodal, A., and O. Pompeiano: The vestibular nuclei in the cat, *J. Anat. 91*:438-454, 1957

Brodal, A., K. Kristiansen, and J. Jansen: Experimental demonstration of a pontine homologue in birds, *J. Comp. Neurol. 92*:23-70, 1950

Brodal, P.: The corticopontine projection from the visual cortex in the cat. I. The total projection and the projection from area 17, *Brain Res. 39*:297-317, 1972a

Brodal, P.: The corticopontine projection from the visual cortex in the cat. II. The projection from areas 18 and 19, *Brain Res. 39*:319-335, 1972b

Brodie, B. B., D. F. Bogdanski, and L. Bonomi: Formation, storage and metabolism of serotonin (5-hydroxytryptamine) and catecholamines in lower vertebrates, in *Comparative Neurochemistry,* D. Richter, ed., Macmillan, New York, 1964

Burr, H. S.: An electro-dynamic theory of development suggested by studies of proliferation rates in the brain of Amblystoma, *J. Comp. Neurol. 56*:347-372, 1932

Cahn, P. H., ed: *Lateral Line Detectors,* Indiana University Press, Bloomington, Ind., 1967

Cajal, S. de R y: *Textura del Sistema Nervioso del Hombre y de los Vertebrados*, N. Moya, Madrid, 1900

Cajal, S. de R y: *Histologie du Système Nerveux de l'Homme et des Vertébrés*, Consejo Superior de Investigaciones Científicas, Madrid, 1909-1911 (reprinted 1952)

Cajal, S. de R y: *The Structure of the Retina*, S. A. Thorpe and M. Glickstein, translators and eds., Thomas, Springfield, Ill., 1972

Calne, D. B., and C. A. Pallis: Vibratory sense: A critical review, *Brain* 89:723-746, 1966

Campa, J. F., and W. K. Engel: Histochemical and functional correlations in anterior horn neurons of the cat spinal cord, *Science* 171:198-199, 1971

Campa, J. F., H. B. Sarnat, and J. M. Lloyd: Comparative histochemistry of spinal motor neurons in vertebrates, Programs and Abstracts, Society for Neuroscience, 3rd Ann Meeting, San Diego, Calif., Nov. 7-10, 1973

Campbell, C. B. G., and W. Hodos: The concept of homology and the evolution of the nervous system, *Brain Behav. Evol.* 3:353-367, 1970

Campbell, C. B. G., J. A. Jane, and D. Yashon: The retinal projections of the tree shrew and hedgehog, *Brain Res.* 5:406-418, 1967

Cantor, F. K.: Vestibulo-temporal connections demonstrated by induced seizures, *Neurology* 21:507-516, 1971

Carpenter, M. B.: Fiber projections from the descending and lateral vestibular nuclei in the cat, *Amer. J. Anat.* 107:1-15, 1960

Carpenter, M. B.: The ascending vestibular system and its relationship to conjugate horizontal eye movements, in *The Vestibular System and Its Diseases*, R. J. Wolfson, ed., University of Pennsylvania Press, Philadelphia, 1966

Carpenter, M. B.: Central oculomotor pathways, in *The Control of Eye Movements*, P. Bach-y-Rita and C. C. Collins, eds., Academic Press, New York, 1971

Carpenter, M. B., F. A. Alling, and D. S. Bard: Lesions of the descending vestibular nucleus in the cat, *J. Comp. Neurol.* 114:39-46, 1960

Carpenter, M. B., G. M. Brittin, and J. Pines: Isolated lesions of the fastigial nuclei in the cat, *J. Comp. Neurol.* 109:65-84, 1958

Carpenter, M. B., and N. L. Strominger: Cerebello-oculomotor fibers in the rhesus monkey, *J. Comp. Neurol.* 123:211-230, 1964

Carpenter, M. B., and N. L. Strominger: Efferent fibers of the subthalamic nucleus in the monkey. A comparison of the efferent projections of the subthalamic nucleus, substantia nigra and globus pallidus, *Amer. J. Anat.* 121:41-72, 1967

Casagrande, V. A., J. K. Harting, W. C. Hall, and I. T. Diamond: Superior colliculus of the tree shrew: A structural and functional subdivision into superficial and deep layers, *Science* 177:444-447, 1972

Charlton, H. H.: Optic tectum and the related fiber tracts in blind fishes. A. Troglichthys rosae and Typhlichthys eigenmanni, *J. Comp. Neurol.* 57:285-325, 1933

Chow, K. L., J. S. Blum, and R. A. Blum: Cell ratios in the thalamo-cortical visual system of Macaca mulatta, *J. Comp. Neurol.* 92:227-240, 1950

Christ, J. F.: Derivation and boundaries of the hypothalamus, with atlas of hypothalamic grisea, in *The Hypothalamus*, W. Haymaker, E. Anderson, and W. J. H. Nauta, eds., Thomas, Springfield, Ill., 1969

Clementi, F., F. Fraschini, E. Mueller, and A. Zanoboni: The pineal gland and the control of electrolyte balance and of gonadotropic secretion: Functional and morphologic observations, *Prog. Brain Res.* 10:585-603, 1965

Close, R. I.: Dynamic properties of mammalian skeletal muscles, *Physiol. Rev. 52*: 129-197, 1972

Coghill, G. E.: The primary ventral roots and somatic motor column of Amblystoma, *J. Comp. Neurol. 19*:121-143, 1913

Coghill, G. E.: Correlated anatomical and physiological studies on the growth of the nervous system of amphibia, *J. Comp. Neurol. 24*:161-233, 1914

Coghill, G. E.: *Anatomy and the Problem of Behavior,* Cambridge University Press, Cambridge, Mass., 1929 (reprinted by Hafner, New York, 1963)

Cohen, B., J. Suzuki, S. Shanzer, and M. Bender: Semicircular canal control of eye movements, in *The Oculomotor System,* M. Bender, ed., Hoeber, New York, 1964

Colmant, H. J.: Ueber die Wandstruktur des dritten Ventrikels der Albinoratte, *Histochemie 11*:40-61, 1967

Cooper, E. R. A.: The development of the substantia nigra, *Brain 69*:22-33, 1946

Courville, J.: Rubrobulbar fibers to the facial nucleus and the lateral reticular nucleus (nucleus of the lateral funiculus). An experimental study in the cat with silver impregnation methods, *Brain Res. 1*:317-337, 1966

Cowan, W. M., G. Raisman, and T. P. S. Powell: The connections of the amygdala, *J. Neurol. Neurosurg. Psychiat. 28*:137-151, 1965

Craigie, E. H.: Observations on the brain of the hummingbird, *J. Comp. Neurol. 45*: 377-481, 1928

Crosby, E. C.: Relations of brain centers to normal and abnormal eye movements in the horizontal plane, *J. Comp. Neurol. 99*:477-480, 1953

Crosby, E. C.: Comparative aspects of cerebellar morphology, in *Neurobiology of Cerebellar Evolution and Development,* R. Llinás, ed., Amer. Med. Assoc., Chicago, 1969

Crosby, E. C., and M. J. Showers: Comparative anatomy of the preoptic and hypothalamic areas, in *The Hypothalamus,* W. Haymaker, E. Anderson, and W. J. H. Nauta, eds., Thomas, Springfield, Ill., 1969

Crosby, E. C., and R. T. Woodburne: The comparative anatomy of the preoptic area and the hypothalamus, *Assoc. Res. Nerv. Ment. Dis. Proc. 20*:52-169, 1940

Crosby, E. C., and R. T. Woodburne: The nuclear pattern of the non-tectal portions of the midbrain and isthmus in the armadillo, *J. Comp. Neurol. 78*:191-212, 1943a

Crosby, E. C., and R. T. Woodburne: The nuclear pattern of the non-tectal portions of the midbrain and isthmus in the shrew and bat, *J. Comp. Neurol. 78*:253-288, 1943b

Crosby, E. C., and R. T. Woodburne: The nuclear pattern of the non-tectal portions of the midbrain and isthmus in primates, *J. Comp. Neurol. 78*:441-482, 1943c

Crosby, E. C., and R. T. Woodburne: The mammalian midbrain and isthmus regions. Part II. The fiber connections. C. The hypothalamo-tegmental pathways, *J. Comp. Neurol. 94*:1-32, 1951

Crosby, E. C., T. Humphrey, and E. W. Lauer: *Correlative Anatomy of the Nervous System,* Macmillan, New York, 1962

Cuenod, M.: Split-brain studies. Functional interaction between bilateral central nervous structures, in *The Structure and Function of Nervous Tissue,* vol. 5, Academic Press, New York, 1972

Curtis, A. H., and H. F. Helmholz: A study of the anterior horn cells of an abrachius and their relation to the development of the extremities, *J. Comp. Neurol. 21*: 323-343, 1911

Dammerman, K. W.: Der Saccus vasculosus der Fische, ein Tiefeorgan, *Ztschr. f. Wissensch. Zool.* 96:654-726, 1910

de la Torre, E., M. G. Netsky, and I. Meschan: Intracranial and extracranial circulations in the dog: anatomic and angiographic studies, *Amer. J. Anat.* 105:343-382, 1959

de Lorenzo, A. J. D.: The olfactory neuron and the blood-brain barrier, in *Taste and Smell in Vertebrates* (Ciba Foundation Symposium), G. E. W. Wolstenholme and J. Knight, eds., Churchill, London, 1970

Dempster, W. T.: The morphology of the amphibian endolymphatic organ, *J. Morphol.* 50:71-120, 1930

Diamond, I. T., and W. C. Hall: Evolution of neocortex, *Science* 184:251-262, 1969.

Diamond, I. T., M. Snyder, H. Killackey, J. A. Jane, and W. C. Hall: Thalamo-cortical projections in the tree shrew (Tupaia glis), *J. Comp. Neurol.* 139: 273-306, 1970

Dijkgraaf, S.: Lokalisationsversuche am Fischgehirn, *Experientia* 5:44-45, 1949

Dijkgraaf, S.: Sound reception in the dogfish, *Nature* 197:93-94, 1963a

Dijkgraaf, S.: The functioning and significance of the lateral line organs, *Biol. Rev.* 38:51-105, 1963b

Dooling, E. C., J. F. Barlow, J. V. Murphy, and E. P. Richardson: Cysts of the cavum septi pellucidi, *Arch. Neurol.* 27:79-84, 1972

Dorn, E.: Der Saccus vasculosus, in *Handbucher mikroscopischen Anatomie des Menschen. Nervensystem,* pp. 140-185, W. von Moellendorff, ed., Springer, Berlin, 1955

Dow, R. S., and G. Moruzzi: *The Physiology and Pathology of the Cerebellum,* University of Minnesota Press, Minneapolis, 1958

Droogleever-Fortuyn, J.: Topographical relations in the telencephalon of the sunfish, Eupomotis gibbosus, *J. Comp. Neurol.* 116:249-263, 1961

DuBois, F. S.: The tractus solitarius and attendant nuclei in the Virginian opossum (Didelphis virginiana), *J. Comp. Neurol.* 47:189-224, 1929

Dubowitz, V.: Comparative studies in mature human and animal muscles, in *Developing and Diseased Muscle* (SIMR Res. Monograph No. 2), Spastics Int. Med. Pub. and Heinemann Med. Books, London, 1969

Eakin, R. M.: Lines of evolution of photoreceptors, *J. Gen. Physiol.* 46:359A-360A, 1962

Eakin, R. M., and J. A. Westfall: Fine structure of the retina in the reptilian third eye, *J. Biophys. Biochem. Cytol.* 6:133-134, 1959

Eakin, R. M., and J. A. Westfall: Further observations on the fine structure of the parietal eye of lizards, *J. Biophys. Biochem. Cytol.* 8:483-499, 1960

Earle, K. M., M. Baldwin, and W. Penfield: Incisural sclerosis and temporal lobe seizures produced by hippocampal herniation at birth, *AMA Arch. Neurol. Psychiat.* 69:27-42, 1953

Ebbesson, S. O. E.: Retinal projections in two teleost fishes (Opsanus tau and Gymnothorax funebris). An experimental study with silver impregnation methods, *Brain Behav. Evol.* 1:134-154, 1968

Ebbesson, S. O. E.: On the organization of central visual pathways in vertebrates, *Brain Behav. Evol.* 3:178-194, 1970

Ebbesson, S. O. E.: A proposal for a common nomenclature for some optic nuclei in vertebrates and the evidence for a common origin of two such cell groups, *Brain Behav. Evol.* 6:75-91, 1972

Ebbesson, S. O. E., and L. Heimer: Projections of the olfactory tract fibers in the nurse shark (Ginglymostoma cirratum), *Brain Res.* 17:47-55, 1970

Ebbesson, S. O. E., J. A. Jane, and D. M. Schroeder: A general overview of major interspecific variations in thalamic organization, *Brain Behav. Evol.* 6:92-130, 1972

Ebbesson, S. O. E., and D. M. Schroeder: Connections of the nurse shark's telencephalon, *Science* 173:254-256, 1971

Eccles, J. C., M. Ito, and J. Szentágothai: *The Cerebellum as a Neuronal Machine,* Springer, New York, 1967

Edds, M. V.: Neuronal specificity in neurogenesis, in *The Neurosciences,* G. C. Quarton, T. Melnechuk, and F. O. Schmitt, eds., Rockefeller University Press, New York, 1967

Edinger, L., and B. Fischer: Ein Mensch ohne Grosshirn, *Arch. f. d. ges. Physiol.* 152:535-561, 1913

Egar, M., and M. Singer: The role of the ependyma in spinal cord regeneration in the urodele, Triturus, *Exp. Neurol.* 37:422-430, 1972

Ellenberger, C., J. Hanaway, and M. G. Netsky: Embryogenesis of the inferior olivary nucleus in the rat: A radioautographic study and re-evaluation of the rhombic lip, *J. Comp. Neurol.* 137:71-88, 1969

Engel, W. K.: The multiplicity of pathologic reactions of human skeletal muscle, Proc. 5th Int. Cong. Neuropath., *Exerpta Med.,* 613-624, 1965

Engel, W. K.: Muscle biopsies in neuromuscular diseases, *Ped. Cl. N. Amer.* 14:963-995, 1967

Enger, P. S.: Hearing in fish, in *Hearing Mechanisms in Vertebrates* (Ciba Foundation Symposium), A. V. S. DeReuck and J. Knight, eds., Little, Brown, Boston, 1968

Erickson, R. R., W. C. Hall, J. A. Jane, M. Snyder, and I. T. Diamond: Organization of the posterior dorsal thalamus of the hedgehog, *J. Comp. Neurol.* 131:103-130, 1967

Erulkar, S. D.: Comparative aspects of spatial localization of sound, *Physiol. Rev.* 52:237-360, 1972

Ettlinger, E. G.: *Functions of the Corpus Callosum* (Ciba Foundation Study Grp. No. 20), Little, Brown, Boston, 1965

Eyzaguirre, C.: Functional organization of neuromuscular spindle in toad, *J. Neurophysiol.* 20:522-542, 1957

Favaro, G.: Contribution à l'étude morphologique de l'hypophyse caudale (crenflement caudal de la moelle épinière téléosteens), *Arch. Ital. Biol.* 75:164-170, 1926

Feldman, M. L., and J. M. Harrison: The projection of the acoustic nerve to the ventral cochlear nucleus of the rat. A Golgi study, *J. Comp. Neurol.* 137:267-294, 1969

Fenichel, G. M., and W. K. Engel: Histochemistry of muscle in infantile spinal muscular atrophy, *Neurology* 13:1059-1066, 1963

Fex, J.: Efferent inhibition in the cochlea by the olivo-cochlear bundle, in *Hearing Mechanisms in Vertebrates,* Ciba Foundation Symposium, A. V. S. De Reuck and J. Knight, eds., Little, Brown, Boston, 1968

Field, E. J., and R. J. Harrison: *Anatomical Terms. Their Origin and Derivation,* 2nd ed., Heffer, Cambridge, 1957

Fleischhauer, K.: Untersuchungen am Ependym des Zwischen- und Mittel-hirns der

Landschildkrote (Testudo agraeca), *Ztschr. Zellforsch u. mikr. Anat.* 46:729-767, 1957

Fleischhauer, K.: Regional differences in the structure of the ependyma and subependymal layers of the cerebral ventricles of the cat, in *Regional Neurochemistry*, S. S. Kety and J. Elkes, eds., Pergamon, London, 1961

Foley, J. M., and D. Baxter: Observations on the morphology of the cells of the locus coeruleus and substantia nigra in infants, *J. Neuropath. Exp. Neurol.* 15:219-221, 1956

Foley, J. M., and D. Baxter: On the nature of pigment granules in the cells of the locus coeruleus and substantia nigra, *J. Neuropath. Exp. Neurol.* 17:586-598, 1958

Fox, C. A.: The mammillary peduncle and ventral tegmental nucleus in the cat, *J. Comp. Neurol.* 75:411-425, 1941

Fox, C. A.: The structure of the cerebellar cortex, in *Correlative Anatomy of the Nervous System*, E. C. Crosby, T. L. Humphrey, and E. W. Lauer, Macmillan, New York, 1962

Fox, C. A., D. Hillman, K. Siegesmund, and C. Dutta: The primate cerebellar cortex: A Golgi and electron miscroscopic study, *Prog. Brain Res.* 25:174-225, 1967

Franz, V.: Haunt, Sinnesorgane und Nervensystem der Akranier, *Jenaische Ztschr. f. Naturw.* 59:401-526, 1923

Fraser, G. R.: Association of congenital deafness with goitre (Pendred's syndrome). A study of 207 families, *Ann. Human Genet.* 28:201-249, 1965

Freeman, J. A.: The cerebellum as a timing device: An experimental study in the frog, in *Neurobiology of Cerebellar Evolution and Development*, R. Llinás, ed., Amer. Med. Assoc., Chicago, 1965

Gamper, E.: Bau und Leistungen eines menschlichen Mitteilhirnwesens (Arhinencephalie mit Encephalocele). Zugleich ein Beitrag zur Teratologie und Fasersystomatik, *Ztschr. f. d. ges. Neurol. u. Psychiat.* 7:154, 1926

Garey, L. J., E. G. Jones, and T. P. S. Powell: Interrelationships of striate and extrastriate cortex with the primary relay sites of the visual pathway, *J. Neurol. Neurosurg. Psychiat* 31:135-157, 1968

Gazzaniga, M. S.: *The Bisected Brain*, Appleton-Century-Crofts, New York, 1970

Gazzaniga, M. S., and H. Freedman: Observations on visual processes after posterior callosal section, *Neurology* 23:1126-1130, 1973

Gershenfeld, H. M., J. H. Tramezzani, and H. DeRobertis: Ultrastructure and function in neurohypophysis of the toad, *Endocrinology* 66:741-768, 1960

Gfeller, E.: Brain pigment and catecholamines (letter to editor), *Lancet* 2:739, 1965

Gillilan, L. A.: The nuclear pattern of the non-tectal portions of the midbrain and isthmus in rodents, *J. Comp. Neurol,* 78:213-252, 1943a

Gillilan, L. A.: The nuclear pattern of the non-tectal portions of the midbrain and isthmus in ungulates, *J. Comp. Neurol.* 78:289-364, 1943b

Gillilan, L. A.: A comparative study of the extrinsic and intrinsic arterial blood supply to the brains of submammalian vertebrates, *J. Comp. Neurol.* 130:175-196, 1967

Gillilan, L. A.: Blood supply to primitive mammalian brains, *J. Comp. Neurol.* 145:209-222, 1972

Glees, P.: *Neuroglia: Morphology and Function*, Blackwell, Oxford, 1955

Glees, P., and P. D. Wall: Commissural fibers of the macaque thalamus, *J. Comp. Neurol.* 88:129-136, 1948

Globus, J. H.: The meningiomas: Their origin, divergence in structure, and relationship to contiguous tissue in the light of the phylogenesis and ontogenesis of the meninges; with a suggestion of a simplified classification of meningeal neoplasms, *Assoc. Res. Nerv. Ment. Dis., Proc. 16*:210-265, 1937

Gooddy, W.: Cerebral representation, *Brain 79*:167-187, 1956

Graeber, R. C., and S. O. E. Ebbesson: Visual discrimination learning in normal and tectal-ablated nurse sharks (Ginglymostoma cirratum), *Comp. Biochem. Physiol. 42A*:131-139, 1972

Graeber, R. C., S. O. E. Ebbesson, and J. A. Jane: Visual discrimination in sharks without optic tectum, *Science 180*:413-415, 1973

Granit, R.: *The Basis of Motor Control,* Academic Press, New York, 1970

Gray, E. G.: The spindle and extrafusal innervation of a frog muscle, *Proc. Roy. Soc. Lond.,* series B, *146*:416-430, 1957

Green, J. D.: The hippocampus, *Physiol. Rev. 44*:561-608, 1964

Greenfield, J. G.: *The Spino-Cerebellar Degenerations,* Thomas, Springfield, Ill., 1954

Gunn, M.: A study of the enteric plexuses in some amphibians, *Quart. J. Micr. Sci. 92*:55-78, 1951

Hall, W. C., and F. F. Ebner: Thalamo-telencephalic projections in a turtle (Pseudemys scripta), *Anat. Rec. 163*:193, 1969

Hampson, J. L., C. R. Harrison, and C. N. Woolsey: Cerebro-cerebellar projections and the somatotopic localization of motor function in the cerebellum, *Assoc. Res. Nerv. Ment. Dis., Proc. 30*:299-316, 1952

Hanaway, J., S. I. Lee, and M. G. Netsky: Pachygyria: relation of findings to modern embryologic concepts, *Neurology 18*:791-799, 1968

Hanaway, J., J. A. McConnell, and M. G. Netsky: Histogenesis of the substantia nigra, ventral tegmental area of Tsai and interpeduncular nucleus: an autoradiographic study of the mesencephalon in the rat, *J. Comp. Neurol. 142*:59-73, 1971

Hanaway, J., and M. G. Netsky: Heterotopias of the inferior olive: Relation to Dandy-Walker malformation and correlation with experimental data, *J. Neuropath. Exp. Neurol. 30*:380-389, 1971

Hansen-Pruss, O. C.: Meninges of birds, with a consideration of the sinus rhomboidalis, *J. Comp. Neurol. 36*:193-217, 1923

Harkmark, W.: The rhombic lip and its derivatives in relation to the theory of neurobiotaxis, in *Aspects of Cerebellar Anatomy,* J. Jansen and A. Brodal, eds., John Grundt Tanum, Oslo, 1954

Harriman, D. G. F., and M. Garland: The pathology of Adie's syndrome, *Brain 91*:401-418, 1968

Harris, G. W., and R. George: Neurohumeral control of the adenohypophysis and the regulation of the secretion of TSH, ACTH, and growth hormone, in *The Hypothalamus,* W. Haymaker, E. Anderson, and W. J. H. Nauta, eds., Thomas, Springfield, Ill., 1969

Harrison, J. M., and R. Irving: The organization of the posterior ventral cochlear nucleus in the rat, *J. Comp. Neurol. 126*:391-402, 1966

Harrison, J. M., and W. B. Warr: A study of the cochlear nuclei and ascending auditory pathways of the medulla, *J. Comp. Neurol. 119*:341-352, 1962

Hart, M. N., N. Malamud and W. G. Ellis: The Dandy-Walker syndrome. A clinicopathologic study based on 28 cases, *Neurology 22*:771-780, 1972

Haymaker, W.: Hypothalamo-pituitary neural pathways and the circulatory system of the pituitary, in *The Hypothalamus,* W. Haymaker, E. Anderson, and W. J. H. Nauta, eds., Thomas, Springfield, Ill., 1969

Heath, C. J., and E. G. Jones: Interhemispheric pathways in the absence of a corpus callosum. An experimental study of commissural connections in the marsupial phalanger, *J. Anat. 109:*253-270, 1971

Hebb, C., and D. Ratković: Choline acetylase in the evolution of the brain in vertebrates, in *Comparative Neurochemistry,* D. Richter, ed., Macmillan, New York, 1964

Heimer, L.: The secondary olfactory connections in mammals, reptiles and sharks, *Ann. N.Y. Acad. Sci. 167:*129-146, 1969

Heisey, S. R.: Brain and choroid plexus blood volumes in vertebrates, *Comp. Biochem. Physiol. 26:*489-498, 1968

Hendrickson, A. E., and D. E. Kelly: Development of the amphibian pineal organ; fine structure during maturation, *Anat. Rec. 170:*129-142, 1971

Hern, J. E. C., C. G. Phillips, and R. Porter: Electrical thresholds of unimpaled corticospinal cells in the cat, *Quart. J. Physiol. 47:*134-140, 1962

Herrick, C. J.: The amphibian forebrain. III. The optic tracts and centers of Amblystoma and the frog, *J. Comp. Neurol. 39:*433-489, 1925

Herrick, C. J.: *Brains in Rats and Men,* University of Chicago Press, Chicago, 1929 (reprinted by Hafner, New York, 1963)

Herrick, C. J.: *The Brain of the Tiger Salamander,* University of Chicago Press, Chicago, 1948

Herrick, C. J., and G. E. Coghill: The development of reflex mechanisms in Amblystoma, *J. Comp. Neurol. 25:*65-85, 1915

Hess, A.: The sarcoplasmic reticulum, the T system, and the motor terminals of slow and twitch muscle fibers in the garter snake, *J. Cell. Biol. 26:*467-476, 1965

Hirano, H.: Ultrastructural study on the morphogenesis of the neuromuscular junction in the skeletal muscle of the chick, *Ztschr. f. Zellforsch. u. mikr. Anat. 79:*198-208, 1967

Hirsch, E. F.: *The Innervation of the Vertebrate Heart,* Thomas, Springfield, Ill., 1970

Hirsch, E. F., and G. C. Kaiser: *The Innervation of the Vertebrate Lung,* Thomas, Springfield, Ill., 1969

Hoffman, H. H.: The olfactory bulb, accessory olfactory bulb and hemisphere of some anurans, *J. Comp. Neurol. 120:*317-336, 1963

Hoffman, C. K.: Zur Entwicklungsgeschichte des Selachierkopfes, *Anat. Anz. 9:*638-653, 1894

Hollinshead, W. H.: The innervation of the adrenal glands, *J. Comp. Neurol. 64:*449-467, 1936

Holmes, W.: The adrenal homologues in the lungfish Protopterus, *Proc. Roy. Soc. Lond.* series B, *137:*549-562, 1950

Horstmann, E.: Die Faserglia des Selachiergehirns, *Ztschr. Zellforsch. u. mikr. Anat. 39:*588-617, 1954

Hubel, D. H., and T. N. Wiesel: Receptive fields of single neurones in the cat's cortex, *J. Physiol. 148:*574-591, 1959

Hubel, D. H., and T. N. Wiesel: Receptive fields, binocular interaction and functional architecture in the cat's visual cortex, *J. Physiol. 160:*106-154, 1962

Hubel, D. H., and T. N. Wiesel: Shape and arrangement of columns in cat's striate cortex, *J. Physiol. 165:*559-568, 1963

Hubel, D. H., and T. N. Wiesel: Receptive fields and functional architecture of monkey striate cortex, *J. Physiol. 195:*215-243, 1968

Huber, G. C., and E. C. Crosby: The nuclei and fiber paths of the avian diencephalon, with consideration of telencephalic and certain mesencephalic centers and connections, *J. Comp. Neurol. 48*:1-225, 1929

Huber, G. C., and E. C. Crosby: The reptilian optic tectum, *J. Comp. Neurol. 57*:57-163, 1933

Hughes, E. B., and W. T. Smith. An unusual tumour histologically resembling a chemodectoma removed surgically from the pineal region, Proc. 2nd Int. Cong. Neuropath., London, *Exerpta Medica* 114-115, 1955

Hughes, R. A., J. W. Kernohan, and W. McK. Craig: Caves and cysts of the septum pellucidum, *Arch. Neurol. Psychiat. 74*:259-266, 1955

Hunter, J., and H. H. Jasper: Effects of thalamic stimulation in unanesthetised animals, *Electroenceph. Clin. Neurophysiol. 1*:305-324, 1949

Igarashi, S., and T. Kamiya: *Atlas of the Vertebrates Brain; Morphologic Evolution from Cyclostomes to Mammals,* University Park Press, Baltimore, 1972

Iwai, E., S. Saito, and S. Tsukahara: Analysis of central mechanism in visual discrimination learning of goldfish, *Tohoku J. Exp. Med. 102*:135-142, 1970

Jacobsohn, L.: Ueber die Kerne des Menschlichen Hirnstamms, *Anhang. zu den Abh. Preuss Akad. Wiss., Physik-Math. Kl.,* 1909

Jackson, J. H.: Croonian lectures, *Brit. Med. J. 1*:501, 660, 703, 1884

Jakob, A.: Die Extrapyramidalen Erkrankungen mit Besonderer Beruchsichtigung der Pathologischen Anatomie und Histologie und der Pathophysiologie der Bewegungstorungen, *Ges. d. Neurol. u. Psychiat. 37*:1-416, 1923

Jane, J. A., N. Levey, and N. J. Carlson: Tectal and cortical function in vision, *Exp. Neurol. 35*:61-77, 1972

Jane, J. A., and D. M. Schroeder: A comparison of dorsal column nuclei and spinal afferents in the European hedgehog (Erinaceus europeaus), *Exp. Neurol. 30*: 1-17, 1971

Jansen, J.: The brain of Myxine glutinosa, *J. Comp. Neurol. 49*:359-507, 1930

Jansen, J.: Experimental studies on the intrinsic fibers of the cerebellum. I. The arcuate fibers, *J. Comp. Neurol. 57*:369-399, 1933

Jansen, J.: On cerebellar evolution and organization from the point of view of a morphologist, in *Neurobiology of Cerebellar Evolution and Development,* R. Llinás, ed., Amer. Med. Assoc., Chicago, 1969

Jansen, J., and A. Brodal: *Aspects of Cerebellar Anatomy,* Gundersen, Oslo, 1954

Jasper, H. H., and J. Kershman: Electroencephalographic classification of the epilepsies, *Arch. Neurol. Psychiat. 45*:903-943, 1941

Jeeves, M. A.: Psychological studies of three cases of congenital agenesis of the corpus callosum, in *Functions of the Corpus Callosum* (Ciba Foundation Study Group No. 20), E. G. Ettlinger, ed., Little, Brown, Boston, 1965

Johnston, J. B.: The brain of Petromyzon, *J. Comp. Neurol. 12*:1-86, 1902

Jones, E. G.: The innervation of muscle spindles in the Australian opossum, Trichosurus vulpecula, with special reference to the motor nerve endings, *J. Anat. 100*:733-759, 1966

Joseph, B. S., and D. G. Whitlock: Central projections of selected dorsal roots in anuran amphibians, *Anat. Rec. 160*:279-288, 1968a

Joseph, B. S., and D. G. Whitlock: Central projections of brachial and lumbar dorsal roots in reptiles, *J. Comp. Neurol. 132*:469-484, 1968b

Jouan, P., and S. Samperez: Etude del al sécrétion des corticostéroides et de l'hormone adrénocorticotrope hypophysaire chez le rat epiphysectomisé, *Prog. Brain Res. 10*:604-611, 1965

Jouvet, M.: Neurophysiology of the states of sleep, in *The Neurosciences*, G. C. Quarton, T. Melnechuk, and F. O. Schmitt, eds., Rockefeller University Press, New York, 1967

Kahn, E. A., E. C. Crosby, R. C. Schneider, and J. A. Taren: *Correlative Neurosurgery*, Thomas, Springfield, Ill., 1969

Kahn, E. A., and E. C. Crosby: Korsakoff's syndrome associated with surgical lesions involving the mammillary bodies, *Neurology 22*:117-125, 1972

Kahn, K.: The natural course of experimental cerebral infarction in the gerbil, *Neurology 22*:510-515, 1972

Kaiserman-Abramof, I. R., and S. L. Palay: Fine structural studies of the cerebellar cortex in a mormyrid fish, in *Neurobiology of Cerebellar Evolution and Development*, R. Llinás, ed., Amer. Med. Assoc., Chicago, 1969

Källén, B.: Embryogenesis of brain nuclei in the chick telencephalon, *Ergebn. Anat. EntwGesch. 36*:62-82, 1962

Kapoor, A. S., and P. P. Ojha: Studies on ventilation of the olfactory chambers of fishes with a critical reevaluation of the role of accessory nasal sacs, *Arch. Biol. 83*:167-178, 1972

Kapoor, A. S., and P. P. Ojha: The olfactory apparatus in the flatfish Cynoglossus oligolepis, *Tr. Amer. Micr. Soc. 92*:298-304, 1973

Kappers, C. U. A.: Weitere Mitteilungen ueber Neurobiotaxis. Die Selektivitat der Zellenwanderung. Die Bedeutung synchronischer Reizverwandtschaft. Verlaug und Endigung der zentralen sogenannten motorischen Bahnen, *Folia. Neurobiol. 1*:507, 1908

Kappers, C. U. A.: Further contributions on neurobiotaxis; an attempt to compare the phenomena of neurobiotaxis with other phenomena of taxis and tropism; the dynamic polarization of the neurone, *J. Comp. Neurol. 27*:261-298, 1916

Kappers, C. U. A., C. G. Huber, and E. C. Crosby: *Comparative Anatomy of the Nervous System of Vertebrates, Including Man*, Macmillan, New York, 1936 (reprinted by Hafner, New York, 1960)

Kappers, C. U. A.: Phenomena of neurobiotaxis as demonstrated by the position of the motor nuclei of the oblongata, *J. Nerv. Ment. Dis. 1*:1-16, 1919

Kappers, C. U. A.: *Anatomie Comparée du Système Nerveux*, De Erven F. Bohn, Haarlem, Masson, Paris, 1947

Kappers, J. A.: The development and structure of the paraphysis cerebri in urodeles with experiments on its function in Amblystoma mexicanum, *J. Comp. Neurol. 92*:93-125, 1950

Kappers, J. A.: The development of the paraphysis cerebri in man with comments on its relationship to the intercolumnar tubercle and its significance for the origin of cystic tumors in the third ventricle, *J. Comp. Neurol. 102*:425-509, 1955

Kappers, J. A.: Survey of the innervation of the epiphysis and the accessory pineal organs of vertebrates. *Prog. Brain Res. 10*:87-153, 1965

Karnovsky, M. J.: The ultrastructural basis of capillary permeability studied with peroxidase as a tracer, *J. Cell. Biol. 35*:213-236, 1967

Karten, H. J.: The organization of the avian telencephalon and some speculations on the phylogeny of the amniote telencephalon, *Ann. N.Y. Acad. Sci. 167*:164-179, 1969

Karten, H. J., and W. Hodos: Telencephalic projections of the nucleus rotundus in the pigeon (Columbia livia), *J. Comp. Neurol. 140*:35-52, 1970

Karten, H. J., and W. J. H. Nauta: Organization of retinothalamic projections in the pigeon and owl, *Anat. Rec. 160*:373, 1968

Kato, M., H. Lakamara, and B. Fujimori: Studies on effects of pyramid stimulation upon flexor and extensor motoneurones and gamma motoneurones, *Jap. J. Physiol. 14*:34-44, 1964

Kemali, M., and V. Braitenberg: *Atlas of the Frog's Brain,* Springer, New York: 1969

Kennedy, B. J., and A. S. Zelickson: Melanoma in an albino, *J.A.M.A. 189*:839-841, 1963

Kirschbaum, W. R.: Agenesis of the corpus callosum and associated malformations, *J. Neuropath. Exp. Neurol. 6*:78-94, 1947

Klatzo, I., and O. Steinwall: Observations on cerebrospinal fluid pathways and behaviour of the blood-brain barrier in sharks, *Acta Neuropathol. 5*:161-175, 1965

Kleerekoper, H.: Some aspects of olfaction in fishes, with special reference to orientation, *Amer. Zool. 7*:385-395, 1967

Kleerkoper, H., and T. Malar: Orientation through sound in fishes, in *Hearing Mechanisms in Vertebrates* (Ciba Foundation Symposium), A. V. S. De Reuck and J. Knight, eds., Little, Brown, Boston, 1968

Kluever, H., and E. Barrera: A method for the combined staining of cells and fibers in the nervous system, *J. Neuropath. Exp. Neurol. 12*:400-403, 1953

Kooy, F. H.: The inferior olive in vertebrates, *Folia Neuro-biol. 10*:205-369, 1916

Korneliussen, H. K.: Cerebellar corticogenesis in Cetacea, with special reference to regional variations, *J. Hirnforsch. 9*:151-185, 1967

Korneliussen, H. K.: On the ontogenetic development of the cerebellum (nuclei, fissures and cortex) of the rat, with special reference to regional variations in corticogenesis, *J. Hirnforsch. 10*:379-412, 1968

Krabbe, K. H.: Development of the pineal organ and a rudimentary parietal eye in some birds, *J. Comp. Neurol. 103*:139-149, 1955

Krnjević, K., and A. Silver: A histochemical study of the cholinergic fibers in the cerebral cortex, *J. Anat. 99*:711-759, 1965

Kuypers, H. G. J. M.: An anatomical analysis of cortico-bulbar connexions to the pons and lower brain stem in the cat, *J. Anat. 92*:198-218, 1958a

Kuypers, H. G. J. M.: Corticobulbar connexions to the pons and lower brain-stem in man. An anatomical study, *Brain 81*:364-387, 1958b

Kuypers, H. G. J. M.: The descending pathways to the spinal cord, their anatomy and function, *Prog. Brain Res. 11*:178-202, 1964

Kuypers, H. G. J. M., and D. G. Lawrence: Cortical projections to the red nucleus and the brain stem in the rhesus monkey, *Brain Res. 4*:151-188, 1967

Lapresle, J., and M. Ben Hamida: The dentato-olivary pathway. Somatotopic relationship between the dentate nucleus and the contralateral inferior olive. *Arch. Neurol. 22*:135-143, 1970

Larramendi, L. M. H.: Analysis of synaptogenesis in the cerebellum of the mouse, in *Neurobiology of Cerebellar Evolution and Development,* R. Llinás, ed., Amer. Med. Assoc., Chicago, 1969

Larroche, J. C.: Maturation morphologique du système nerveux central: ses rapports avec le developpement pondéral du foetus et son age gestationnel, in *Regional Development of the Brain in Early Life,* A. Minkowski, ed., F. A. Davis, Philadelphia, 1967

Larroche, J. C., and J. Baudey: Cavum septi pellucidi, cavum Vergae, cavum veli interpositi: Cavités de la ligne médiane. Etude anatomique et pneumonencéphalographique dans la période néonatale, *Biol. Neonate. 3*:193-236, 1961

Larsell, O.: The differentiation of the peripheral and central acoustic apparatus in the frog, *J. Comp. Neurol. 60*:473-527, 1934

Larsell, O.: The cerebellum of myxinoids and petromyzonts including developmental stages in the lampreys, *J. Comp. Neurol. 86*:395-445, 1947a

Larsell, O.: The nucleus of the IVth nerve in petromyzonts, *J. Comp. Neurol. 86*: 447-466, 1947b

Larsell, O.: *The Comparative Anatomy and Histology of the Cerebellum from Myxinoids through Birds,* J. Jansen, ed., University of Minnesota Press, Minneapolis, 1967

Larsell, O.: *The Comparative Anatomy and Histology of the Cerebellum from Monotremes through Apes,* J. Jansen, ed., University of Minnesota Press, Minneapolis, 1970

Larsell, O., and J. Jansen: *The Comparative Anatomy and Histology of the Cerebellum. The Human Cerebellum, Cerebellar Connections, and Cerebellar Cortex,* University of Minnesota Press, Minneapolis, 1972

Larsen, J. R., and A. Broadbent: The neurosecretory cells of the brain of Aedes aegypti in relation to larval molt, metamorphosis and ovarian development, *Tr. Amer. Micr. Soc. 87*:395-410, 1968

Lasek, R., B. S. Joseph, and D. G. Whitlock: Evaluation of a radioautographic neuroanatomical tracing method, *Brain Res. 8*:319-336, 1968

LeGros Clark, W. E.: The projection of the olfactory epithelium on the olfactory bulb in the rabbit, *J. Neurol. Neurosurg. Psychiat. 14*:1-10, 1951

LeGros Clark, W. E., and D. W. C. Northfield: The cortical projection of the pulvinar in the macaque monkey, *Brain 60*:126-142, 1937

Lemmcn, L. J., E. R. Davis, and L. L. Radnor: Observations on stimulation of the human frontal eye field, *J. Comp. Neurol. 112*:163-168, 1959

Lende, R. A.: A comparative approach to the neocortex: localization in monotremes, marsupials and insectivores, *Ann. N.Y. Acad. Sci. 167*:262-276, 1969

Lettvin, J. Y., H. R. Maturanna, W. S. McCulloch, and W. H. Pitts: What the frog's eye tells the frog's brain, *Proc. Inst. Radio Engrs.* (New York) *47*:1940-1957, 1959

Levi-Montalcini, R.: Events in the developing nervous system, *Prog. Brain Res. 4*:1-29, 1964

Levine, S., and D. Sohn: Cerebral ischemia in infant and adult gerbils, *Arch. Pathol. 87*:315-317, 1969

Licht, P., and C. S. Nicoll: Localization of prolactin in the reptilian pars distalis, *Gen. Comp. Endocrinol. 12*:526-535, 1969

Lin, H., and W. R. Ingram: Probable absence of connections between the retina and the hypothalamus in the cat, *Exp. Neurol. 37*:23-36, 1972

Lindström, T.: On the cranial nerves of the cyclostomes with special reference to the nervus trigeminus, *Acta Zool. 30*:315-458, 1949

Liss, L., and L. Mervis: The ependymal lining of the cavum septi pellucidi: A histological and histochemical study, *J. Neuropath. Exp. Neurol. 23*:355-367, 1964

Llinás, R., and D. E. Hillman: Physiological and morphological organization of the cerebellar circuits in various vertebrates, in *Neurobiology of Cerebellar Evolution and Development,* R. Llinás, ed., Amer. Med. Assoc., Chicago, 1969

Lofgren, F.: The infundibular recess, a component in the hypothalamo-adenohypophyseal system, *Acta Morphol. Neerl. Scandin. 3*:55-78, 1959

Loken, A. C., and A. Brodal: A somatotopic pattern in the human lateral vestibular nucleus, *Arch. Neurol.* 23:350-357, 1970

Lumley, J. S. P.: The role of the massa intermedia in motor performance in the rhesus monkey, *Brain* 95:347-356, 1972

Lundberg, A., and P. E. Voorhoeve: Pyramidal activation of interneurones of various spinal reflex arcs in the cat, *Experientia* 1-5, 1961

MacLean, P. D.: The hypothalamus and emotional behavior, in *The Hypothalamus*, W. Haymaker, E. Anderson, and W. J. H. Nauta, eds., Thomas, Springfield, Ill., 1969

Malamud, N.: *Atlas of Neuropathology*, University of California Press, Los Angeles, 1957

Marsden, C. D.: Pigmentation in the nucleus substantiae nigrae of mammals, *J. Anat.* 95:256-261, 1961

Marsden, C. D.: Brain pigment and its relation to brain catecholamines, *Lancet* 2:475-476, 1244, 1965

Martin, P.: Role of the vestibular system in the control of posture and movement in man, in *Myotatic, Kinesthetic and Vestibular Mechanisms* (Ciba Foundation Symposium), A. V. S. de Reuck and J. Knight, eds., Little, Brown, Boston, 1967

Martin, A. R., and G. Pilar: Dual mode of synaptic transmission in the avian ciliary ganglion, *J. Physiol.* 168:443-463, 1963

Massopust, L. C., and R. Thompson: A new interpedunculo-diencephalic pathway in rats and cats, *J. Comp. Neurol.* 118:97-105, 1962

McKibben, P. S.: The nervus terminalis in urodele amphibians, *J. Comp. Neurol.* 21:261-309, 1911

Meller, K., and P. Glees: The development of the mouse cerebellum. A Golgi and electron microscopical study, in *Neurobiology of Cerebellar Evolution and Development*, R. Llinás, ed., Amer. Med. Assoc., Chicago, 1969

Mettler, F. A.: Supratentorial mechanisms influencing the oculomotor apparatus, in *The Oculomotor System*, M. B. Bender, ed., Hoeber, New York, 1964

Michael, C. R.: Visual receptive fields of single neurons in superior colliculus of the ground squirrel, *J. Neurophysiol.* 35:815-832, 1972a

Michael, C. R.: Functional organization of cells in superior colliculus of the ground squirrel, *J. Neurophysiol.* 35:833-846, 1972b

Mittag, T. W., J. S. Mindel, and J. P. Green: Choline acetyltransferase in familial dysautonomia, N.Y. Acad. Sci. Conf. on the Trophic Function of the Neuron, Mar. 5-7, 1973, in press

Mollgaard, K., and M. Moller: On the innervation of the human fetal pineal gland, *Brain Res.* 52:428-432, 1973

Morrison, R. S., and E. W. Dempsey: Study of the thalamocortical relations, *Amer. J. Physiol.* 135:281-292, 1942

Moruzzi, G.: Reticular influences on the EEG, *Electroenceph. Clin. Neurophysiol.* 16:2-17, 1964

Moruzzi, G., and H. W. Magoun: Brain stem reticular formation and activation of the EEG, *Electroenceph. Clin. Neurophysiol.* 1:455-473, 1949

Moskowitz, N.: Comparative aspects of some features of the central auditory system of primates, *Ann. N.Y. Acad. Sci.* 167:357-369, 1969

Moszkowska, A.: Contribution à l'etude du mécanisme de l'antagonisme epiphyso-hypophysaire, *Prog. Brain Res.* 10:564-576, 1965

Moulton, D. G.: Olfaction in mammals, *Amer. Zool.* 7:421-429, 1967

Moulton, J. M., A. Jurand, and H. Fox: A cytological study of Mauthner's cells in Xenopus laevis and Rana temporaria during metamorphosis, *J. Embryol. Exp. Morphol. 19*:415-431, 1968

Mueller, E.: Studien ueber Neuroglia, *Arch. mikroskop. Anat. 60*:11-62, 1900

Mugnaini, E.: Ultrastructural studies on the cerebellar histogenesis. II. Maturation of nerve cell populations and establishment of synaptic connections in the cerebellar cortex of the chick, in *Neurobiology of Cerebellar Evolution and Development*, R. Llinás, ed., Amer. Med. Assoc., Chicago, 1969

Murphy, M. G., and J. L. O'Leary: Hanging and climbing functions in raccoon and sloth after total cerebellectomy, *Arch. Neurol. 28*:111-117, 1973

Murphy, M. G., J. L. O'Leary, and D. Cornblath: Axoplasmic flow in cerebellar mossy and climbing fibers, *Arch. Neurol. 28*:118-123, 1973

Myers, R. D.: Temperature regulation: Neurochemical systems in the hypothalamus, in *The Hypothalamus*, W. Haymaker, E. Anderson, and W. J. H. Nauta, eds., Thomas, Springfield, Ill., 1969

Nalbandov, A. V., and J. W. Graber: Neural control of the anterior and the posterior pituitary gland in birds, in *The Hypothalamus*, W. Haymaker, E. Anderson, and W. J. H. Nauta, eds., Thomas, Springfield, Ill., 1969

Nathan, P. W., and M. C. Smith: Long descending tracts in man. I. Review of present knowledge, *Brain 78*:248-303, 1955

Nauta, W. J. H., and W. Haymaker: Hypothalamic nuclei and fiber connections, in *The Hypothalamus*, W. Haymaker, E. Anderson, and W. J. H. Nauta, eds., Thomas, Springfield, Ill., 1969

Nauta, W. J. H., and H. G. J. M. Kuypers: Some ascending pathways in the brain stem reticular formation, in *Reticular Formation of the Brain*, H. H. Jasper et al., eds., Little, Brown, Boston, 1958

Nelson, D. R., and R. H. Johnson: Acoustic attraction of Pacific reef sharks: Effect of pulse intermittency and variability, *Comp. Biochem. Physiol. 42A*:85-95, 1972

Netsky, M. G., Degenerations of the cerebellum and its pathways, in *Pathology of the Nervous System*, vol. 1, J. Minckler ed., McGraw-Hill, New York, 1968

Netsky, M. G., and S. Shuangshoti: Studies on the choroid plexus, *Neurosci. Res. 3*:131-173, 1970

Nicol, J. A. C.: Autonomic nervous system in lower chordates, *Biol. Rev. 27*:1-49, 1952

Nicoll, C. S., and H. A. Bern: Further analysis of the occurrence of pigeon crop sac-stimulating activity (prolactin) in the vertebrate adenohypophysis, *Gen. Comp. Endocrinol. 11*:5-20, 1968

Niewenhuys, R.: Comparative anatomy of the spinal cord, *Prog. Brain Res. 11*:1-57, 1964

Nieuwenhuys, R.: Comparative anatomy of the cerebellum, *Prog. Brain Res. 25*:1-93, 1967

Nieuwenhys, R.: A survey of the structure of the forebrain in higher bony fishes (Osteichthyes), *Ann. N.Y. Acad. Sci. 167*:31-64, 1969

Nieuwenhuys, R., and C. Nicholson: A survey of the general morphology, the fiber connections, and the possible functional significance of the gigantocerebellum of mormyrid fishes, in *Neurobiology of Cerebellar Evolution and Development*, R. Llinás, ed., Amer. Med. Assoc., Chicago, 1969

Norman, R. M., and H. Urich: Cerebellar hypoplasia associated with systemic degeneration in early life, *J. Neurol. Neurosurg. Psychiat. 21*:159-166, 1958

Norman, R. M., D. R. Oppenheimer, and A. H. Tingey: Histological and chemical findings in Krabbe's leukodystrophy, *J. Neurol. Neurosurg. Psychiat.* 24:223-232, 1961

Norton, A. C.: *The Dorsal Column System of the Spinal Cord: Its Anatomy, Physiology, Phylogeny and Sensory Function,* an updated review, U.S. Dept. of HEW, Washington, D.C., 1969-1971

Novales, R. R., and B. J. Novales: Analysis of antagonisms between pineal melatonin and other agents which act on the amphibian melanophore, *Prog. Brain Res.* 10:507-519, 1965

Nyberg-Hansen, R.: Origin and termination of fibers from the vestibular nuclei descending in the medial longitudinal fasciculus. An experimental study with silver impregnation methods in the cat, *J. Comp. Neurol.* 122:355-364, 1964

Nyberg-Hansen, R., and A. Brodal: Sites of termination of corticospinal fibers in the cat, *J. Comp. Neurol.* 120:369-391, 1963

Nyberg-Hansen, R., and T. A. Mascitti: Sites and mode of termination of fibers of the vestibulospinal tract in the cat. An experimental study with silver impregnation techniques, *J. Comp. Neurol.* 122:369-387, 1964

Ocker and Crane: *Blind Flight in Theory and Practice,* quoted by R. Blodget, *Flying,* p. 57, Jan. 1972

Ogata, T., and M. Mori: Histochemical study of oxidative enzymes in vertebrate muscles, *J. Histochem. Cytochem.* 12:171-182, 1964

Ohloff, G., and A. F. Thomas, eds.: *Gustation and Olfaction,* Academic Press, New York, 1971

Ojemann, G. A., and A. A. Ward: Speech representation in ventrolateral thalamus, *Brain,* 94:669-680, 1971

Oksche, A.: Histologische Untersuchungen ueber die Bedeutung des Ependyms, der Glia und der Plexus chorioidei fur den Kohlenhydratsoffwechsel des ZNS, *Ztschr. Zellforsch. u. mikr. Anat.* 48:74-129, 1958

Oksche, A.: Histologische, histochemische und experimentelle Studien am Subkommissural organ von Anuren (Mit Hinweisen auf den Epiphysenkomplex), *Ztschr. Zellforsch. u. mikr. Anat.* 57:240-326, 1962

Oksche, A.: Survey of the development and comparative morphology of the pineal organ, *Prog. Brain Res.* 10:3-29, 1965

Oksche, A., and M. von Harnack: Elektronenmikroskopische Untersuchungen am Stirnorgan von Anuran (Zur Frage der Lichtrezeptoren), *Ztschr. Zellforsch. u. mikr. Anat.* 59:239-288, 1963

Oppelt, W. W., L. Bunim and D. P. Rall: Distribution of glucose in the spiny dogfish (S. acanthius) and the brier skate (R. eglanteria), *Life Sci.* 7:497-503, 1963

Ortman, R.: Parietal eye and nerve in Anolis carolinenis, *Anat. Rec.* 137:386, 1960

Palkovits, M.: Participation of the epithalamo-epiphyseal system in the regulation of water and electrolytes metabolism, *Prog. Brain Res.* 10:627-634, 1965

Pantin, C. F. A.: The elementary nervous system, *Proc. Roy. Soc.,* series B, 140:147-168, 1952

Papez, J. W., *Comparative Neurology,* Crowell, New York, 1929

Papez, J. W.: A proposed mechanism of emotion, *Arch. Neurol. Psychiat.* 38:725-743, 1937

Parsons, T. S.: Evolution of the nasal structure in the lower tetrapods, *Amer. Zool.* 7:397-413, 1967

Pasik, P., and T. Pasik: Oculomotor functions in monkeys with lesions of the cerebrum and the superior colliculi, in *The Oculomotor System,* M. B. Bender, ed., Hoeber, New York, 1964

Patton, H. D.: Physiology of smell and taste, *Ann. Rev. Physiol. 12*:469-484, 1950

Paul, E.: Ueber die Typen der Ependymzellen und ihre regionale Verteilung bei Rana temporaria L, *Ztschr. Zellforsch. u. mikr. Anat. 80*:461-487, 1967

Peachey, L. D.: Structure and function of slow striated muscle, in *Biophysics of Physiological and Pharmacological Actions,* pp. 391-411, Amer. Assoc. Advance. Science, Washington, D.C., 1961

Peachey, L.: The structure of the extraocular muscle fibers of mammals, in *The Control of Eye Movements,* P. Bach-y-Rita, C. C. Collins, and J. E. Hyde, eds., Academic Press, New York, 1971

Pearson, J., G. Budzilovich, and M. J. Finegold: Sensory, motor and autonomic dysfunction: The nervous system in familial dysautonomia, *Neurology 21*:486-493, 1971

Pearson, J., J. Dancis, and F. Axelrod: Current concepts of dysautonomia: neuropathological defects, N.Y. Acad. Sci. Conf. on the Trophic Function of the Neuron, Mar. 5-7, 1973, in press.

Pearson, R.: *The Avian Brain,* Academic Press, New York, 1972

Pfaffmann, C., ed.: *Olfaction and Taste,* Rockefeller University Press, New York, 1969

Piatt, J.: A study of the factors controlling the differentiation of Mauthner's cell in Amblystoma, *J. Comp. Neurol. 86*:199-223, 1947

Pick, J.: *The Autonomic Nervous System: Morphological, Comparative, Clinical, and Surgical Aspects,* Lippincott, Philadelphia, 1970

Plante, S.: The comparative anatomy of the interpeduncular nucleus in the brain of the rat, cat and monkey, *J. Neurol. Sci. 16*:155-163, 1972

Polak, M., and J. E. Azcoaga: Morphology and distribution of the neuroglia in the hypothalamus and neurohypophysis, in *The Hypothalamus,* W. Haymaker, E. Anderson, and W. J. H. Nauta, eds., Thomas, Springfield, Ill., 1969

Pollen, D. A.: Experimental spike and wave responses and petit mal epilepsy, *Epilepsia 9*:221-232, 1968

Polyak, S.: *The Vertebrate Visual System,* University of Chicago Press, Chicago, 1957

Pompeiano, O., and A. Brodal: The origin of vestibulospinal fibers in the cat. An experimental study with comments on the descending medial longitudinal fasciculus, *Arch. Ital. Biol. 95*:166-195, 1957a

Pompeiano, O., and A. Brodal: Spino-vestibular fibers in the cat. An experimental study, *J. Comp. Neurol. 108*:353-382, 1957b

Pompeiano, O., and A. Brodal: Experimental demonstration of a somatotopical origin of rubrospinal fibers in the cat, *J. Comp. Neurol. 108*:225-252, 1957c

Preston, J. B., and D. G. Whitlock: Precentral facilitation and inhibition of motoneurones, *J. Neurophysiol. 23*:154-170, 1960

Pye, J. D.: Hearing in bats, in *Hearing Mechanisms in Vertebrates* (Ciba Foundation Symposium), A. V. S. DeReuck and J. Knight, eds., Little, Brown, Boston, 1968

Quay, W. B.: Histological structure and cytology of the pineal organ in birds and mammals, *Prog. Brain Res. 10*:49-86, 1965a

Quay, W. B.: Experimental evidence for pineal participation in homeostasis of brain composition, *Prog. Brain Res. 10*:646-653, 1965b

Raisman, G.: The connexions of the septum, *Brain* 89:317-348, 1966

Rakic, P., and P. I. Yakovlev: Development of the corpus callosum and cavum septi in man, *J. Comp. Neurol.* 132:45-72, 1968

Rasmussen, G. L.: Efferent fibers of the cochlear nerve and cochlear nucleus, in *Neural Mechanisms of the Auditory and Vestibular Systems*, G. L. Rasmussen and W. F. Windle, eds., Thomas, Springfield, Ill., 1960

Rasmussen, G. L., and R. Gacek: Concerning the question of an efferent fiber component of the vestibular nerve in the cat, *Anat. Rec.* 130:361-362, 1958

Rayner, M. D., and M. J. Keenan: Role of red and white muscles in swimming of the skipjack tuna, *Nature* 214:392-393, 1967

Rechtschaffen, A., E. A. Wolpert, W. C. Dement, S. A. Mitchell, and C. Fischer: Nocturnal sleep of narcoleptics, *Electroenceph. Clin. Neurophysiol.* 15:599-609, 1963

Reese, T. S., and M. J. Karnovsky: Fine structural localization of a blood-brain barrier to exogenous peroxidase, *J. Cell. Biol.* 34:207-217, 1967

Reger, J. F.: The fine structure of neuromuscular synapses of gastrocnemii from mouse and frog, *Anat. Rec.* 130:7-24, 1958

Retzius, G.: Zur Kenntnis des centralen Nervensystems von Amphioxus lanceolatus, *Biol. Untersuch.* 2:29-46, 1891

Retzlaff, E.: A mechanism for excitation and inhibition of the Manthner's cells in teleosts: A histological and neurophysiological study, *J. Comp. Neurol.* 107:209-225, 1957

Rexed, B.: The cytoarchitectonic organization of the spinal cord in the cat, *J. Comp. Neurol.* 96:415-496, 1952

Rexed, B.: A cytoarchitectonic atlas of the spinal cord in the cat, *J. Comp. Neurol.* 100:297-380, 1954

Rexed, B.: Some aspects of the cytoarchitectonics and synaptology of the spinal cord, *Prog. Brain Res.* 11:58-92, 1964

Robertson, J. D.: The ultrastructure of a reptilian myoneural junction, *J. Biophys. Biochem. Cytol.* 2:381-394, 1956

Robin, E. D.: The evolutionary advantages of being stupid, *Perspectives Biol. Med.* 16:369-380, 1973

Rockel, A. J., C. J. Heath, and E. G. Jones: Afferent connections to the diencephalon in the marsupial phalanger and the question of sensory convergence in the "posterior group" of the thalamus, *J. Comp. Neurol.* 145:105-130, 1972

Rohde, E.: Histologische Untersuchungen ueber das Nervensystem von Amphioxus, *Zool. Anz.* 11:190-196, 1888a

Rohde, E.: Histologische Untersuchungen ueber das Nervensystem von Amphioxus lanceolatus, *Schneiders Zool. Beitr.* 2:169-211, 1888b

Romer, A. S.: *The Vertebrate Body*, 4th ed., Saunders, Philadelphia, 1970

Rorke, L. B., and H. E. Riggs: *Myelination of the Brain in the Newborn*, Lippincott, Philadelphia, 1969

Rosales, R. K., M. J. Lemay, and P. I. Yakovlev: The development and involution of the massa intermedia with regard to age and sex, *J. Neuropath. Exp. Neurol.* 27:166, 1968

Rose, M.: Der Allocortex bei Tier und Mensch, *J. Psychol. Neurol.* 34:1-112, 1927

Ross, M. D.: The general visceral efferent component of the eighth cranial nerve, *J. Comp. Neurol.* 135:453-478, 1969

Roth, W. D.: Metabolic and morphologic studies on the rat pineal organ during puberty, *Prog. Brain Res.* 10:552-563, 1965

Rovainen, C. M., G. E. Lemcoe, and A. Peterson: Structure and chemistry of glucose producing cells in meningeal tissue of the lamprey, *Brain Res.* 30:99-118, 1971

Russell, D. S., and L. C. Rubinstein: *Pathology of Tumours of the Nervous System*, 3rd ed., Williams and Wilkins, Baltimore, 1971

Russell, G. V.: The nucleus locus coeruleus (dorsolateralis tegmenti), *Texas Rep. Biol. Med.* 13:939-988, 1955

Sanides, F.: Comparative architectonics of the neocortex of mammals and their evolutionary interpretation, *Ann. N.Y. Acad. Sci.* 167:404-423, 1969

Sarnat, H. B.: Occurrence of fluorescent granules in the Purkinje cells of the cerebellum, *Anat. Rec.* 162:25-32, 1968

Sarnat, H. B., J. F. Campa, and J. Lloyd: Relation of ependyma, neuroglia and vessels in the nutrition of the spinal cord of vertebrates: A comparative histochemical study, *Neurology* 23:443, 1973

Sarnat, H. B., J. F. Campa, and J. M. Lloyd: Comparative histochemical study of ependymal and glial processes in the spinal cord of vertebrates, and the inverse relation to vascularity, *Amer. J. Anat.*, in press, 1974.

Sawyer, C. H.: Regulatory mechanisms of secretion of gonadotropic hormones, in *The Hypothalamus*, W. Haymaker, E. Anderson, and W. J. H. Nauta, eds., Thomas, Springfield, Ill., 1969

Sawyer, W. H.: Comparative physiology and pharmacology of the neurohypophysis, *Recent Prog. Hormone Res.* 17:437-465, 1961

Scalia, F.: A review of recent experimental studies on the distribution of the olfactory tracts of mammals, *Brain Behav. Evol.* 1:101-123, 1968

Scalia, F.: The termination of retinal axons in the pretectal region of mammals, *J. Comp. Neurol.* 145:223-258, 1972

Scalia, F., M. Halpern, H. Knapp, and W. Riss: The efferent connections of the olfactory bulb in the frog: A study in degenerating unmyelinated fibres, *J. Anat.* 103:245-262, 1968

Schally, A. V., A. Arimura, and A. J. Kastin: Hypothalamic regulatory hormones, *Science* 179:341-348, 1973

Scharrer, E., and B. Scharrer: Neurosecretion, *Physiol. Rev.* 25:171-181, 1945

Scheibel, M. E., and A. B. Scheibel: Structural substrates for integrative patterns in the brain stem reticular formation, in *Reticular Formation of the Brain*, H. H. Jasper, ed., Little, Brown, Boston, 1958

Scherer, H. J.: Melanin pigmentation of the substantia nigra in primates, *J. Comp. Neurol.* 71:91-98, 1939

Schneider, A.: *Beitrage zur vergleichenden Anatomie und Entwicklungsgeschichte der Wirbelthiere*, Berlin, 1879

Schneider, R. C., E. C. Crosby, and E. A. Kahn: Certain afferent cortical connections of the rhinencephalon, *Prog. Brain Res.* 3:191-217, 1963

Schnitzlein, H. N.: The habenula and the dorsal thalamus of some teleosts, *J. Comp. Neurol.* 118:225-267, 1962

Schnitzlein, H. N., and J. R. Faucette: General morphology of the fish cerebellum, in *Neurobiology of Cerebellar Evolution and Development*, R. Llinás, ed., Amer. Med. Assoc., Chicago, 1969

Schoen, J. H. R.: Comparative aspects of the descending fibre systems in the spinal cord, *Prog. Brain Res.* 11:203-222, 1964

Schroeder, D. M., J. A. Jane, and W. J. H. Nauta: Thalamic projections from the dorsal column and cerebellar nuclei and tectum in the hedgehog, Erinacens europaeus, *Anat. Rec. 166*:374, 1970

Schwartzkopff, J.: Discussion in *Hearing Mechanisms in Vertebrates* (Ciba Foundation Symposium), A. V. S. DeReuck and J. Knight, eds., Little, Brown, Boston, 1968

Schwarz, G. A.: The orthostatic hypotension syndrome of Shy-Drager, *Arch. Neurol. 16*:123-138, 1967

Shaner, R. F.: The development of the nuclei and tracts related to the acoustic nerve in the pig, *J. Comp. Neurol. 60*:5-19, 1934

Shaner, R. F.: Development of the finer structure and fiber connections of the globus pallidus, corpus of Luys and substantia nigra in the pig, *J. Comp. Neurol. 64*:213-225, 1936

Shanklin, W. M.: On diencephalic and mesencephalic nuclei and fiber paths in the brains of deep sea fish, *Phil. Tr. Roy. Soc. Lond.*, series B, *224*:361-419, 1935

Shepherd, G. M.: Synaptic organization of the mammalian olfactory bulb, *Physiol. Rev. 52*:864-917, 1972

Shuangshoti, S., and M. G. Netsky: Choroid plexus and paraphysis in lower vertebrates, *J. Morphol. 120*:157-188, 1966a

Shuangshoti, S., and M. G. Netsky: Histogenesis of choroid plexus in man, *Amer. J. Anat. 118*:283-316, 1966b

Shy, G. M., and G. A. Drager: A neurological syndrome associated with orthostatic hypotension. A clinical-pathological study, *Arch. Neurol. 2*:511-527, 1960

Sidman, R. L., and J. B. Angevine: Autoradiographic analysis of time of origin of nuclear versus cortical components of mouse telencephalon, *Anat. Rec. 142*: 326, 1962

Silén, L.: On the nervous system of Glossobalanus marginatus Meek, *Acta. Zool. 31*:149-175, 1950

Sinclair, D.: *Cutaneous Sensation*, Oxford University Press, London, 1967

Singer, P. A., J. Cate, D. G. Ross, and M. G. Netsky: Melanosis of the dentate nucleus, *Neurology*, in press, 1974

Smith, A. A., T. Taylor, and S. B. Wortis: Abnormal catecholamine metabolism in familial dysautonomia, *New Eng. J. Med. 268*:705-707, 1964

Smith, G. E.: The origin of the corpus callosum; a comparative study of the hippocampal region of the cerebrum of Marsupialia and certain Chiroptera, *Trans. Linn. Soc. Lond.* 2nd series, *Zool. 7*:47-69, 1897

Smith, G. E.: Some problems relating to the evolution of the brain, *Lancet.* 1-6, 147-155, 221-227, 1910

Smith, G. E.: A preliminary note on the morphology of the corpus striatum and the origin of the neopallium, *J. Anat. 53*:271-291, 1919

Snider, R. S., and E. Eldred: Cerebo-cerebellar relationship in the monkey, *J. Neurophysiol. 15*:27-40, 1952

Snyder, M., and I. T. Diamond: The organization and function of the visual cortex in the tree shrew, *Brain Behav. Evol. 1*:244-288, 1968

Sotelo, C.: Ultrastructural aspects of the cerebellar cortex of the frog, in *Neurobiology of Cerebellar Evolution and Development*, R. Llinás, ed., Amer. Med. Assoc., Chicago, 1969

Speidel, C. C.: Gland-cells of internal secretion in the spinal cord of the skates, thesis, Princeton University, 1917

Sperry, R. P.: Optic nerve regeneration with return of vision in anurans, *J. Neurophysiol. 7*:57-69, 1944

Sperry, R. P.: Mechanisms of neural maturation, in *Handbook of Experimental Psychology*, S. S. Stevens, ed., Wiley, New York, 1951

Stager, K. E.: Avian olfaction, *Amer. Zool.* 7:415-419, 1967

Stauffer, H. M., L. B. Snow, and A. B. Adams: Roentgenologic recognition of habenular calcification as distinct from calcification in the pineal body, *Amer. J. Roentgenol.* 70:83-92, 1953

Stefanelli, A.: The mauthnerian apparatus in the Ichthyopsida; its nature and function and correlated problems of neurohistogenesis, *Quart. Rev. Biol.* 26:17-34, 1951

Stell, W. K.: The structure and morphologic relations of rods and cones in the retina of the spiny dogfish, Squalus, *Comp. Biochem. Physiol.* 42A:141-151, 1972

Sterzi, G.: Ricerche intorno all' anatomia comparata ed all ontogenesi delle meningi, e considerazioni sulla filogenesi, *Atti. d. r. Ist. Veneto di. Sc., Lett. ed. Arti.* 60:1101, 1901

Sterzi, G.: Recherches sur l'anatomie comparée et sur l'ontogénèse des meninges. I. Méninges médullaires, *Arch. Ital. Biol.* 37:257-269, 1902

Stevenson, J. A. F.: Neural control of food and water intake, in *The Hypothalamus*, W. Haymaker, E. Anderson, and W. J. H. Nauta, eds., Thomas, Springfield, Ill., 1969

Steyne, W., Observations on the ultrastructure of the pineal eye, *J. Roy. Micr. Soc.* 79:47-58, 1960a

Steyne, W.: Electron miscroscopic observations on the epiphysial sensory cells in lizards and the pineal sensory cell problem, *Ztschr. Zellforsch. u. mikr. Anat.* 51:735-747, 1960b

Stingelin, W., and D. G. Senn: Morphologic studies on the brain of sauropsida, *Ann. N.Y. Acad. Sci.* 167:156-163, 1969

Stone, L. S.: Polarization of the retina and development of vision, *J. Exp. Zool.* 145:85-95, 1960

Studnička, R. K.: Untersuchungen ueber Bau der Schnerven der Wirbeltiere, *Jena Ztschr. f. Naturwiss.* 31:1-28, 1898

Szentágothai, J.: Die innere Gliederung des Oculomotoriuskernes, *Arch. Psychiat.* 115:127-135, 1942

Szentágothai, J.: Propriospinal pathways and their synapses, *Prog. Brain Res.* 11:155-177, 1964a

Szentágothai, J.: Pathways and synaptic articulation patterns connecting vestibular receptors and oculomotor nuclei, in *The Oculomotor System*, M. Bender, ed., Hoeber, New York, 1964b

Taft, A. E.: A comparison of anterior horn cells in the normal spinal cord and after amputation, *Arch. Neurol. Psychiat.* 3:41-48, 1920

Tahmoush, A. J., J. E. Brooks, and J. L. Keltner: Palatal myoclonus associated with abnormal ocular and extremity movements, *Arch. Neurol.* 27:431-440, 1972

Talbot, S. A.: A lateral localization in cat's visual cortex, *Fed. Proc.* 1:84, 1942

Tarlov, E. C., and R. Y. Moore: The tecto thalamic connections in the brain of the rabbit, *J. Comp. Neurol.* 126:403-421, 1966

Ten Cate, J.: Zur Physiologie des Zentralnervensystems des Amphioxus (Brachiostoma lanceolatus). I. Die reflektorische Tatigkeit des Amphioxus, *Arch. Neerl. Physiol.* 23:409-415, 1938

Tennyson, V. M., and G. D. Pappas: An electron microscope study of ependymal cells of the fetal, early postnatal and adult rabbit, *Ztschr. f. Zellforsch. u. mikr. Anat.* 56:595-618, 1962

Teravainen, H.: Development of the myoneural junction in the rat, *Ztschr. f. Zell-forsch. u. mikr. Anat.* 87:249-265, 1968

Terni, T.: Sul nucleo accessorio d'origine del nervo abducente nei rettili, *Monitore Zool. Ital.* (Firenze), 32:67-76, 1921

Terni, T.: Ricerche sul nervo abducente e in special modo intorno al significato del suo nucleo accessorio d'origine, *Arch. Fisiol.* 20:305, 1922

Thieblot, L.: Physiology of the pineal body, *Prog. Brain Res.* 10:479-488, 1965

Thieblot, L., and S. Blaise: Influence de la glande pinéale sur la sphère génitale, *Prog. Brain Res.* 10:577-584, 1965

Thompson, D. W.: *On Growth and Form,* 2nd ed., Cambridge University Press, New York, 1959

Thompson, E. L.: The dorsal longitudinal fasciculus in Didelphis virginiana, *J. Comp. Neurol.* 76:239-281, 1942

Thompson, I. MacL.: On the cavum septi pellucidi, *J. Anat.* 67:59-77, 1932

Tilney, F., and L. F. Warren: The morphology and evolutionary significance of the pineal body, *Amer. Anat. Mem.,* no. 9, Wistar, Philadelphia, 1919

Toncray, J. E., and W. J. S. Krieg: The nuclei of the human thalamus: a comparative approach, *J. Comp. Neurol.* 85:421-459, 1946

Torack, R. M.: Area postrema: A feedback control of choroid plexus function?, *Prog. Neuropath.* 2:115-127, 1973

Tretjakoff, D.: Das Nervensystem von Ammocoetes. I. Das Rueckenmark, *Arch. f. mikr. Anat.* 73:607-680, 1909a

Tretjakoff, D.: Das Nervensystem von Ammocoetes. II. Gehirn, *Arch. f. mikr. Anat.* 74:636-779, 1909b

Troost, B. T., R. B. Weber, and R. B. Daroff: Hemispheric control of eye movements. I. Quantitative analysis of refixation saccades in a hemispherectomy patient, *Arch. Neurol.* 27:441-448, 1972a

Troost, B. T., R. B. Daroff, R. B. Weber, and L. F. Dell'Osso: Hemispheric control of eye movements. II. Quantitative analysis of smooth pursuit in a hemispherectomy patient, *Arch. Neurol.* 27:449-452, 1972b

Truex, R. C., and M. B. Carpenter: *Human Neuroanatomy,* 6th ed., Williams and Wilkins, Baltimore, 1970

Tumarkin, A.: The pelycosaur, the whale and the golden mole, *J. Otol. Laryngol.* 79:667-694, 1965

Tumarkin, A.: Evolution of the auditory conducting apparatus in terrestrial vertebrates, in *Hearing Mechanisms in Vertebrates* (Ciba Foundation Symposium), A. V. S. de Reuck and J. Knight, eds., Little, Brown, Boston, 1968

Tumarkin, A.: A biologist looks at psycho-accoustics, *J. Sound Vibr.* 21:1-12, 1972

Uchizono, K.: Synaptic organization of the mammalian cerebellum, in *Neurobiology of Cerebellar Evolution and Development,* R. Llinás, ed., Amer. Med. Assoc., Chicago, 1969

van Bergeijk, W. A.: Evolution of the sense of hearing in vertebrates, *Amer. Zool.* 6:371-377, 1966

van de Kamer, J. C.: Histological structure and cytology of the pineal complex in fishes, amphibians and reptiles, *Prog. Brain Res.* 10:30-48, 1965

van den Akker, L. M.: *An Anatomical Outline of the Spinal Cord of the Pigeon,* van Gorcum, Assen, The Netherlands, 1970

van Rijnberk, G.: Sur l'innervation segmentale de la peau de la nageoire thoracique chez le requin (Scyllium catalus), *Folia Neuro-biol.* 10:423-427, 1916

Vesselkin, N. P., A. L. Agoyan, and L. M. Nomokonova: A study of thalamotelen-cephalic afferent systems in the frog, *Brain Behav. Evol. 4*:295-306, 1971

von Baumbarten, R., and G. C. Salmoiraghi: Respiratory neurons in the goldfish, *Arch. Ital. Biol. 100*:31-47, 1962

von Bonin, G., and G. A. Shariff: Extrapyramidal nuclei among mammals, *J. Comp. Neurol. 94*:427-438, 1951

von Ledebur, J. F.: Ueber die Sekretion und Resorption von Gasen in der Fischschwimmblase, *Biol. Rev. 12*:217-244, 1937

von Lenhossék, M.: Zur Kenntnis der Neuroglia des menschlichen Rueckenmarkes, *Vernhandl. d. anat. Gesellsch. 5*:193-221, 1891

Votaw, C. L.: Certain functional and anatomical relations of the cornu ammonis of the Macaque monkey, *J. Comp. Neurol. 114*:283-293, 1960

Wagman, I. H.: Eye movements induced by electric stimulation of cerebrum in monkeys and their relationship to bodily movements, in *The Oculomotor System*, M. B. Bender, ed., Hoeber, New York, 1964

Walberg, F.: Do the motor nuclei of the cranial nerves receive corticofugal fibers? An experimental study in the cat, *Brain 80*:597-605, 1957

Walberg, F., D. Bowsher, and A. Brodal: The termination of primary vestibular fibers in the vestibular nuclei in the cat. An experimental study with silver methods, *J. Comp. Neurol. 110*:391-415, 1958

Walker, A. E.: Internal structure and afferent-efferent relations of the thalamus, in *The Thalamus*, D. P. Purpura and M. D. Yahr, eds., Columbia University Press, New York, 1966

Walker, A. E., and T. A. Weaver, Jr.: Ocular movements from the occipital lobe in the monkey, *J. Neurophysiol. 3*:353-357, 1940

Walls, G. L.: *The Vertebrate Eye and Its Adaptive Radiation*, Cranbrook Inst. Sci., Bloomfield Hills, Mich., 1942

Warwick, R.: Representation of the extra-ocular muscles in the oculomotor nuclei of the monkey, *J. Comp. Neurol. 98*:449-504, 1953

Warwick, R.: Oculomotor organization, in *The Oculomotor System*, M. B. Bender, ed., Hoeber, New York, 1964

Weindl, A., and R. J. Joynt: Ultrastructure of the ventricular walls, *Arch. Neurol. 26*:420-427, 1972

Weinshilboum, R. M., and J. Axelrod: Reduced plasma dopamine-beta-hydroxylase activity in familial dysautonomia, *New Eng. J. Med. 285*:938-942, 1971

Welker, W. I., and S. Seidenstein: Somatic sensory representation in the cerebral cortex of the racoon (Procyon lotor), *J. Comp. Neurol. 111*:469-501, 1959

Welsch, J. H.: The quantitative distribution of 5-hydroxytryptamine in the nervous system, eyes and other organs of some vertebrates, in *Comparative Neuro-chemistry*, D. Richter, ed. Macmillan, New York, 1964

Wever, E. G.: The mechanics of hair-cell stimulation, *Ann. Otol. Rhinol. Laryngol. 80*:786-804, 1971

Winkler, C.: A case of olive-pontine cerebellar atrophy and our conceptions of neo- and palaio-cerebellum, *Schweiz Arch. f. Neurol. u. Psychiat. 13*:684-702, 1923

Wolstenholme, G. E. W., and J. Knight: *Taste and Smell in Vertebrates* (Ciba Foundation Symposium), Churchill, London, 1970

Woodard, J. S.: Origin of the external granule layer of the cerebellar cortex, *J. Comp. Neurol. 115*:65-73, 1960

Woodworth, J. A., R. S. Beckett, and M. G. Netsky: A composite of hereditary ataxias: a familial disorder with features of olive-ponto-cerebellar atrophy, Leber's optic atrophy, and Friedrich's ataxia, *A.M.A. Arch. Int. Med. 104*: 595-606, 1959

Wurtman, R. J., and J. Axelrod: The formation, metabolism and physiologic effects of melatonin in mammals, *Prog. Brain Res., 10*:520-529, 1965

Yakovlev, P. I.: Pathoarchitectonic studies of cerebral malformations. III. arrhinencephalies (holotelencephalies), *J. Neuropath. Exp. Neurol. 18*:22-55, 1959

Yakovlev, P. I., and A. Lecours: The myelogenetic cycles of regional maturation of the brain, in *Regional Development of the Brain in Early Life*, A. Minkowski, ed., F. A. Davis, Philadelphia, 1967

Yoon, M. G.: Transposition of the visual projection from the nasal hemiretina onto the foreign rostral zone of the optic tectum in goldfish, *Exp. Neurol. 37*:451-462, 1972

Young, J. Z.: On the autonomic nervous system of the teleostean fish Uranoscopus scaber, *Quart. J. Micr. Sci. 74*:491-535, 1931a

Young, J. Z.: The pupillary mechanism of the teleostean fish Uranoscopus scaber, *Proc. Roy. Soc.*, series B, *107*:464-485, 1931b

Young, J. Z.: The autonomic nervous system of selachians, *Quart. J. Micr. Sci. 75*: 571-624, 1933

Zeman, W., and J. R. M. Innes: *Craigie's Neuroanatomy of the Rat*, Academic Press, New York, 1963

Zettner, A., and M. G. Netsky: Lipoma of the corpus callosum, *J. Neuropath. Exp. Neurol. 19*:305-319, 1960

Zimmerman, E. A., W. W. Chambers, and C. N. Liu: An experimental study of the anatomical organization of the cortico-bulbar system in the albino rat, *J. Comp. Neurol. 123*:301-324, 1964

Zingesser, L. H., M. M. Schechter, and A. Medina: Angiographic and pneumoencephalographic features of holoprosencephaly, *Amer. J. Roentgenol. 97*:561-574, 1966

Zitko, B. A., J. F. Howes, R. K. Razdan, B. C. Dalzell, H. C. Dalzell, J. C. Sheehan, and H. G. Pars: Brain and body temperatures in a panting lizard, *Science 177*:431-433, 1972

Atlas of comparative sections of central nervous system in selected vertebrates

Several good atlases are available for identifying structures in the brains of many mammals commonly used in the laboratory. Many of these atlases have stereotaxic coordinates. Relatively few such pictorial displays of the brains of submammalian vertebrates are available. Notable exceptions are the atlases of the salamander (Herrick, 1948), frog (Kemali and Braitenberg, 1969), and the recent representative survey of all classes of vertebrates by Igarashi and Kamiya (1972). An atlas of the spinal cord of the pigeon also has been published (van den Akker, 1970). Older works, such as those of Cajal (1909-1911), Papez (1929), Kappers, Huber and Crosby (1936) and Larsell (1967) are richly illustrated with line drawings of sections of particular interest.

The following atlas is designed to be used, not for the meticulous identification of all structures described in the text of this book, but rather to compare relations of structures at similar levels in several vertebrates. For this purpose, we have adopted a different format than is used in other atlases: cerebral sections of six different species, each of a different class of vertebrate, are depicted on facing pages. These species are not necessarily the same in all plates, but were selected because they contrast with other species in a particular part of the brain. Man, however, is the sixth species in all plates. The larval form of the lamprey (*Ammocoetes*) is used as representative of the most primitive condition of the vertebrate brain.

Brains of normal animals, and human brains of patients dying with disease unrelated to the nervous system, were fixed in formalin. The small animal brains and human brainstem were then embedded in paraffin and cut at 8 microns. Sections were then processed with luxol fast blue and cresyl violet to stain both myelinated fibers and neurons. Each photograph was magnified differently because of discrepancies in the size of the brains.

PLATE 1   SPINAL CORD

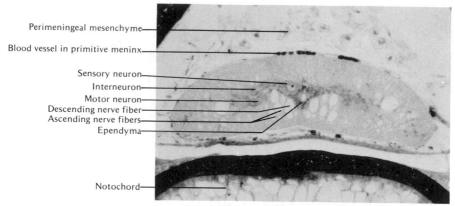

Perimeningeal mesenchyme

Blood vessel in primitive meninx

Sensory neuron
Interneuron
Motor neuron
Descending nerve fiber
Ascending nerve fibers
Ependyma

Notochord

Figure 1 Larval lamprey *(Ammocoetes)*

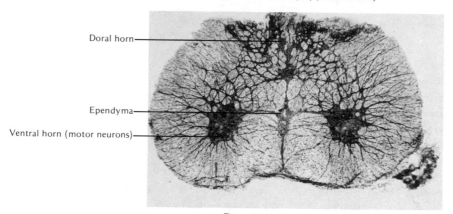

Doral horn

Ependyma

Ventral horn (motor neurons)

Figure 2 Shark *(Squalus acanthias)*

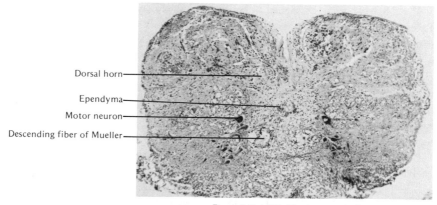

Dorsal horn

Ependyma

Motor neuron

Descending fiber of Mueller

Figure 3 Goldfish *(Cassius aureatus)*

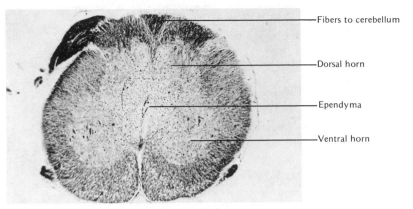

—Fibers to cerebellum

—Dorsal horn

—Ependyma

—Ventral horn

Figure 4 Frog *(Rana pipiens)*

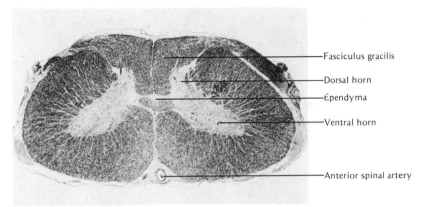

—Fasciculus gracilis

—Dorsal horn

—Ependyma

—Ventral horn

—Anterior spinal artery

Figure 5 Lizard *(Iguana iguana)*

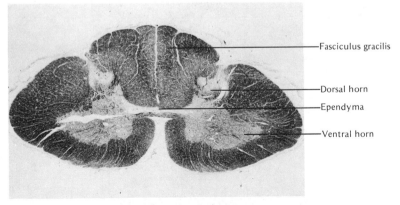

—Fasciculus gracilis

—Dorsal horn

—Ependyma

—Ventral horn

Figure 6 Man *(Homo sapiens)*

PLATE 2   LOWER MEDULLA

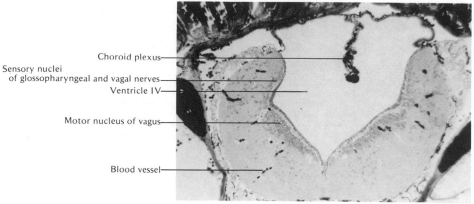

Choroid plexus

Sensory nuclei
of glossopharyngeal and vagal nerves

Ventricle IV

Motor nucleus of vagus

Blood vessel

Figure 1 Larval lamprey *(Ammocoetes)*

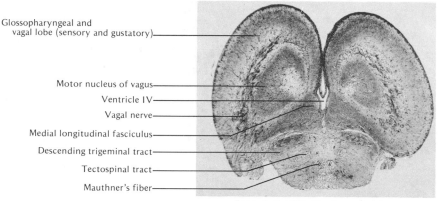

Glossopharyngeal and
vagal lobe (sensory and gustatory)

Motor nucleus of vagus

Ventricle IV

Vagal nerve

Medial longitudinal fasciculus

Descending trigeminal tract

Tectospinal tract

Mauthner's fiber

Figure 2 Goldfish *(Cassius aureatus)*

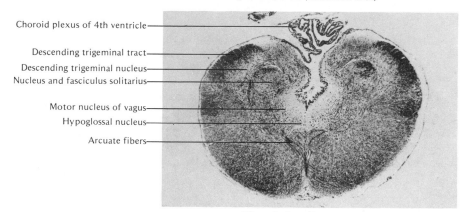

Choroid plexus of 4th ventricle

Descending trigeminal tract

Descending trigeminal nucleus

Nucleus and fasciculus solitarius

Motor nucleus of vagus

Hypoglossal nucleus

Arcuate fibers

Figure 3 Frog *(Rana pipiens)*

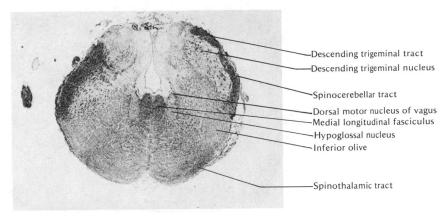

Figure 4 Alligator *(Alligator mississippiensis)*

- —Descending trigeminal tract
- —Descending trigeminal nucleus
- —Spinocerebellar tract
- —Dorsal motor nucleus of vagus
- —Medial longitudinal fasciculus
- —Hypoglossal nucleus
- —Inferior olive
- —Spinothalamic tract

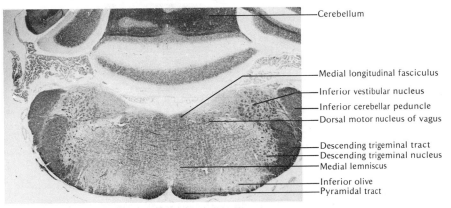

Figure 5 Opossum *(Didelphis virginiana)*

- —Cerebellum
- —Medial longitudinal fasciculus
- —Inferior vestibular nucleus
- —Inferior cerebellar peduncle
- —Dorsal motor nucleus of vagus
- —Descending trigeminal tract
- —Descending trigeminal nucleus
- —Medial lemniscus
- —Inferior olive
- —Pyramidal tract

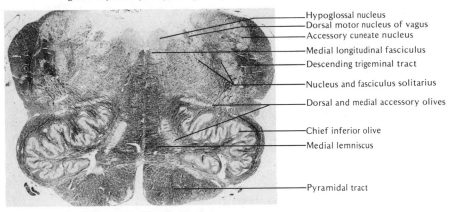

Figure 6 Man *(Homo sapiens)*

- —Hypoglossal nucleus
- —Dorsal motor nucleus of vagus
- —Accessory cuneate nucleus
- —Medial longitudinal fasciculus
- —Descending trigeminal tract
- —Nucleus and fasciculus solitarius
- —Dorsal and medial accessory olives
- —Chief inferior olive
- —Medial lemniscus
- —Pyramidal tract

PLATE 3   UPPER MEDULLA (PONS)

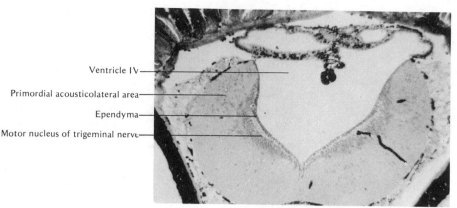

Ventricle IV

Primordial acousticolateral area

Ependyma

Motor nucleus of trigeminal nerve

Figure 1 Larval lamprey *(Ammocoetes)*

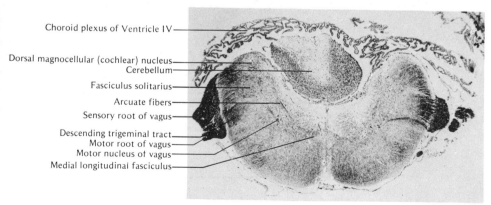

Cerebellum

Mesencephalocerebellar tract

Cerebellar crest (eminentia granularis)

Lateral line lobe

Vestibular area
Descending trigeminal tract
Medial longitudinal fasciculus
Secondary gustatory tract
Vestibular and lateral line nerves
Decussation of vestibulospinal tract
Tectobulbar and tectospinal tract

Figure 2 Goldfish *(Cassius aureatus)*

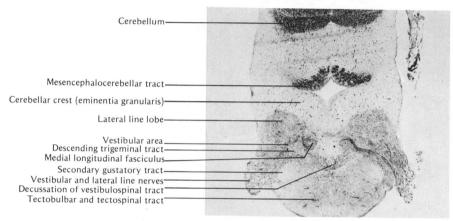

Choroid plexus of Ventricle IV

Dorsal magnocellular (cochlear) nucleus
Cerebellum

Fasciculus solitarius

Arcuate fibers

Sensory root of vagus

Descending trigeminal tract
Motor root of vagus
Motor nucleus of vagus
Medial longitudinal fasciculus

Figure 3 Frog *(Rana pipiens)*

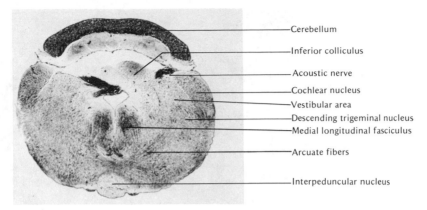

Figure 4 Lizard *(Anolis carolinensis)*

- Cerebellum
- Inferior colliculus
- Acoustic nerve
- Cochlear nucleus
- Vestibular area
- Descending trigeminal nucleus
- Medial longitudinal fasciculus
- Arcuate fibers
- Interpeduncular nucleus

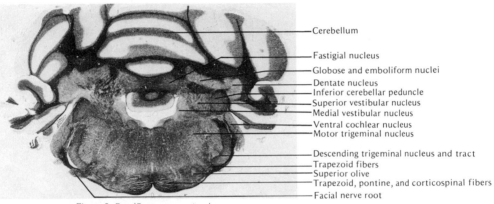

Figure 5 Rat *(Rattus norvegicus)*

- Cerebellum
- Fastigial nucleus
- Globose and emboliform nuclei
- Dentate nucleus
- Inferior cerebellar peduncle
- Superior vestibular nucleus
- Medial vestibular nucleus
- Ventral cochlear nucleus
- Motor trigeminal nucleus
- Descending trigeminal nucleus and tract
- Trapezoid fibers
- Superior olive
- Trapezoid, pontine, and corticospinal fibers
- Facial nerve root

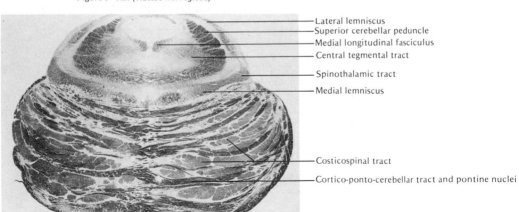

Figure 6 Man *(Homo sapiens)*

- Lateral lemniscus
- Superior cerebellar peduncle
- Medial longitudinal fasciculus
- Central tegmental tract
- Spinothalamic tract
- Medial lemniscus
- Costicospinal tract
- Cortico-ponto-cerebellar tract and pontine nuclei

PLATE 4   MIDBRAIN

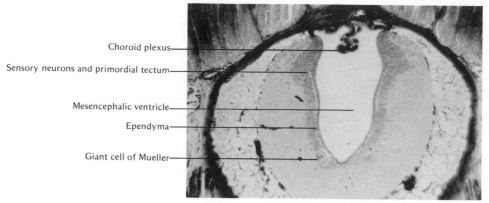

Choroid plexus

Sensory neurons and primordial tectum

Mesencephalic ventricle

Ependyma

Giant cell of Mueller

Figure 1 Larval lamprey *(Ammocoetes)*

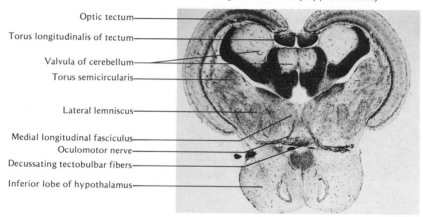

Optic tectum

Torus longitudinalis of tectum

Valvula of cerebellum

Torus semicircularis

Lateral lemniscus

Medial longitudinal fasciculus

Oculomotor nerve

Decussating tectobulbar fibers

Inferior lobe of hypothalamus

Figure 2 Goldfish *(Cassius aureatus)*

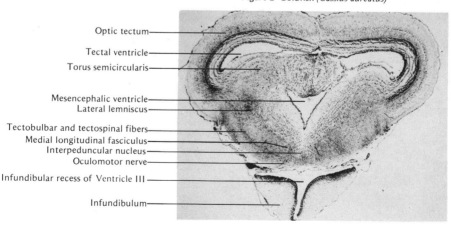

Optic tectum

Tectal ventricle

Torus semicircularis

Mesencephalic ventricle
Lateral lemniscus

Tectobulbar and tectospinal fibers
Medial longitudinal fasciculus
Interpeduncular nucleus
Oculomotor nerve

Infundibular recess of Ventricle III

Infundibulum

Figure 3 Frog *(Rana pipiens)*

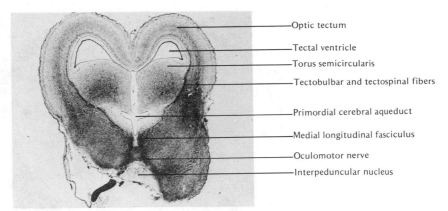

Optic tectum

Tectal ventricle

Torus semicircularis

Tectobulbar and tectospinal fibers

Primordial cerebral aqueduct

Medial longitudinal fasciculus

Oculomotor nerve

Interpeduncular nucleus

Figure 4 young Alligator *(Alligator mississippiensis)*

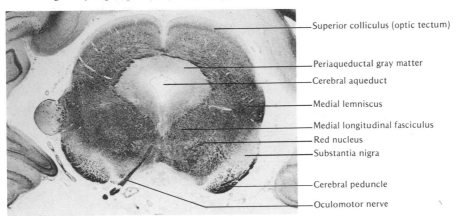

Superior colliculus (optic tectum)

Periaqueductal gray matter

Cerebral aqueduct

Medial lemniscus

Medial longitudinal fasciculus

Red nucleus

Substantia nigra

Cerebral peduncle

Oculomotor nerve

Figure 5 Opossum *(Didelphis virginiana)*

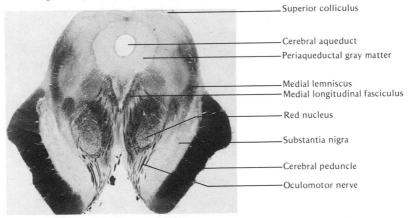

Superior colliculus

Cerebral aqueduct

Periaqueductal gray matter

Medial lemniscus

Medial longitudinal fasciculus

Red nucleus

Substantia nigra

Cerebral peduncle

Oculomotor nerve

Figure 6 Man *(Homo sapiens)*

PLATE 5   DIENCEPHALON

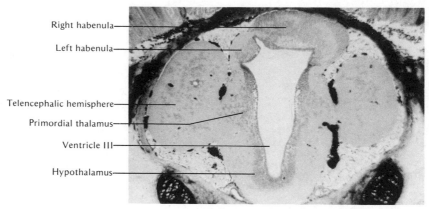

Right habenula—

Left habenula—

Telencephalic hemisphere—

Primordial thalamus—

Ventricle III—

Hypothalamus—

Figure 1 Larval lamprey *(Ammocoetes)*

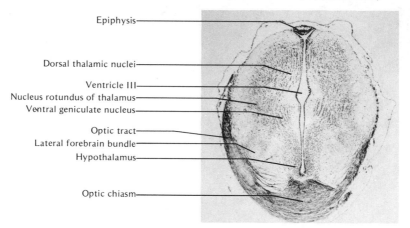

Epiphysis—

Dorsal thalamic nuclei—

Ventricle III—
Nucleus rotundus of thalamus—
Ventral geniculate nucleus—

Optic tract—
Lateral forebrain bundle—
Hypothalamus—

Optic chiasm—

Figure 2 Frog *(Rana pipiens)*

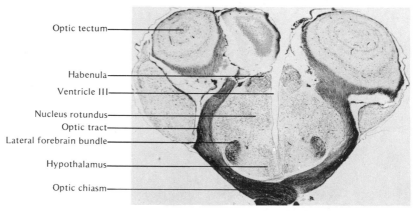

Optic tectum—

Habenula—
Ventricle III—

Nucleus rotundus—
Optic tract—
Lateral forebrain bundle—

Hypothalamus—

Optic chiasm—

Figure 3 Lizard *(Anolis carolinensis)*

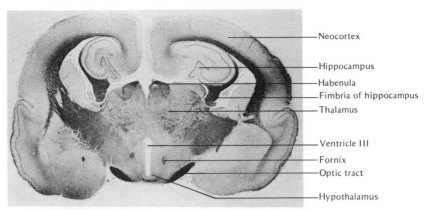

Figure 4 Opossum *(Didelphis virginiana)*

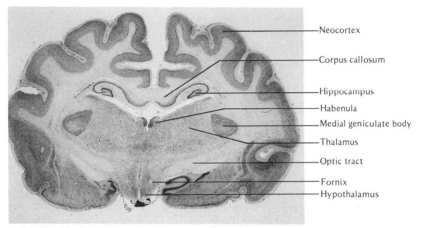

Figure 5 Cat *(Felis domesticus)*

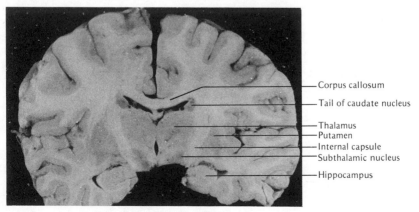

Figure 6 Man *(Homo sapiens)*

PLATE 6   FOREBRAIN

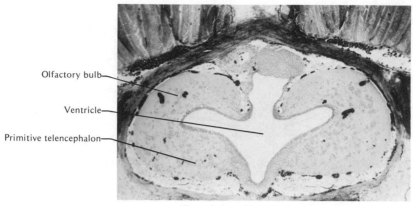

Olfactory bulb

Ventricle

Primitive telencephalon

Figure 1   Larval lamprey *(Ammocoetes)*

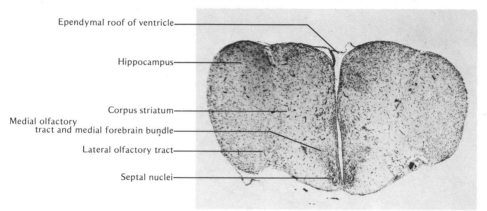

Ependymal roof of ventricle

Hippocampus

Corpus striatum

Medial olfactory
tract and medial forebrain bundle

Lateral olfactory tract

Septal nuclei

Figure 2   Goldfish *(Cassius aureatus)*

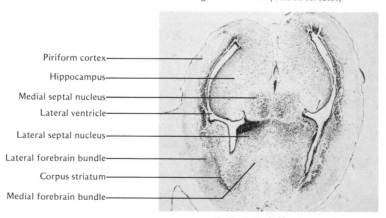

Piriform cortex

Hippocampus

Medial septal nucleus

Lateral ventricle

Lateral septal nucleus

Lateral forebrain bundle

Corpus striatum

Medial forebrain bundle

Figure 3   Frog *(Rana pipiens)*

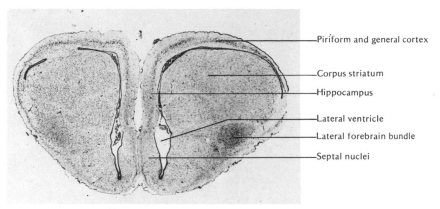

Figure 4 Young alligator *(Alligator mississippiensis)*

—Piriform and general cortex

—Corpus striatum

—Hippocampus

—Lateral ventricle

—Lateral forebrain bundle

—Septal nuclei

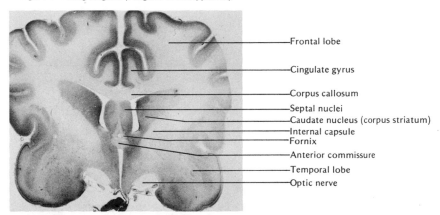

Figure 5 Dog *(Canis familiaris)*

—Frontal lobe

—Cingulate gyrus

—Corpus callosum

—Septal nuclei

—Caudate nucleus (corpus striatum)

—Internal capsule

—Fornix

—Anterior commissure

—Temporal lobe

—Optic nerve

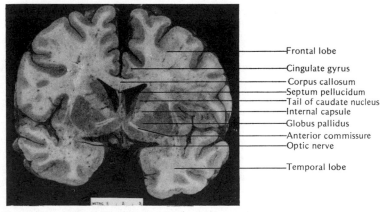

Figure 6 Man *(Homo sapiens)*

—Frontal lobe

—Cingulate gyrus

—Corpus callosum

—Septum pellucidum

—Tail of caudate nucleus

—Internal capsule

—Globus pallidus

—Anterior commissure

—Optic nerve

—Temporal lobe

Index

Italicized page number indicates principal discussion.